Elementary
principles of
laboratory
instruments

Elementary principles of laboratory instruments

LESLIE W. LEE

B.S., M.T. (ASCP)

Assistant Director of Laboratories,
Orange Memorial Hospital, Orlando, Florida;
Clinical Assistant Professor of Allied Health Sciences,
Florida Technological University, Orlando

THIRD EDITION

with 176 illustrations

THE C. V. MOSBY COMPANY

SAINT LOUIS   1974

THIRD EDITION

Copyright © 1974 by The C. V. Mosby Company

Second edition copyrighted 1970

First edition published privately by Mr. Leslie W. Lee

Printed in the United States of America

Distributed in Great Britain by Henry Kimpton, London

Library of Congress Cataloging in Publication Data

Lee, Leslie W
  Elementary principles of laboratory instruments.

  First ed. published in 1967 under title: Elementary principles of instruments.
  1. Medical instruments and apparatus. I. Title.
[DNLM: 1. Equipment and supplies. 2. Laboratories. 3. Technology, Medical—Instrumentation. W26 L478e 1974]
R856.L39 1974   616.07′56′028   73-14509
ISBN 0-8016-2916-0

VH/VH/VH 9 8 7 6 5 4 3 2 1

Preface

During the past 10 years, instruments have come to play such an important part in laboratory techniques that a thorough understanding of their operation is essential for anyone who works in this field. Until recently, very little attempt has been made to teach the principles of instruments in detail. Most laboratory workers have acquired a sketchy idea of the instruments they use by hastily perusing the operating manuals. A number of commercially oriented workshops have been given which were helpful but which hardly fill the need for complete training.

Because of my concern about the general lack of knowledge regarding the principles of instruments, I have presented a number of workshops and classes to students and medical technologists. This book is an outgrowth of a manual prepared for use in these programs. Several good texts are available to cover the more sophisticated analytical methods; however, there seems to be a need for a book that explains the elementary principles of a number of instruments without involving the reader in a discouraging amount of technical detail. It is hoped that this book will fill that need.

The book will prove useful in teaching biology and chemistry students as well as medical technologists. The material is presented in such a way that the student need not have a heavy background in physics, mathematics, or electronics to gain a basic knowledge of the instruments used. Obviously all the analytical tools discussed here have more sophisticated aspects; indeed, any one means of analysis, such as electrophoresis, may represent an entire discipline in itself. It is hoped that this presentation will give enough of an understanding for the student to orient himself in the laboratory and begin his accumulation of the facts and skills.

The reader will notice that no attempt is made to teach the detailed operation of any equipment. The intent instead is to explain the principles of operation. With the aid of an operating manual or other instruction, the necessary operating skills are easily acquired. The principles involved should really be taught before the instrument is handled.

This material might serve as a text for a course in instruments, for medical technology training, or for workshops. It can also be of value as a reference in the working laboratory.

I am indebted to the many instrument manufacturers and their representatives who have so generously given their permission for reproduction of materials. Many friends and associates have also been helpful with their advice and encouragement.

Leslie W. Lee
January, 1967

v

Introduction
to third edition

The first edition, *Elementary Principles of Instruments,* was published in early 1967. At that time the Preface carried a comment about the rapid increase in instrumentation during the previous 10 years. Within the intervening years the introduction of sophisticated equipment has accelerated at a rate that few people would have imagined a decade ago. This veritable revolution in the methods of analysis in the clinical laboratory has drastically changed the role of the technologist. Training programs in the medical sciences have had to adjust to these changes.

The second edition, *Elementary Principles of Laboratory Instruments,* introduced in 1970, precipitated changes in the teaching of instrumentation that seemed significant at the time. Now, however, still much more time must be given to this vital subject if the challenge of technological change is to be met.

Whether we look at the figures in terms of total tests, revenue generated, or clinical effect, it is patently apparent that perhaps as many as three fourths of all laboratory tests are done with the substantial help of some sort of instruments and the majority of these by totally automated procedures.

There is every reason to believe that in the next few years a much larger percentage of laboratory tests will be totally automated. One company is claiming that within a few months two pieces of their equipment will be able to totally automate 70% of all tests done in the average laboratory. Means are under consideration at the present time for automation of nearly every laboratory test now being performed.

In the face of this technological revolution it is imperative that the training of the medical laboratory worker be altered considerably. Medical technology curriculums in most schools devote far too little time to preparing students to understand, operate, and maintain instruments and instrument systems. Hopefully this third edition will provide help in revising curriculums and updating course outlines. It furnishes more information about automated systems and data handling, describes many new instruments, and anticipates some of the instruments that are not yet in routine use.

As time goes on, instruments become obsolete. Some approaches to analysis are discarded in favor of newer and better methods. Yesterday's specific lesson material may seem to be irrelevant and today's material may seem that way tomorrow. Still, we cannot wait for tomorrow to find out what will then be relevant. Since much of what we do today is based on yesterday's mistakes and inadequacies, the learning is not lost.

In the current edition, principles are explained in such a way that the material learned will have some lasting usefulness and that the student will think about the problem rather than simply accept a device because it is new.

Those thoroughly trained in the science of electronics may become impatient with many of the simplified explanations, but the intent is to give students some comprehension of the logic of electricity without unduly burdening them with technical detail.

Leslie W. Lee

Contents

ix

Elementary principles of laboratory instruments

1

Matter and energy

A great many of the instruments that will be discussed in this book are made to measure changes that occur in matter. The change in question may be the absorption of light energy by a liquid, the light energy emitted when an element is burned in a flame, the freezing point of a liquid, or some other change. These changes involve *energy* and *matter*. Before starting to talk about instruments let us review briefly some concepts of matter and energy.

All matter is made up of *atoms*. The atoms are composed of an electrically positive *nucleus*, around which *electrons* move in orbits at varying distances. The simplest element is helium, which has only one *proton* or positive charge in the nucleus and one electron or negative charge orbiting around it. Other elements have a larger number of protons in the nucleus and always an equal number of electrons in orbit around it. There may also be electrically neutral *neutrons* in the nucleus but the net charge of the stable atom is neutral. Each element has a characteristic number of electrons and protons. The proton has a measurable weight and all protons weigh the same. Almost all the weight of the atom is in its protons and neutrons. The electrons have a great deal of energy and represent practically the entire energy of the atom but they have essentially no weight.

The electrons are characteristically arranged in *shells*, or orbits, around the nucleus. These shells are designated as K, L, M, N, etc., lettering from the center outward. Each shell has a maximum number of electrons that it can hold, and these shell capacities are indicated in Fig. 1-1. Each shell's capacity must be satisfied before electrons will be found in the next more distant shell. Thus sodium, with eleven electrons, will have two electrons in

the K shell, eight in the L shell, and its one remaining electron in the M shell. There will be no electrons in the shells farther out.

The *atomic number* is the number of protons in the atom; the *atomic weight* is roughly the number of protons and neutrons combined. See table on p. 261 for a list of the elements, giving for each element its atomic number, approximate atomic weight, and chemical symbol.

As the temperature of an atom increases, the electrons move farther from the nucleus and the distance between atoms increase. When the atoms become far apart, the substance becomes a gas. If the atoms approach each other to the point where

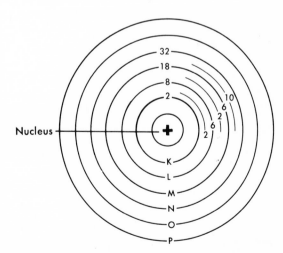

Fig. 1-1. Schematic representation of an atom, showing electron shells and their capacities. Note subshells of L and M.

the distance between nuclei is about the same as the diameter of the atom, the substance will become a liquid. As the atoms get still closer together, their outer electron orbits begin to overlap and a solid is formed. These outer electrons are called *valence electrons.* If the valence electrons match each other, as do the parts of a puzzle, a series of atoms occurs, with atoms connected in each plane in the same way, and a crystal is formed. This crystal will be *symmetrical* and, since the same configuration occurs over and over, we say it is *periodic* in nature. The outer electron orbit of most atoms has a radius in the order of 1 angstrom (Å) (about 1 ten millionth of a millimeter). Since the outer orbits of electrons in a crystal overlap, we would expect the atoms in a crystal to be about 2 Å apart. These distances may vary somewhat and orbits may be distorted and overlapped to the point that no single electron can be identified as belonging to a specific atom. Electrons may be shared and may adopt some new systematic pattern of motion.

In metals there are usually many electrons in the valence orbit. In the solid state, then, many of the electrons are located in the overlapping, distorted outer shells and many electrons are shared. As many as 10^{23} electrons may be present in a cubic centimeter of metal. We usually think of the electrons, in such a situation, as an *electron cloud* or sea of electrons in motion. When these electrons move under the influence of an electric or magnetic field, we say an electric current is conducted.

Substances having electrons that are easily displaced from their atomic structures are good conductors of electricity. Most metals are good conductors. Substances that give up their electrons only under great stress are nonconductors and may be called *insulators, resistors,* or *dielectrics.* As noted above, the valence electrons of atoms in a crystal are tied together in a bonding arrangement; this does not allow them to be displaced easily. Hence pure crystals are, in general, poor conductors of electricity.

Anyone who has played with magnets knows that the like poles of a magnet repel each other and the unlike poles attract. The negative pole of a magnet will repel electrons, since they are negative charged. The positive pole will attract these negative-charged electrons. If the negative pole of a magnet is moved along a wire, the electrons are repelled within the wire and move away from the magnet. Such a flow of electrons through a conductor is an electric current. One may also produce electricity in other ways.

In an *electrochemical cell,* or "battery," a metal is exposed to the effect of an electrolyte such as a strong acid. The chemical reaction leaves an excess of electrons, on the surface of the metal, at the same time that the carbon electrode is losing electrons. When a conductor provides a pathway for them, electrons will pass from the metal to the carbon, producing an electric current. Fig. 1-2 shows the internal detail of the familiar *zinc-acid dry cell.* Various types of electrochemical cells will be considered later.

In a *photovoltaic cell,* or *photocell,* electrons may be dislodged from certain substances, such as oxides or selenides of metals, by light energy and made to flow to a metal base, which in turn gives up its electrons to replace those in the original photosensitive oxide or selenide layer. Such an arrangement is known as a *photoemissive cell.* (See Fig. 1-3.) The effect of light on electron flow will be given attention throughout this book, since *photoelectric devices* are involved in a large percentage of the instruments discussed.

When metals are heated, their electrons move faster and begin to escape from their orbits. The number of electrons that escape at a given temperature is different for different metals. If two metals are brought

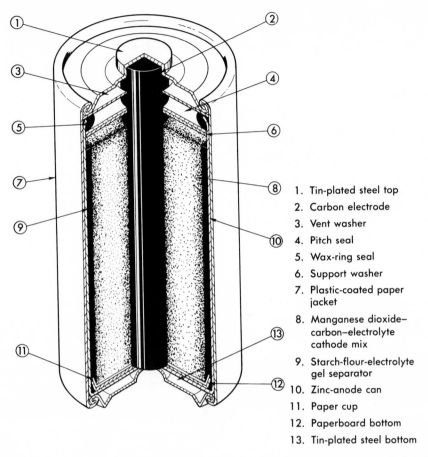

1. Tin-plated steel top
2. Carbon electrode
3. Vent washer
4. Pitch seal
5. Wax-ring seal
6. Support washer
7. Plastic-coated paper jacket
8. Manganese dioxide–carbon–electrolyte cathode mix
9. Starch-flour-electrolyte gel separator
10. Zinc-anode can
11. Paper cup
12. Paperboard bottom
13. Tin-plated steel bottom

Fig. 1-2. Cross section of an electrochemical cell or "dry battery." (Courtesy RCA, Electronic Components.)

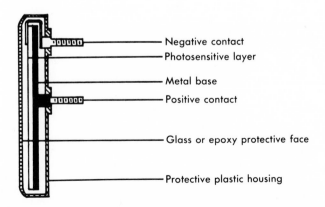

— Negative contact
— Photosensitive layer

— Metal base
— Positive contact

— Glass or epoxy protective face

— Protective plastic housing

Fig. 1-3. Cross section of a photoemissive cell or photocell.

into contact and are heated, a potential difference, or a difference in concentration of electrons, will appear at their interface. This potential difference can be measured. A device for measuring temperature in this way is called a *thermocouple.*

When the electrons are flowing from a steady source, such as a chemical cell, in the same direction through a circuit, they constitute what is said to be a *direct current* (DC).

Most electricity in use in the home and laboratory is produced by *generators.* A generator is a coil of wire that is mechanically turned in a magnetic field. Electrons in the coil are driven first in one direction in the wire, then in the opposite direction. Thus an *alternating current* (AC) is produced. If we were to plot this flow of electricity versus time on a graph, we would find momentarily no flow of electricity. There would then be a flow in one direction, increasing to a maximum before dropping back to zero. The current would then begin to flow in the opposite direction, increasing by the same amount and again dropping back to zero. This pattern is a *sine wave.* (See Fig. 1-4.)

Most house current is alternating at 60 cycles per second (cps). The newer termi-nology for cycles per second is *hertz,* which is abbreviated Hz. This is its *frequency.* The potential of house current is nominally 110 volts (v). Actually the *effective voltage* of house current is usually regulated at 117 v. Effective voltage is also called the *rms* value or *root mean square.* If an infinite number of values along the curve of the sine wave were squared and av-eraged and the root of this average derived, the answer would give the *rms* or *effective* voltage. The effective voltage × 1.414 is equal to the *peak* or *maximum* voltage. The effective voltage of alternating current is equal to the DC voltage that would be required to do the same work.

Alternating current in instruments may be in forms other than sine waves such as square waves or saw-toothed waves. These forms may be demonstrated and studied on an *oscilloscope* screen. In the discussion of thermionic emission and vacuum tubes, we shall see how the oscilloscope works.

Two alternating currents may be passed together through the same conductor. They are said to be *in phase* if they have the same frequency and their positive and negative voltages exactly coincide. If this is not the case, they are said to be *out of phase.* The current produced is the total

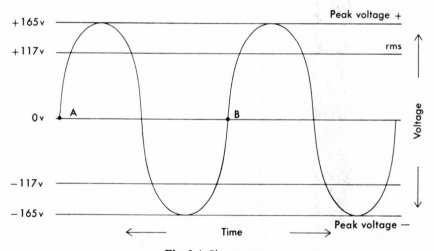

Fig. 1-4. Sine wave.

of the two currents at any instant. Two equal currents exactly 180 degrees out of phase would exactly oppose each other and would completely cancel each other. The result would be no current flow.

When an electric current flows through a wire, a magnetic field is produced around the wire. If the voltage in the wire is quite high, this magnetic field may be very strong. If another wire is run parallel to the one carrying the current, a current is *induced* in this second wire. The magnetic field mentioned above is called the *field of induction* and the current induced in the parallel wire is called an *induction current*. The magnetic force in the field of induction is called its *magnetic flux*. The strength of this magnetic flux decreases as one moves farther from the wire. Induction is an important electrical phenomenon and will be discussed further during consideration of transformers, relays, induction coils, and meters.

As electrons pass through a conductor, they collide with other electrons, pass through the force fields of molecules, etc. and are thus slowed down or impeded in their flow. This *resistance* varies between materials. Generally resistance of wire increases as the temperature rises. (This characteristic may be used to measure temperature.) When electrons meet resistance, some electrical energy is lost; it is converted to heat energy. The rate of flow of current is reduced and heat is produced. Resistance is an important consideration both in the alteration and control of electric currents and in the production of heat, as we shall see in subsequent chapters.

UNITS OF MEASUREMENT OF ELECTRICITY

Electricity can, in some ways, be compared to water. The volume of water flowing through a pipe may be measured in gallons; the electricity flowing through a wire may be measured in *coulombs*. One coulomb of electricity is 6.28×10^{18} electrons, or 6.28 billion billion electrons. This is an awkward expression, and it is easier to speak in terms of *amperes*. One ampere (amp) is the flow of 1 coulomb of electricity past a point in 1 second. Obviously the larger the pipe, the more water can flow through it. By the same token, the larger the wire or the lower the resistance to flow, the more coulombs can flow or the more amperes it can carry.

If we force a larger volume of water through a small pipe, we can say we increase the pressure. With electricity, the same thing occurs. We call this pressure *electromotive force* or EMF, and we measure it in *volts*. A volt is the force required to move 1 coulomb through a resistance of 1 ohm; or, to express it another way, 1 v of force is present when 1 *joule* of work is accomplished in moving 1 coulomb from one point to another.

In the case of electricity (unlike water), electrons cannot flow unless they can follow a conductor. When electrical pressure (or EMF) exists but electrons cannot flow, we say there is a *difference in potential* present. Such a potential difference will flow off to the earth if contact is made. The potential of *ground* (a contact to the earth) is zero. Occasionally in electrical equipment, induction, static electricity, or shorts may cause unwanted potential in the instrument and may cause shocks or erratic instrument responses. For this reason instruments' frames, or other points, may be "grounded" to drain off any potential difference. We might make an analogy with water by saying the water in a clamped hose on a water bottle has the potential to produce a stream that would flow to the ground if the clamp were removed.

In most modern buildings a three-pronged plug is used for electrical devices. One of the flat prongs contacts a wire in the receptacle that has zero potential. The second flat prong has a potential of about 117 v. When contact is established between the two through a lamp, a heater, or an instrument, electricity will flow. The third prong on the electric plug is used as a ground and is usually connected to any nonconducting metal surface of the appliance. When plugged into the wall, this prong makes contact with a wire that is connected to a water pipe or other conductor having immediate and good contact with the earth under the building. By this route, unwanted electric charges are released to the earth, which has an infinite capacity to absorb either negative or positive charges.

We say that water moving through a pipe encounters resistance if a section of the pipe is smaller or if there are filters, valves, etc. to impede its flow. Electricity also encounters *resistance,* as we have seen. Various types of material offer more resistance to the flow of electricity than others. Copper has a very low resistance whereas Nichrome wire has considerable resistance. The smaller the wire, the more resistance is offered if other conditions are equal. A hot wire generally offers more resistance than a cold one. Resistance is measured in *ohms*. One ohm, often indicated in diagrams by the Greek letter *omega* (Ω), is approximately the resistance offered by a column of mercury 1 meter long and 1 millimeter in diameter at room temperature. One ohm of resistance is said to be present when 1 volt is required to move 1 coulomb of electricity.

As mentioned earlier, resistance to the flow of current causes electrical energy to be converted to heat energy. This energy can be expressed as power in terms of *watts*. A watt (w) is defined as the power required to produce 1 joule of work in 1 second. In terms of electricity, a watt of power is consumed when 1 ampere flows from one point to another in 1 second, under the pressure of 1 volt.

Electrical energy loss may also be by conversion into mechanical energy, as in a motor. The electromotive force (in volts) times the volume of current (in amperes) gives the power (in watts, or joules per second) that is produced.

As we examine electrical phenomena, we will find other definitions and terms of measurement used in electricity, but those just mentioned are the basic ones necessary to an understanding of the material to follow.

DYNAMICS OF ELECTRICITY

It might be well at this point to discuss the flow of electricity. As has already been mentioned, an electric current is assumed to be the flow or forward movement of electrons through a conductor. Although the mechanism of this movement is still not well understood, it seems apparent that a sort of "falling domino" effect is involved. When an electron moves in a conductor, the electrical effect seems to move forward very rapidly (3×10^{10} cm/sec in a vacuum), whereas the electron itself may drift forward at about 1 cm/sec.

Before the nature of electricity was as well understood as it is today, we assumed that electricity moved from the positive to the negative pole. This was accepted by convention and has never been changed. Although it will prove convenient for us to think in terms of electrons moving from the negative to the positive pole, *conventional flow* (positive to negative) is still assumed in most wiring diagrams and electrical symbols. This is less confusing than it would at first seem, since the actual direction of flow is seldom of much significance to the effect produced.

Joule's law ($W = EI$) says that power in watts is equal to volts times amperes. From this expression, another (Ohm's law) may be derived. Ohm's law ($E = IR$) says that voltage is equal to the product of current volume in amperes times resistance in ohms.

The voltage mentioned pertains to the voltage drop across any "resistance" where electromotive force is converted to power. By derivation, Ohm's law can also be ex-

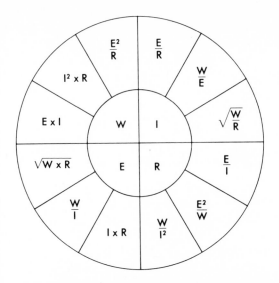

Fig. 1-5. Equations derived from Ohm's and Joule's laws.

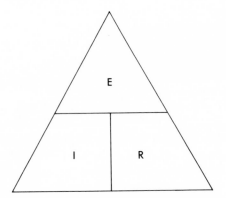

Fig. 1-6. Diagrammatic representation of Ohm's law.

pressed as $I = E/R$ or $R = E/I$. All the normally used variations of Ohm's and Joule's laws are expressed in the circular diagram of Fig. 1-5. In each quadrant the factor in the inner circle is equal to each of the expressions in the outer circle. For example, $E = I \times R$ and $I = W/E$.

Another expression of Ohm's law can be seen in the triangular arrangement of Fig. 1-6. Any single value is equal to the other two, in the relationship that they hold in the triangle. Thus $E = IR$, $I = E/R$, and $R = E/I$. The implications of these relationships will become more ap-

parent as we progress. The diagrams presented here make it easier to remember the relationships without deriving the appropriate equation each time.

SERIES AND PARALLEL CIRCUITS

All devices, in electric circuits, that produce power in any form may be considered as *resistors*. Resistors may be built into a circuit in either of two ways. If they are connected in an end-to-end fashion, we say they are *in series*. If they are connected in such a way that all their left ends are connected to one side of the circuit and their right ends to the other, we say they are *in parallel*. (See Fig. 1-7.)

When resistances are arranged in series, their values add, as we would suppose. For example, the 40-ohm and 60-ohm resistors in the series circuit in Fig. 1-7 would add to produce a total of 100 ohms of resistance for the whole circuit.

In the parallel circuit the situation is somewhat different. Here the current has a choice of several pathways, and the total resistance is less than that of any single resistor. The resistance for the entire circuit can be expressed by the following equation:

$$\frac{1}{R_T} = \frac{1}{R_1} + \frac{1}{R_2} + \frac{1}{R_3} \cdots$$

or

$$R_T = \frac{1}{\dfrac{1}{R_1} + \dfrac{1}{R_2} + \dfrac{1}{R_3} \cdots}$$

In the series circuit the voltage drops each time a resistance is encountered. These voltage drops may be called *IR drops,* since E (the voltage loss) is equal to I × R in each case. The total of the IR drops is the total voltage of the circuit. Therefore we can say that in a series circuit the voltage drops as it goes through each resistor but the amperage is constant.

In the parallel circuit voltage is constant throughout the circuit, but the amperage through each resistor will depend on its

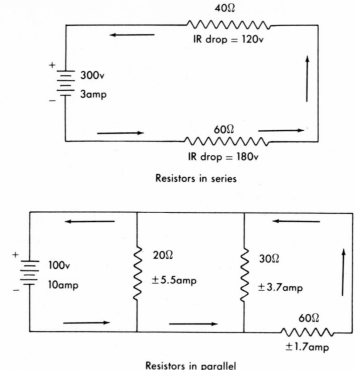

Fig. 1-7. Series and parallel circuits. Arrows indicate the direction of electron flow.

value in ohms. We shall see later that voltage may be read on a voltmeter by placing the meter in parallel with the circuit; but to measure amperes, we must actually disconnect the circuit at some point so that the ammeter can be placed in series with other elements.

In an actual instrument it is not often that we see either a simple parallel or a simple series circuit. Rather there will be an intermixing of the two, with some elements in series and others in parallel. In Fig. 1-8 resistors *7, 8,* and *9* are in parallel with each other but the *group* of resistors is in series with resistors *5, 6,* and *10.* The motor *(1)* and the lamp *(2)* are in series with each other but are both parallel to resistors *3* and *4.* This sort of arrangement can become complicated but can be resolved easily if each part of the circuit is considered separately. If we were to "draw a box around" resistors *7, 8,* and *9* and

were to consider them as a separate situation, we could use our basic equation $(1/R_T = 1/R_1 + 1/R_2 + 1/R_3)$ to determine what resistance this group adds to the others in the series. In a similar way we could calculate the overall resistance inserted by the components *1 + 2* (in parallel with *3 + 4).*

MEASUREMENT OF ELECTRICITY

Current passing through a wire causes a field of magnetic induction to be built up around the wire. This magnetic field has a direction and is generally considered to rotate around the wire. If the current is moving away from you (conventional direction), the direction of the field of force will be counterclockwise.

Now, if we wrap the conducting wire into a coil and reexamine the field of force, we find that all the lines of force are pointing in the same direction in the center of

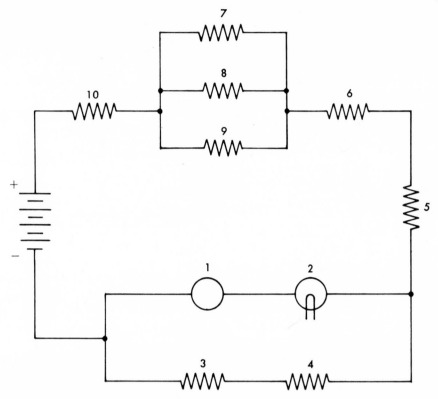

Fig. 1-8. Circuit showing components in series and parallel.

the coil. These lines come together to form a strong magnetic force in the center of the coil. In fact, the coil of wire constitutes an *electromagnet*. If we supply a core of some magnetizable metal, such as iron, we can enhance the magnetic properties of this field. When current is flowing through the coil, one end of the metal core will become the positive pole of the magnet and the other end will become the negative pole.

When an electromagnet, such as the one we have just described, is suspended between the poles of a permanent magnet, we produce a device that is capable of measuring electricity. When no current is flowing through it, the coil, has no magnetic field and can rest comfortably with its ends adjacent to the poles of the magnet. When current flows through the coil, however, the positive pole of the permanent magnet will repel the positive pole

of the coil (electromagnet), which will swing away if it is able to do so.

This is essentially the idea of the *d'Arsonval movement,* used in ammeters and galvanometers. In an ordinary ammeter the coil is attached to a *spindle,* which is mounted between rubies or hard metal surfaces so that the coil can turn freely. A pointer is attached to the coil in such a way that it can move over the face of a *calibrated scale.* (See Fig. 1-9.) The larger the current passing through the coil, the farther the pole of the coil is deflected and the farther the needle will sweep over the calibrated scale.

When we want the meter to be able to read very small currents, we use very fine wire and a small coil in a relatively weak magnetic field. If we wish to measure larger currents, we resort to a series of closely calibrated resistors that act as *shunts* to route all but a measured fraction of the

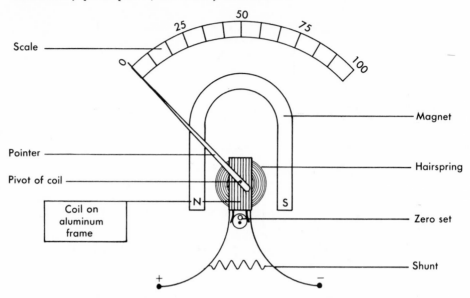

Fig. 1-9. Basic d'Arsonval movement.

current around the meter movement. For instance, if the meter movement presented a resistance of 1000 ohms, a resistor of 100 ohms in parallel would carry about 9/10 of the current around the meter and only about 1/10 would pass through the meter. Similarly a 10-ohm resistor would allow only 1/100 of the current to go through the coil. If we multiply the meter reading by the factor we have used, we can read the values for a very heavy current. In practice, separate scales may be provided on the meter to avoid the necessity of multiplying.

One other detail is necessary to make the meter workable. A *horsehair spring* is attached to the spindle to allow us to apply slight tension to return the coil to its resting position opposite the pole of the magnet (and the pointer to zero). If the zero setting is disturbed, we can correct it by turning a small screw that changes the tension of the spring.

These parts are diagrammatically illustrated in Fig. 1-9. Many ammeter covers are constructed of clear plastic so that the parts can be seen.

The d'Arsonval movement was originally designed to measure current flow in amperes. The same device can be used to measure volts if we place a very large resistor ahead of the meter to bring the amperage down to meter sensitivity. For example, if the meter movement is designed to deflect full scale with 1 milliampere of current and we wish 100 v to move our meter full scale, we apply Ohm's law as follows:

$$R = \frac{E}{I}$$

$$R = \frac{100 \text{ v}}{0.001 \text{ amp}}$$

R = 100,000 ohms, or 100 K ohms

In this case a resistor of 100 K ohms is required (K is used as a symbol meaning 1000). A voltage divider network with different resistors and a multiposition switch can be used to give a choice of voltage scales. A meter so equipped is called a *DC voltmeter*.

The voltmeter that we have described can also be used to measure alternating current if we add a *rectifier*, which is a device for converting alternating current to direct current. Rectifiers and the process

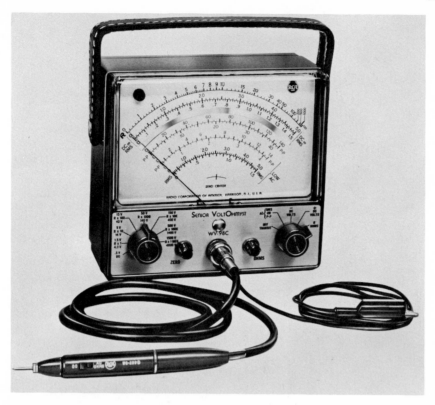

Fig. 1-10. VTVM multimeter. (Courtesy RCA, Electronic Components.)

of rectification will be discussed in more detail a little later.

The only electrical unit we have not yet seen how to measure is the ohm. The same d'Arsonval movement may be used in an *ohmmeter* if we simply supply a very accurate source of electricity that will deflect the meter exactly full scale. Each ohm of resistance introduced will reduce the current flow and the needle will fall back. The ohm scale is therefore numbered from right to left. (The ampere and volt scales are from left to right, of course.) This is not a straight-line function, and the ohm scale becomes much more concentrated as it approaches infinity at the left end of the scale. The accurate source of electricity provided for the ohmmeter is usually an electrochemical cell and is called a "reference cell," since it is capable of producing a very constant voltage. Electro-

chemical cells, or "batteries," are discussed on pp. 20 to 22.

If all the above functions—voltmeter, ohmmeter, and milliammeter—are combined into one measuring device, we call the instrument a *VOM* or *multimeter.* Another type of multimeter, called a *vacuum-tube voltmeter* or *VTVM,* is available. (See Fig. 1-10.) It is more sensitive than the VOM. In the VOM the current to move the meter must come from the source being measured; there is some *internal resistance,* therefore, and this causes some error. In the VTVM the source being measured serves only to control the *gain* of a *vacuum tube* that supplies the current to move the meter. This process is discussed on p. 17.

The *oscilloscope* is a voltage-measuring device that allows us to study the wave pattern as a function of time on an illu-

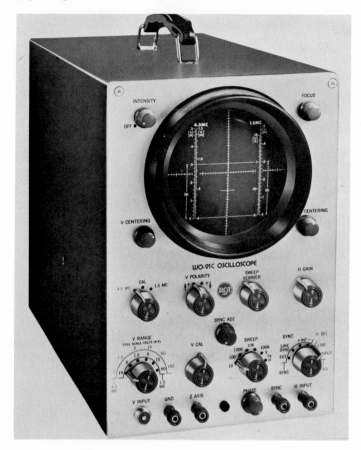

Fig. 1-11. Oscilloscope. (Courtesy RCA, Electronic Components.)

minated screen. It is also capable of many other measurements. Fig. 1-11 shows an oscilloscope. Understanding of this device depends on an understanding of the cathode-ray tube, which is a fairly complicated component. It too will be discussed, in connection with thermionic emission and vacuum tubes.

The oscilloscope is an extremely useful device in electronics, and we can learn much from it. It is a sturdy instrument that is not easily damaged in normal use. The student who wants to seriously study electronics would do well to become thoroughly acquainted with this test instrument.

In most laboratory instruments the measuring system required is quite simple, compared to that of the multimeter we have just studied. Usually a milliammeter or microammeter with the capability of reading a single range is sufficient. The meter dial may be calibrated in percent transmittance, absorbance, milliequivalents per liter, or some other parameter; but what is actually being measured by the meter is amperage or voltage.

There are several variations on the common milliammeter we have examined. One of the commonest is the string galvanometer. As noted above, the basic d'Arsonval movement does present some resistance. The pointed ends of the spindle bearing the coil produce friction as they turn against the ruby or metal surfaces, and some power is consumed in moving the

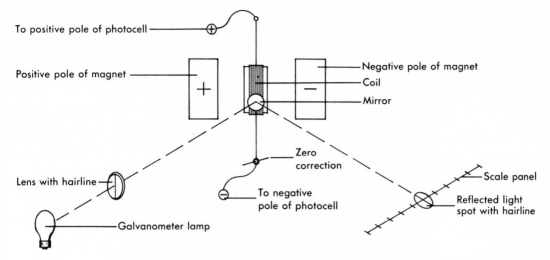

To positive pole of photocell

Positive pole of magnet

Negative pole of magnet

Coil

Mirror

Zero correction

Lens with hairline

To negative pole of photocell

Scale panel

Reflected light spot with hairline

Galvanometer lamp

Fig. 1-12. Diagrammatic representation of a string galvanometer.

needle. In addition to these disadvantages, there may be some *parallax* error in reading the hand in front of the dial. Furthermore, there is no provision made for reading a negative current. The string galvanometer, as used in many instruments, almost eliminates these problems. The coil is suspended on a small phosphor-bronze string or wire, which provides both suspension and electrical connections for the coil. The torque force required to twist the suspending string is negligible for most applications. A small mirror is attached to the coil and a beam of light is directed into it. As the coil is rotated, the mirror image of the light travels along a translucent scale panel. A hairline shadow in the light image provides for accurate reading. Reflection of the light image consumes no power, of course; and since the light (with the small shadow) falls directly on the scale, no parallax error is possible. Fig. 1-12 is a diagrammatical representation. Offsetting the advantages of the string galvanometer is the fact that this kind of measuring device is less linear over a wide range than is the more common ammeter configuration.

By shifting the position of the mirror image to the center of the scale we can make the string galvanometer into a *null-balance instrument,* capable of deflection in either direction. By causing two currents to oppose each other and modifying one by varying resistance, the meter can be made to read zero; the difference between the two currents will be proportional to the resistance needed to bring them into balance.

As equipment becomes more sophisticated, the *digital voltmeter* is becoming more and more common. Most of these devices work on a *null-balancing principle,* using a servomotor to move the digit wheels forward or backward as needed. These ideas need some explaining. In a null-balancing system a *reference source* such as a flashlight battery is balanced against the unknown signal. Let us look at this idea first. In Fig. 1-13 a reference cell is connected to a meter to provide a signal to drive the meter to the right. The unknown signal from a photocell is connected to the meter backward so as to oppose the reference cell and drive the meter needle to the left. When the two electric signals are equal, the meter will stand at exactly zero with the needle in the center of the scale. If the signal from the photocell (*photosignal*) is weaker, the needle will move right; and

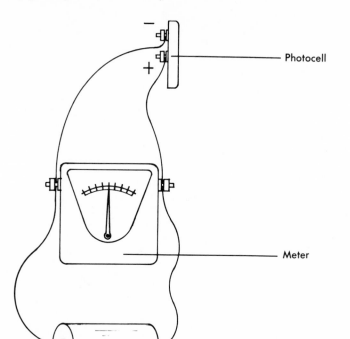

Fig. 1-13. Null-balance system with a reference source opposing a photocell.

if it is stronger than the reference, the needle will move left. The imbalance between these two signals is called an *error signal,* and it can be either positive or negative. From the section on voltmeters you will remember that a resistance must be placed in the line to reduce voltage to the level at which amperage can be measured. Can you calculate the resistance needed here to balance the two sources? (Assume that one milliampere moves the meter full scale.)

There is a device that works like a small direct current motor (to be discussed later) called a *servomotor,* which can move either forward or backward, depending on the direction of current flow. This servomotor, driven by the error signal, turns a variable resistor to bring the two currents into balance by introducing resistance into the pathway of the stronger of the two. The resistance thus introduced is relative to the original unknown voltage, and a digital readout can be made to register this

voltage or some related parameter such as milliequivalents or absorbance units. Servomotors are used a great deal in more sophisticated laboratory instruments, and they will be discussed again.

In addition to the devices for measuring electricity that have already been noted, there are a few others that deserve mention. Recorders, which make some sort of continuous or intermittent record on paper, may work on any of several different principles that will be described more completely in a later chapter. In general, we can say that most recorders fall into one of two categories already mentioned. The first includes the recorders that use a d'Arsonval movement and in some way substitute a writing arm and pen for the pointer. In the second are those that use a servomotor to drive a pen across the paper.

Still another type of measuring device uses the capacitance of glow tubes, Nixie tubes, or bar tubes to indicate current flow.

These are the glowing spots or lighted numbers that are used on such instruments as the newer Coulter counters and the Orion pH meters. They require more background explanation and will be discussed in the next chapter. More recently, *light-emitting diodes* or LEDs have gained wide acceptance as numerical indicators. These are interesting and will be mentioned again when we consider semiconductor devices.

CARE AND USE OF METERS

A multimeter such as the VOM or VTVM is strongly recommended as a working tool in the clinical laboratory. These instruments are rugged and well built, but certain sensible precautions must be taken when using them.

It should be obvious from the description of the d'Arsonval movement that meters incorporating this movement are sensitive to mechanical shock. They should never be handled roughly.

The switches on the front of the instrument tell which parameter and what range you will read. If 115 v is applied to the meter with the range switch set on 3 v, the tiny coil in the meter movement may be completely burned up and the instrument ruined. A fuse is provided to keep this from happening. To discover the fuse you may have to remove the instrument from its case. Usually the fuse is soldered to its leads to reduce the internal resistance of the meter. You should always set the range switch higher than the expected value and decrease the settings as necessary to read accurately.

Voltage is measured in parallel; that is, the leads can be contacted to the circuit at two points and the difference in potential between the two points will be indicated on the dial.

To measure amperage with the ordinary VOM, you must pass the current through the instrument. In other words, the instrument must be in series in the circuit that is to be measured; so the circuit must actually be broken at some point to allow the meter to be connected.

When measuring ohms, you are passing the current from a battery in the multimeter through the resistance you wish to measure. If the battery deteriorates so much that you can no longer zero the meter when the leads are connected, you obviously cannot get an accurate reading. Care must be taken that an old corroding battery does not leak and damage the circuits of the meter. An alkaline or mercury battery is less likely to have this problem.

When measuring a resistance in a circuit, be sure that one end of the circuit is open so that you are not measuring resistance of more than one pathway at a time. Never try to measure resistance when current is passing through the circuit.

Be sure to read the instructions that come with your VOM or VTVM and become familiar with the instrument before starting to use it.

Do not store the instrument with the switch set to read ohms. If the lead wires make contact, the battery may be discharged as it sits on the shelf.

REVIEW QUESTIONS

1. What is electricity?
2. How do AC and DC differ?
3. List three ways electricity can be produced.
4. Write Ohm's law three ways to express the values of voltage, amperage, and resistance —each in terms of the other two parameters.
5. Why are metals good conductors?
6. A circuit contains four resistors: 30 ohms, 2.2 K ohms, 51 megohms, and 0.2 K ohms. They are in series. What is the total resistance?
7. If the resistors in question 6 were all in parallel, what would be the total resistance of the circuit?
8. How does an ohmmeter work?
9. What is induction?
10. What is an ampere?

2
Electrical components and circuits

In the first chapter we have briefly reviewed the nature of electricity and how it is measured. Let us now look at the devices or components used to make electrical energy do what we want it to do. Electronics is a vast field that people spend their lives studying. In these few pages we can consider only a very simplified version. Hopefully, however, you will get a better insight into the way instruments work by understanding what each component is able to do.

During the past decade, semiconductor diodes and transistors have been developed to replace vacuum tubes for nearly all functions. Semiconductors have many advantages, as we shall see presently. Vacuum tubes have nearly disappeared from newer instruments—with a couple of important exceptions. To understand these important exceptions we need to understand vacuum tubes and thermionic electron emission.

VACUUM TUBES AND THERMIONIC ELECTRON EMISSION

All vacuum tubes have at least two electrodes. The negative electrode is the cathode or emitter of electrons. The positive electrode is the anode or plate. The plate is maintained at a higher positive voltage than the cathode so that electrons will have a tendency to be attracted to it. With such a voltage differential a stream of electrons can be made to flow from the cathode

to the plate. This current is greatly enhanced if (1) the system is in a vacuum, (2) the cathode is heated, and (3) the proper selection of cathode material is made. Within limits, the greater the voltage differential between the electrodes, the greater is the flow of electrons.

Half-wave rectifiers. A vacuum tube with only a heated cathode and a plate is called a *diode*. If alternating current is presented to a diode, electrons will pass from the cathode to the plate during the positive (forward) half of a cycle. When electrons try to flow in the other direction (negative half of the cycle), they are repelled by the negative cathode and cannot pass. Thus the current that passes is direct current, since it is flowing in only one direction, but it is intermittent. We can say that alternating current is *rectified* to produce direct current and we can call this tube a *rectifier*. It retains only half of the sine wave, however, so we call it a half-wave rectifier. Fig. 2-1 shows the symbol used for a tube of this sort.

Full-wave rectifiers. If two plates are inserted in the tube and given appropriate charges (Fig. 2-2), the positive part of the alternating current will flow to one of the

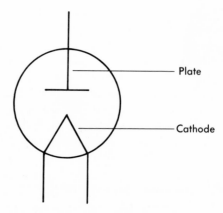

Fig. 2-1. Diagrammatic half-wave rectifier.

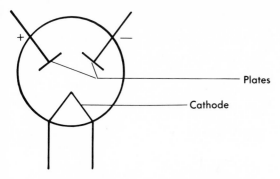

Fig. 2-2. Diagrammatic full-wave rectifier.

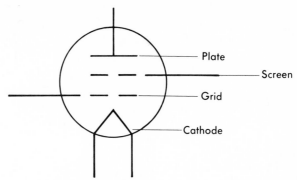

Fig. 2-4. Tetrode (symbol).

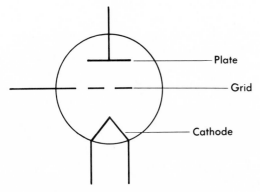

Fig. 2-3. Triode (symbol).

plates and the negative part will flow to the other. By reversing polarity and combining the two currents, we obtain a direct current varying from zero to peak voltage twice as often as the frequency. The full-wave rectifier is, in effect, two half-wave rectifiers in one envelope using a common emitter. (Further modification of this signal will be discussed later.)

Triodes. Triodes are similar to diodes but with a third element introduced (Fig. 2-3). This element is a loose coil of wire or a screen, positioned between the cathode and the plate but close to the cathode, called the *grid*. The grid is maintained at a negative voltage, which tends to counteract the attraction of the plate for the emitted (negative) electrons. If the grid voltage is entirely closed off (that is, made zero), all the electrons will flow to the plate. If

grid voltage is increased to a maximum, the flow of electrons will effectively cease. In this way the small grid voltage can control a much larger current in a linear fashion, and changes in the grid voltage are greatly amplified. (Thus the triode is an amplifier tube.) As can be seen from the above, the amplification depends on the grid voltage. When the grid voltage is decreased, we say we have increased the *gain;* this means that we have increased the amplification. Sometimes it is expedient to take the output of one tube and use it as the grid voltage for a second tube to achieve a second *stage* of amplification.

Tetrodes. A tetrode is a triode that is further modified by the addition of a *screen* between the grid and the plate (Fig. 2-4). The screen is given a positive charge somewhat lower than that of the plate. The screen makes the tube more stable, by lowering the capacitance, and allows higher amplification. Tetrodes are not often used.

Pentodes. The pentode has still another element added—the *suppressor grid* (Fig. 2-5). Electrons from the cathode (primary emission) may strike the plate with sufficient force to dislodge other electrons from the plate. This is called *secondary emission.* When the positive-charged screen is present (in the tetrode), there is a tendency for these dislodged electrons (the secondary emission) to be attracted back to the screen and to collide with the electrons being at-

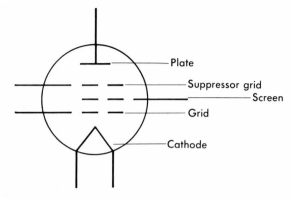

Fig. 2-5. Pentode (symbol).

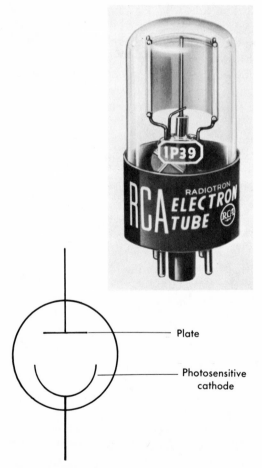

Fig. 2-6. Phototube (courtesy RCA, Electronic Components) and its symbol.

tracted to the plate. The suppressor grid is connected directly to the cathode and therefore presents a negative charge that repels the "secondary emmission" of electrons from the plate. Pentodes give high amplification but have somewhat greater signal distortion than do triodes.

There are a variety of special-purpose and combination tubes available, having different functions. For example, some tubes combine two functions in one envelope. These may be shown on wiring diagrams as two half tubes, their functions and their schematic representations being widely separated. This is true, for example, of the 12AX7 tube in the wiring diagram of the Spectronic 20. (See Fig. 4-15.)

Phototubes or photoemissive tubes (Fig. 2-6). These are vacuum tubes that have a cathode composed of a material such as rubidium or lithium that will act as a resistor in the dark but will emit electrons in quantity when exposed to light. The rate of emission of electrons is a linear function of the amount of light striking the cathode within a fairly wide range of light intensity. The light acts in almost the same manner as grid voltage, allowing a large current change with a small change in light intensity. The cathode usually has a large surface area designed to catch the maximum amount of light. Varying the cathode materials changes the wavelength at which the phototube gives its highest response. The addition of a small amount of inert gas to the vacuum tube enhances its amplification. The electrons traveling from cathode to plate dislodge electrons from the gas molecules, producing an *avalanche effect* as more gas atoms are ionized. There is a practical limit to amplification by this process, since too high a voltage will produce a permanent ionization of the gas and destroy the tube.

Photomultiplier tubes (Fig. 2-7). The photomultiplier tube is a photoemissive tube with the ability to amplify the primary emission. The cathode catching the

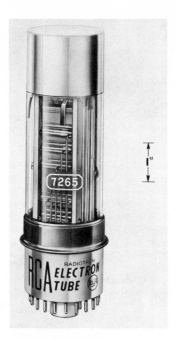

Fig. 2-7. Photomultiplier tube. (Courtesy RCA, Electronic Components.)

light signal emits a stream of electrons, which is attracted first to one *dynode,* with a charge of perhaps +100 v, and then to a second dynode with a charge of +200 v. This process continues through several dynodes. The signal is then taken off on the collector electrode or plate. The voltage jump of 100 v per dynode is about the maximum allowable and the jump between the last dynode and the collector should not exceed 45 v for good tube life and stability.

The gain or amplifying power of the photomultiplier is increased by increasing the voltage increment of the dynodes and the plate. Similarly, by reduction of the primary voltage at the transformer, all voltages are reduced proportionately and the amplification factor reduced. Photomultiplier tubes can provide an amplification factor of 2,000,000 × and can detect a light signal 1/100 the intensity of that measurable by a phototube. Even when the light lasts for only a millionth of a sec-

ond, as may be the case in scintillation counters, the photomultiplier can detect it.

RCA, one of the largest manufacturers of photomultiplier tubes, recently announced a breakthrough that will increase amplification another tenfold by the use of a gallium phosphide dynode. The company claims that it will now be possible to differentiate between light-producing phenomena that generate one, two, three, four, or more primary electrons.*

Cathode-ray tube, or CRT. Newer instruments are using cathode-ray tubes for various purposes. On the Coulter counter the screen, showing peaks corresponding to cells of various sizes, is the front of a CRT. On the Technicon AutoAnalyzer, SMA-12/60, CRTs are used to show colorimeter response to each channel. On the gamma camera, two CRTs provide visualization of isotope distribution in the patient. On the oscilloscope, which was discussed under measurement of electricity, the CRT is the heart of the instrument. During the next several years we will certainly see much heavier use of these convenient devices.

Fig. 2-8 shows a cross section through an oscilloscope tube. This is a vacuum tube utilizing the principle of thermionic emission discussed above. CRTs may have slightly different internal arrangements but have several features in common. The cathode is located at the back of the tube. It is heated by a filament. There is a very high charge on the anode elements to pull the electrons from the cathode and hurl them against the phosphor-coated screen, which is the front of the tube. The coating of the screen itself acts as the plate where electrons, hitting at high velocity, cause the phosphor to glow. Just in front of the cathode is a negative-charged grid that controls the brightness of the spot on the screen by slowing down the stream of elec-

*Laboratory Equipment, vol. 5, p. 1, January, 1969.

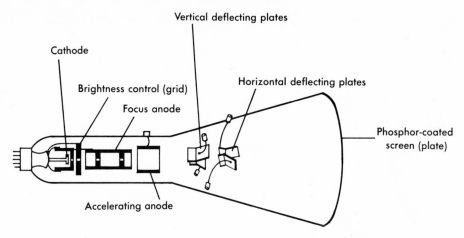

Fig. 2-8. Cross section through a cathode-ray tube (CRT).

trons just as a grid controls electron flow in the triode discussed above.

Between the grid and the screen are focusing and accelerating anode rings through which the electron beam is directed. Also there are two sets of deflecting plates. One of these sets is able, by the application of voltage, to deflect the beam of electrons to the right or left. The other set of plates, by the same mechanism, directs the beam higher or lower on the screen.

The oscilloscope has a sweep circuit that applies an alternating current to the horizontal deflecting plates, causing the beam to move from left to right as a function of time. The vertical deflection plates cause the beam to move from bottom to top as voltage increases. If 60-cycle alternating current is presented to the oscilloscope and the horizontal sweep control is set at 60 sweeps a second, a sine wave will be traced on the screen. Since the phosphor on the inside of the screen will continue to glow for a little while and the stream of electrons will retrace its path 60 times a second, the trace appears to stand still. The sweep circuit can be adjusted to correspond with any wave frequency. The vertical controls can be varied likewise to increase or decrease the height of the trace.

Most oscilloscopes have other refine-ments. The period of time that the phosphor will glow can be controlled on some models. Most have a base line control with which the base voltage can be adjusted to raise or lower the pattern on the screen. Many instruments can stretch out the trace horizontally so that one small part of a wave form can be studied in detail. Some instruments have a triggering device that causes a given point in a wave form to make the horizontal sweep move back to the left and repeat the trace each time the point is reached. This sort of mechanism is used, for example, with patient-monitoring electrocardiographic equipment.

Some CRTs have two or more separate "electron guns" in one tube so that two or more wave forms from different circuits or parts of a circuit can be compared simultaneously.

A special electronic switch on some oscilloscopes enables them to monitor several different circuits in fast succession, placing the traces one below the other on the screen. This switching has to be extremely fast, of course.

OTHER ELECTRICAL COMPONENTS

Electrochemical cells and batteries. When two dissimilar metals, such as zinc and copper, are immersed in an electro-

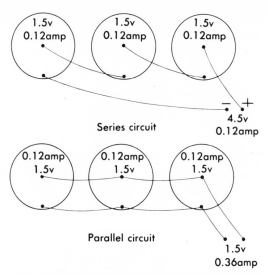

Fig. 2-9. "Batteries" in series and in parallel. Circuit voltage and amperage.

lyte, such as a solution of sulfuric acid, a difference in electron concentration on the two metals occurs. In this case, zinc ions go into solution, leaving electrons on the zinc plate. The positive-charged hydrogen ions migrate to the copper to combine with free electrons from the copper. If the two metal strips, which we may call *electrodes,* are connected by a wire and if a meter is introduced into this circuit, an electric current can be demonstrated. In effect, we have constructed a simple primary cell. (See Fig. 1-2.)

Carbon-zinc cells. The familiar flashlight battery is essentially a simple primary cell. It uses zinc and carbon in a matrix of graphite moistened with an electrolyte. Eventually the zinc deteriorates to the point where the cell ceases to function. There is no way to rejuvenate a "battery" of this kind. The carbon-zinc cell develops about 1.5 v. The amperage or capacity depends upon the size of the cell. As we can see from Fig. 2-9, these cells may be wired in series to add voltage or in parallel to add amperage or capacity. It is often undesirable, from the point of space required, to wire thirty separate cells of this sort in

series to get 45 v. For this reason, if limited amperage is needed, cells are packed inside one jacket and connected in series to produce the high voltage. This may be achieved by simply stacking a carbon plate, electrolyte mix, and a zinc plate, followed by another series of carbon, electrolyte, zinc, etc., for as many layers as are required for the desired voltage. In other types the individual cells are wrapped in a plastic material, connected in series by short wires, and stacked into a tight bundle. This arrangement of several cells into one unit is a true *battery*. The word "battery" is commonly used in error to describe a cell.

Alkaline cells and batteries. These have become common during the past few years. They work on a principle very similar to that of the carbon-zinc cell, but manganese dioxide and zinc are used as electrodes and the electrolyte is potassium hydroxide (which accounts for the name). The arrangement of the cell is physically somewhat different, providing more interface. The capacity of these cells is much higher and their shelf life is considerably longer than those of carbon-zinc cells. The price is considerably higher, but these cells are becoming more economical as they are sold in greater quantity.

Mercury cells and batteries. These cells have a zinc amalgam for one electrode and a mercuric oxide–zinc material for the other. The physical arrangement is different from both the carbon-zinc cell and the alkaline battery. The output is an exact and reproducible 1.35 v, which is a highly desirable feature when this is used as a reference cell. The capacity of this cell is somewhat more than that of the alkaline battery. The price is also quite high in comparison to the other two. Since it does not break down as the carbon-zinc cell does, with loss of electrolyte, it is much safer for use close to delicate circuitry. Compound (stacked) batteries of mercury cells are made with voltages up to around 50 v.

Electrolytic-cell, secondary-cell, or wet-

cell batteries. These are what we commonly refer to as "car batteries." In their commonest form they contain several cells arranged in a battery to produce 6, 12, or 24 v. Each cell will produce about 2.1 v; therefore three cells are necessary to produce 6 v. Each cell, of these lead-acid batteries, contains two electrodes, one that is lead and the other oxide. The lead is converted to lead sulfate by the electrolytic action of the liquid sulfuric acid. Two electrons are released to the lead electrode for each molecule of lead sulfate formed. The lead oxide electrode is reduced to lead sulfate, taking up two electrons. When current is applied to recharge the battery, the lead sulfate is reconverted to lead and lead oxide. This reversible process can be repeated many times during the life of the battery. The state of discharge can be measured by the specific gravity of the sulfuric acid containing the lead sulfate. Eventually the electrodes deteriorate so much that the battery is no longer functional, but the cycle of discharging and charging can be repeated many hundreds of times before this happens. A lead-acid battery provides a copious supply of constant direct current at an economical price. It is, of course, quite heavy and rather messy because of the sulfuric acid.

At one time these batteries were commonly used as a power source in clinical laboratories. They are no longer used to any extent. Their economy is negligible compared to the cost of today's laboratory instruments. At best, they are cumbersome and space consuming and, at worst, dangerous around delicate electrical and optical components because of the damaging acid and acid fumes.

Nickle-cadmium batteries. Another type of rechargeable battery that is becoming popular in the United States is the nickle-cadmium battery. This unit is completely sealed and requires no servicing other than recharging. The positive electrode is nickle hydroxide and the negative electrode is cadmium. When the battery is discharging, the nickle hydroxide is converted to nickle and the cadmium is oxidized. When it is recharging, the process is reversed. Each cell produces about 1.3 v and has fairly high capacity. These batteries can be stored for long periods of time either charged or discharged. They are quite expensive, but are a practical source of constant current and are quite trouble-free.

Photovoltaic cells or photoemissive cells. These devices have the ability to produce an electric current in the presence of light. Some oxides, selenides, etc. of certain metals have the ability to give up electrons under the influence of light energy. (See Fig. 1-3.) The photocell is composed of a film of light-sensitive material on a plate of metal. When it is exposed to light, electrons flow from the oxide, through the circuit, to the metal. The common light meter used in photography is simply a cell of this type coupled to a milliammeter. The current produced is proportional to the light throughout a workable zone of light intensity. Many laboratory colorimeters and spectrophotometers use a photocell to read the intensity of the transmitted light.

Photoconductive cells. Some compounds, such as cadmium sulfide, act as resistors when in the dark but become good conductors when exposed to light. This is the principle of the photoconductive cell. Such cells are often used to open and close circuits by *relays* (which will be described presently). Several of the newer colorimeters and spectrophotometers are using the photoconductive cell as a detector. Other light-sensitive components will be discussed later.

Transformers. As noted earlier, we can pass current through one wire and produce a current in a parallel wire by *induction*. A transformer is composed of two parallel coils of wire wound around a metal core. One coil, called the *primary winding*, conducts the current that is supplied to it. The other coil, called the *secondary winding*, carries the induction current produced. The voltage of the induction current will vary with the ratio of windings in the secondary coil compared to the primary. Amperage in the secondary is relatively small. Transformers may furnish either a lower voltage than the initial voltage *(step-down transformer)* or a higher voltage *(step-up transformer)*. Occasionally a transformer with the same number of turns in the primary and secondary coils is used; hence it gives out the same voltage that was put into it. This is called an *isolating transformer.* Its main function is to stabilize voltage and protect the instrument from sudden power surges. In this case both coils act as *choke* or *induction coils.* (These components will be explained presently.) All transformers tend to protect the induced current from fast fluctuations in the primary current. Often several taps will be placed on the secondary winding to furnish several voltages from one transformer. A *center-tap transformer* gives positive voltage to one side of the center tap and negative voltage to the other side. In most laboratory instruments the necessary voltages to operate the instruments are furnished by transformers.

Resistors. Resistors, as the name implies, are components introduced into a circuit to resist the flow of current. If we review Ohm's law ($E = IR$), we will note that altering resistance causes either voltage or amperage to change. When placed in a series circuit, resistors caused voltage to drop. The amperage between any two points will be equal, however. In such a series circuit the resistance of the whole circuit is the total of individual resistances, and the amperage $\times$ the total resistance gives the total voltage in the circuit. The voltage drop *(IR drop)* for each resistor may be calculated in the same way. For example, if a current of 3 amp is passed through a 40-ohm and a 60-ohm resistor in series, the total resistance is 100 ohms and the total voltage is 100×3 amp or

300 v. The IR drop across the 40-ohm resistor is 40×3 or 120 v and, likewise, across the 60-ohm resistor is 60×3, or 180 v. (See Fig. 1-7.)

If all the resistors are placed in parallel in the circuit, the current is provided with several divergent pathways and the total resistance offered is less than that of any single resistor. The total resistance of the circuit may be figured according to the formula $1/R_T = 1/R_1 + 1/R_2 + 1/R_3$, etc. For example a 20-ohm resistor, a 30-ohm resistor, and a 60-ohm resistor in parallel:

$$\frac{1}{R_T} = \frac{1}{20} + \frac{1}{30} + \frac{1}{60}$$
$$= \frac{3}{60} + \frac{2}{60} + \frac{1}{60}$$
$$= \frac{6}{60} \text{ or } \frac{1}{10}$$

The total resistance in the circuit is 10 ohms. In this case the voltage remains constant for the entire circuit but the amperage through the resistors varies, with the most current passing through the resistor of lowest value and a proportional amount passing through the others.

Fixed resistors. There are two common types. *Composition* resistors are made of powdered graphite and a binding material packed into a plastic shell. They are generally used for small currents and are rated in watts of heat energy that can be dissipated by them. Their physical size determines their wattage, and the ohms of resistance and tolerance value can be read from the color code on the resistor. See resistor code explanation in Fig. 2-10. Special resistors may have their values printed on them. Larger wattages are usually handled through *wire-wound* resistors. These are coils of high-resistance wire, usually embedded in ceramic to enhance their heat dissipation.

Variable resistors. In some situations the resistance in a circuit may need to be varied. The simplest variable resistance is a coil of resistant wire with one contact at

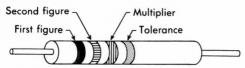

Fig. 2-10. Resistor code explanation. Colors of bands represent numbers:

0 = Black	5 = Green
1 = Brown	6 = Blue
2 = Red	7 = Violet
3 = Orange	8 = Gray
4 = Yellow	9 = White

A. Write down numbers corresponding to first two bands.
B. Add as many zeros as indicated by third band.
C. This number represents the value of the resistor in ohms.
D. If the fourth band is silver, tolerance is 10%. If it is gold, 5%.

Example: Bands are red, orange, yellow, gold. Red = 2, orange = 3, yellow = 4. Value is 230,000 ohms, or 230 K ohms, and should test within ± 5%.

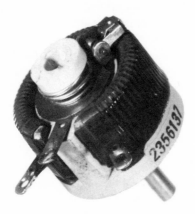

Fig. 2-11. Rheostat.

the end and the other in the form of a "wiper" that can be moved along the coil. Increasing the length of the conducting wire increases the resistance. This sort of arrangement may be called a *rheostat*. (See Fig. 2-11.)

A *potentiometer* is a variable resistor, such as the rheostat. It may consist of a coil of high-resistance wire with a contact on either end and a wiper or sliding contact that can be moved along the coil so as to vary the amount of resistance through which the current must travel. In this way the wiper can be used as a common contact (0 v) for the two currents, the positive sides of which may be passed through either side of the potentiometer. Thus two currents can be balanced, and, if a scale is provided on the potentiometer, the resistance required to balance the currents can be determined. *Pots,* as they are often called, usually are calibrated to give an arbitrary, reproducible resistance. On the null-balance colorimeter previously mentioned the resistance needed to balance two signals is proportional to the signal difference and a calibrated potentiometer gives the necessary information.

In many pots, the coil of high-resistance wire is replaced by a band of graphite containing a given concentration of electrolyte that causes it to have a given resistance per centimeter. When potentiometers are made in this way, they are called *composition pots*. These are cheaper, generally less accurate, and more widely used than the wire-wound variety.

SEMICONDUCTORS

Development of the science of electronics has been completely revolutionized during recent years by the discoveries in the behavior of *semiconductor materials*. Components utilizing semiconductor materials have replaced nearly all types of vacuum tubes and have replaced or modified several other devices. These new components are generally quite small, operate at much lower voltages, produce little heat, and may allow consolidation of various functions into one tiny package. They are cheap to produce and are mechanically sturdy. A thorough understanding of semiconductor physics is far beyond the scope of this text, but some basic knowledge of the subject should prove both interesting and helpful.

The two most common semiconductor elements are *silicon* and *germanium*. Each has four electrons in the outer orbits and

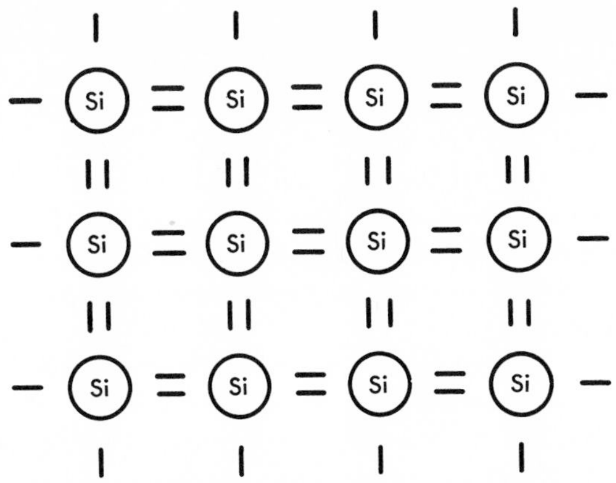

Fig. 2-12. Silicon crystal showing each atom with four valence electrons. Each of these is shared with a neighboring atom in covalent bonding.

forms a sort of crystal lattice or periodic arrangement. In the crystal each of the four valence electrons participates with an electron from a neighboring atom in a covalent bond. (See Fig. 2-12.) At absolute zero temperature this structure should be a perfect insulator, since there are no free electrons available to conduct. At normal temperatures, however, a very few electrons increase in energy enough to free themselves from their bond and become *charge carriers.* Since there are only a few of these, the crystal is still a very poor conductor or a *semiconductor.* Small temperature changes cause considerable change in relative conductivity, however.

If a potential is applied across this semiconductor crystal, the electrons will be drawn to the positive side. When an electron is thus removed from its atom, there is a net positive charge left behind, since the atom was originally in electrical balance. This net positive charge (or vacant position on the atom) is sometimes called a *hole.* The hole may be filled by an electron from a neighboring atom, but this produces a new hole in the atom that gave up its electron. Thus the hole *migrates* or moves in a random manner when it is affected by an electric potential. The elec-

trons and "holes" that migrate under the influence of an electric field are referred to as *carriers.* This can be called *intrinsic conduction* and the flow of electrons be termed a *leakage current.*

Intrinsic conduction is very slight (although sometimes important); in semiconductor electronics we are more interested in *extrinsic conduction,* which is the result of adding an impurity to the semiconductor material.

You will recall that silicon and germanium each has four valence electrons. If one of these crystals is *doped* with an infinitesimal amount of *antimony* (which has five valence electrons), there will be one electron that cannot be matched up in the covalent bonding of the lattice. It represents a spare electron that gives the doped crystal a *net negative* charge. This type of crystal is referred to as an *N-type* semiconductor. (See Fig. 2-13.)

If, instead of using antimony, we now dope the crystal with *indium,* which has three valence electrons, there will be a "hole" where an electron is lacking. The material will hence have a net positive charge and will be called *P-type* material. (See Fig. 2-14.) These N-type and P-type materials have considerable extrinsic conductivity and they are the building blocks used in semiconductor electronics.

When a small N-type crystal is fused to one of P-type, a few of the electrons from the N-type material combine with a few "holes" from the P-type crystal along the interface between them. This produces a tiny zone of material that is in electrical balance and, hence, is a poor conductor. When we try to pass a current through this interface, a small amount of energy must be applied before conduction will occur. This energy may be an electrical potential, heat, light, or other radiation.

SOLID-STATE COMPONENTS

Semiconductor diodes, transistors, and similar devices are generally called *solid-*

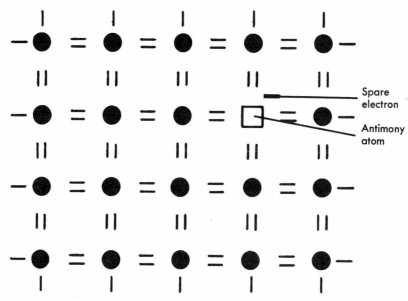

Fig. 2-13. N-type material silicon crystal doped with antimony. The square symbol indicates an atom of antimony and the neighboring heavy bar represents an extra electron that causes the crystal to have a negative charge.

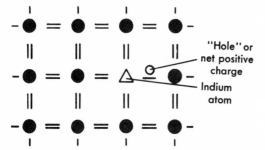

Fig. 2-14. P-type semiconductor material silicon crystal doped with indium, which has three valence electrons. Triangle is indium; and circle represents a "hole," or net positive charge, caused by shortage of one electron in bonding structure.

state components, since there are no vacuum tubes, gas tubes, etc. in which electrons must travel through space.

Semiconductor diodes. By fusing an N-type and a P-type crystal we produce a *diode.* Let us look at some of its characteristics and possible functions.

Rectifier. If a battery is connected to the diode so that the positive terminal is applied to the N side and the negative terminal to the P side, the N carriers will move to the positive terminal and the "holes" in the P side will move to the negative terminal. This increases the effect of the zone of resistance at the juncture, and current will not flow unless a very high voltage is applied. We say we have *reverse-biased* the diode.

If we reverse the poles of the battery, current will flow easily and the diode is now said to be biased in a *forward* direction. Notice that the diode is behaving like a vacuum tube diode and that it can be used as a *rectifier,* since current will pass easily in one direction but will not normally flow in the other.

Zener diode. If we reverse-bias a diode and apply to it a very high voltage, it will, at some point, start to conduct. The voltage at which it does this is called its *Zener breakdown voltage* or simply *Zener voltage.* Once this Zener voltage has been reached, any further increase in voltage causes the resistance of the diode to increase also so

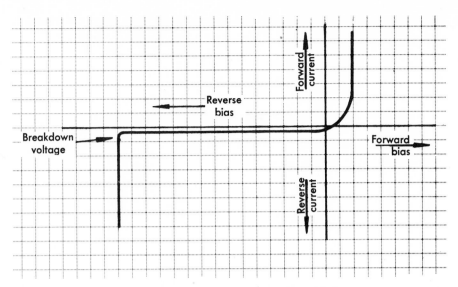

Fig. 2-15. Current flow through Zener diode.

that the flow of current in amperes remains constant. Most diodes would be damaged if used in this way, but *Zener diodes* are produced for the specific purpose of withstanding the high reverse voltage and thus they act as excellent amperage control devices. If too heavy a load is placed on them, they will burn out, of course. The Zener voltage of a diode is abbreviated as V_Z and the amperage above which the diode will break down is indicated as I_{MAX}. (See Fig. 2-15.)

Thermistors. As mentioned earlier, semiconductors are sensitive to temperature change, since bondings are inclined to break at higher temperatures, thus providing free electrons and "holes" to act as carriers. If we forward-bias a diode and apply a current to it, we will find that temperature change will effect the current flow. We can calibrate this *thermistor* and will find it to be highly accurate. Thermistor thermometers may consist of a battery, a thermistor, and an ammeter. Many laboratory devices are now making use of the thermistor. The current flowing through the diode may be used to control heating or cooling mechanisms and to correct the temperature back to its original point.

Photodiodes. Some semiconductor diodes are designed in such a way as to conduct current only when light energy falling on the junction causes valence electrons to absorb energy and become carriers.

Light-emitting diodes or LEDs. Some diodes have been designed to give up energy in the form of light when current passes. These LEDs have now come into common use. The diode may be formed into the shape of a number that lights when the necessary current flows through it. The red-colored readout numbers on many new instruments are of this type.

Semiconductor diodes may also be used in other, more technical functions. They may be tiny and still be quite functional. Since they can be accurate at low currents and voltages, they are extremely versatile. The symbol used for a diode may be either of the two shown in Fig. 2-16.

Transistors. If we sandwich a thin layer of P-type material between two N-type crystals we produce an NPN transistor. Notice that there are two junctions involved and that the total transistor behaves, in many ways, like two separate semiconductor diodes. We normally refer to one of

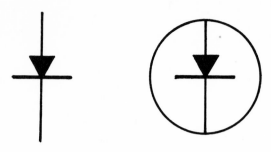

Fig. 2-16. Symbols for semiconductor diodes. Either symbol may be used.

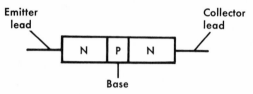

Fig. 2-17. NPN transistor consists of a P-type crystal fused between two N-type crystals. One of the N-type crystals is the emitter and the other, the collector. The P-type crystal is the base.

the N crystals as the emitter and to the other as the collector. The P-type material would be the base. (See Fig. 2-17.)

If we forward-bias the emitter-to-base (E to B) section and reverse-bias the base-to-collector (B to C) section, we will find little resistance in the first case but heavy resistance in the second. If a constant current is passed through the transistor now, the voltage will rise markedly when the current encounters the increased resistance. Ohm's law (E = I × R) predicts this. In the case of the NPN transistor the electrons are the principal carriers.

Placing a small crystal of N material between two crystals of P material produces a PNP transistor that will function much as an NPN transistor does, but with the holes acting as the principal carrier. Symbols for the two types of transistors are given in Fig. 2-19. Arrows point in the direction of "hole" movement, not electron movement. NPN-type transistors are used more commonly than PNPs. Both NPN

and PNP transistors are principally used as amplifiers and may be compared to the triode vacuum tube.

By changes in the biasing and configuration of the wiring detail, transistors can be made to amplify either voltage or current, differentially, or both. Three common configurations are shown in Fig. 2-18, *A* to *C*.

Transistors are sensitive to temperature change. At higher temperatures their function may be distorted and they may be destroyed. *Heat sinks,* generally in the form of metal radiators with thin fins, are often provided for transistors that carry large amounts of currents. The metal case of the transistor (Fig. 2-20) is often fitted tightly into the heat sink to give good heat conduction and dissipation.

If an excessive amount of current is passed through a transistor, much heat is produced. This heat increases conductivity in semiconductor materials, and a destructive cycle known as *thermal runaway* follows. A dead short in a circuit will often burn out transistors in this manner.

A specific type of transistor amplifier that is worth special mention here is the *field-effect transistor,* or FET. As mentioned elsewhere, vacuum tube amplifiers cannot amplify direct current without *drift* or gradual change in the amplification factor. Development of the FET has made it possible to do this now. Since most detectors—photocells, thermocouples, pH electrodes, etc.—give some gradual change in a DC signal, *choppers* are used to convert a direct current signal to alternating current for amplification. Since choppers are often rather troublesome and expensive components, the use of FETs is beginning to make significant changes in the design of many instruments. (Choppers will be discussed in more detail elsewhere.)

Many specialized transistors have been developed, and the science of semiconductors has become extremely sophisticated. It is beyond the scope of this text to do more

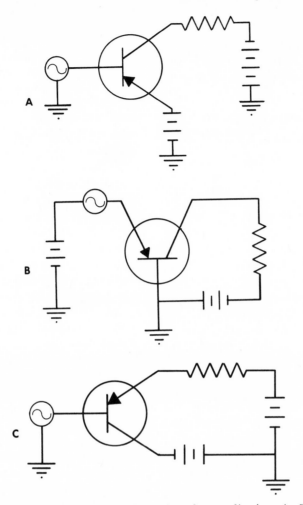

Fig. 2-18. PNP transistor in various configurations for amplication. **A,** Common emitter configuration. Both sides of the transistor are reverse-biased. Voltage and current are both amplified. **B,** Grounded-base configuration. Emitter to base is forward-biased but base to collector is reverse-biased. Voltage is amplified but current is unchanged. **C,** Emitter follower configuration. Emitter to base is reverse-biased. Base to collector is forward-biased. Current only is amplified.

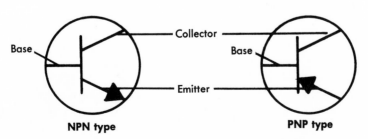

Fig. 2-19. Symbols for NPN and PNP transistors.

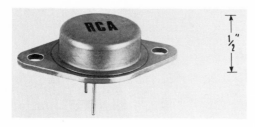

Fig. 2-20. Power transistor. (Courtesy RCA, Electronic Components.)

than acquaint the student briefly with a few of the more important ideas involved in their use.

Many of the functions of components can be integrated with those of similar components and an entire circuit arrangement placed in a tiny capsule. For example, an alternating current could be rectified by the use of two or four rectifiers and the resultant current controlled by a Zener diode. All of these components could be combined into a tiny crystalline structure housed in a small envelope. Much more complicated functions are combined in this way. The combined circuits, often no larger than a pencil eraser, are called *integrated circuits.*

Making use of integrated circuits has become a science, and designing equipment in the form of such components has become a new specialty that has made possible fantastically sophisticated electronic devices—of small size and at low cost. The pocket electronic calculator and the desk top computer are examples. The full impact of these devices has not yet been felt in the medical laboratory instrument field, but many devices are now on the drawing boards that will revolutionize laboratory instrumentation.

For several years now components such as those discussed have been mounted on *printed circuit boards.* These are fiber or plastic boards onto which strips of metal foil have been printed or pressed. Electricity is conducted through these strips rather than through conventional wires.

The entire board, representing one or several individual circuits, can be pushed into a receptacle that makes all of the necessary contacts with other parts of the instrument: detectors, meters, etc. If an element in a circuit becomes defective, it is thus possible to replace the entire circuit and analyze the component failure at some later time after the instrument is again in operation.

OTHER CIRCUIT ELEMENTS

Capacitors. These are components consisting of two conducting plates separated by a resistance or dielectric material. The plates have a capacity for storing electrons (electric charge). This capacity is measured in *farads* (f) and is called capacitance. A farad is a capacitance of 1 coulomb when under the pressure of 1 volt. The farad is a very large charge, so we more often talk in terms of microfarads (μf).

When the capacitor plate is completely charged, any increase in voltage will cause it to discharge across the dielectric onto the other plate. This ability to store electric charge and to discharge when a given capacitance is reached may be used in any of several ways.

Capacitors when used in a parallel circuit serve as temporary reservoirs for electrons at moments of high voltage. As voltage drops, the electrons are released. In this way the capacitor serves to stabilize current flow when voltage is varying. This process will be examined more carefully in a later discussion of rectification.

If the capacitor is used in a series circuit, its function is somewhat different. The capacitor plate will store a charge until it reaches its capacitance. When it exceeds this level, it will discharge across the dielectric. This electrical impulse can be sensed as a separate electrical event. Since we know the charge that can be stored before it will discharge and we can count discharges, we can compute the current. This is the general idea used in electronic integrators. The circuit configuration may be such that the capacitor will discharge only when an electrical impulse exceeds a certain level. Thus it becomes the central component in *counting circuits.*

In some instances we want to store a large charge of electricity and discharge it at one time for some reason. A capacitor, when used in this way, may be called a *condenser.*

Capacitors may be made in any of several ways. One type consists of a sandwich of two long strips of metal foil with a piece of waxed paper, rolled up tightly. One end of each metallic sheet is connected to one of the external contacts and the whole roll is sealed in a ceramic envelope or metal can. Another type of capacitor consists of a metal plate, covered by a thin layer of its oxide, immersed in an electrolyte solution or paste. The metal and the electrolyte are the two plates and the thin oxide layer acts as the dielectric or insulating layer. This is called an *electrolytic capacitor.* In the electrolytic capacitor, current must always be charged onto the metal plate, rather than into the electrolyte. If the polarity is reversed, the oxide is broken down and the capacitor may be ruined. Occasionally an electrolytic capacitor may leak its electrolyte onto a printed circuit or into delicate parts and ruin an instrument.

Some capacitors consist of two metal plates separated by air. These may be *variable capacitors* or *trimming capacitors,* since the plates can be adjusted and brought closer together, thus reducing their capacitance.

Induction coils. We have seen earlier that a conductor, such as a wire, has a field of induction around it. As pointed out in the section describing the d'Arsonval movement, a coil of wire has an enhanced field of induction. Any coil, when used in such a way as to make use of this induction, is called an *induction* coil or simply an *in-*

ductor. If a current flowing through a coil is suddenly cut off, the field of induction takes an instant to collapse. As a result, the current flow ceases somewhat less suddenly than it would if the inductor were not present. Similarly, any time that a sudden change in the current occurs, the inductor resists the change, making it more gradual. Inductance is measured in henries or in millihenries. One henry is said to be present when a current change of 1 amp/ sec causes 1 v of counter-EMF to form. Inductors are often called *chokes.*

The use of inductors and calculation of their effect is complicated by the resistance and capacitance that may be present in the coil and by other technical considerations. For our purposes here, it is sufficient to understand the concept.

Relays. As has been noted earlier, when a current is passed through a coil, a field of induction or magnetic flux is set up in such a way that one side of the coil is positive and the other is negative. If the coil has an iron core, the core will be similarly polarized. This electromagnetism may be used to open or close a switch or perform other work whenever a current is passed through the coil. Such a device is called a *relay* or *solenoid.* Often it is desirable to have an occurrence, such as a flash of light in a photocell or the discharging of a capacitor, start some process that requires much more electric current. The relay can accomplish this by closing a switch in a much heavier circuit. Various types of counters and many other pieces of laboratory equipment use relays. We generally call this component a *solenoid* when it is used to perform mechanical work such as closing a valve, moving a lever, or stretching a spring. The term *relay* is generally reserved for such a component when it is used as an electric switch.

Choppers. The output from most types of detectors (photocells, for example) is direct current. This current is often small and must be amplified to activate a recorder or servomotor. It is nearly impossible, as noted earlier, to amplify a direct current linearly and consistently. For this reason direct current is often broken up, to make alternating current, by means of a chopper. Choppers work in a number of ways. In a colorimeter a fan may be installed so that the blades of the fan interrupt the beam of light several times a second, causing the photocurrent from the phototube to drop to zero each time the light is cut off. This sort of device is called a *light chopper*.

The photocurrent may be mechanically interrupted by a relay that opens and closes with each cycle of ordinary 60-cycle house current. This kind of device is called a *mechanical chopper* or *oscillator*. (The subject of oscillators is interesting but can be quite technical in nature and is of only slight interest here. Oscillators are of paramount importance in radio and TV work.)

The *neon chopper* is still another type. In this device the direct current to be chopped is passed through a photoconductive cell that is intermittently illuminated by a neon light (which glows only during the positive phase of the AC cycle). The direct current can pass the photoconductive cell only when it is lighted and will be effectively cut off during the fraction of a second that the cell is in darkness.

A transistor can be used as a chopper when properly configured. An alternating current is applied to the base, and bias is arranged in such a way that during one half cycle of the base current the DC signal shorts out through the transistor and during the other half cycle it goes directly to the amplifier.

The chopper current produced by any of these devices may properly be said to be an intermittent direct current, since it varies between 0 v and its peak. If one were to select a reference point midway between zero and the peak voltage, the voltage excursions would then become pos-

itive and negative in relation to this arbitrary point of reference. Hence it would be, in effect, alternating current.

Electric motors. Electric motors have become so common in the world about us that nearly everything we do involves the use of a motor in some way. In the laboratory we are particularly likely to run afoul of an electric motor that is not working or not working properly. A little elementary knowledge of motors and some small attention to maintenance can save a great deal of time and trouble.

In general, all kinds of electric motors work in essentially the same way, which can be readily understood by referring back to the d'Arsonal movement of meters. You will remember that a coil was suspended between the poles of a permanent magnet. When current was passed through the coil, it became an electromagnet and its positive pole was repelled by the positive pole of the permanent magnet. Now, if you can imagine a second coil wound around the same core, which receives a flow of current and becomes magnetized just as the other coil is pushed 90 degrees, you can easily see that the core with the two coils will continue to turn. By alternating the two coils and reversing the polarity, the coil can be made to spin. This, in a very general way, is how motors are made to turn. You may recognize this as essentially a generator—but one in which electricity is producing power instead of power producing electricity. There are two or three common types of motors used in the clinical laboratory.

AC motors. The most frequent is the *induction motor*. In this motor there are two coils wrapped, at right angles, around a spindle. This is called an *armature*. It turns on small bearings, one at each end of the spindle. The armature rotates inside two field coils that are also at 90-degree angles to each other. Alternating current (usually 117 v, 60 cps) is fed to one of the coils while the other, which is 90 degrees out of phase, receives the same supply. Induction fields are produced in the armature coils; these interact with the two electromagnetic coils, causing the armature to turn. As long as the two field coils are 90 degrees out of phase, the rotor (armature) will turn in counterclockwise direction. If the two currents are 180 degrees out of phase, the direction of rotation is reversed.

Induction electric motors are used for many functions in laboratory instruments. Paper-drive motors in recorders, servomotors in tissue-processing equipment, and slit-control motors in spectrophotometers are all this type. Often these small motors have gear trains built into the same housing, to provide different rates of speed. Eventually the gear trains wear out or the bearings freeze. Occasionally some other mechanism freezes, and the motor overloads and burns out. In such cases most motors are easily replaced; many of them are standard. Speeds in the most common configurations are available at electrical supply houses.

Motors such as those used in tabletop centrifuges are made in much the same way as induction motors, with some significant differences. Most of these motors, instead of having only two coils on the armature, have several coils. Also, the magnet fields of the armature are produced by current flowing through the coils rather than by induction. To move this heavy a load with only the induction current field interacting with that of the field coils is not practical.

The problem of alternately providing each of the armature coils with current in sequence is solved by the use of two carbon brushes contacting the *commutator* on the armature (Fig. 2-21). The commutator is a series of arc-shaped brass plates assembled in a circle but separated by mica insulation. Each opposing set of plates is attached to the terminals of one of the armature coils. As the armature turns, the current flows through the brushes and, by way of the brass commutator plates, through one of the coils. An induction field opposing that of the field coil is produced

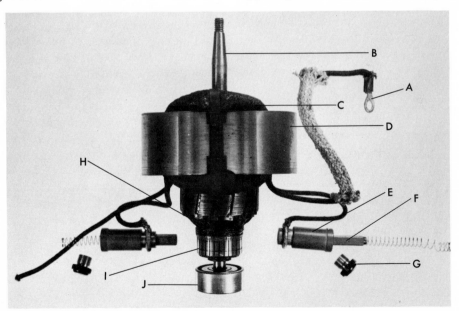

Fig. 2-21. Parts of an electric motor. With the cover removed to expose all parts, the motor will look like this: *A,* instrument ground wire; *B,* motor spindle; *C,* field coils; *D,* magnet; *E,* brush holder; *F,* graphite brush; *G,* brush cover; *H,* lower edge of armature windings; *I,* commutator; *J,* lower bearing.

and causes the armature to rotate. This rotation brings another set of brass commutator plates into contact with the brushes, and the process is repeated.

The use of several coils on the armature allows the centrifuge to move a heavier load. Once the load is moving, more speed can be attained by reducing the number of coils involved. A top speed of 3600 rpm can theoretically be attained if only two poles are used.

Heavily used motors of this type require some maintenance. Although there are "lifetime" bearings in use, most motors of this type need to have the top and bottom bearings lubricated every 2 or 3 months. A light cup grease, which is usually provided with the centrifuge, is indicated.

Brushes should be checked regularly. If the brush is worn more than halfway down, it should be discarded and replaced. Buying brushes is much cheaper than refinishing the commutator. The inside of the brush holder should be cleaned as well as possible and deposits of carbon removed. Some solvent, such as switch cleaner, may help to remove deposits of caked carbon in and around the brush holders. Be sure that new brushes are in straight and can slide freely and that brush springs are long enough to give positive tension. Be sure also that the caps are properly seated and screwed into the brush holders.

The surface of the commutator should be examined occasionally for scratches, pitting, or unusual wear. If the brushes are being used up quickly, the commutator probably needs attention. If the brushes are properly seated and there is still excessive sparking, the surface may be getting rough. The armature can be removed and sent to a motor shop, where the brass commutator ring will be turned down on a lathe, providing a new, smoother surface. This can be done only two or three times before the brass is cut down to the mica separators. Then the armature must be rebuilt.

Field coils or armature coils may short out or develop breaks. They may be rewound, but in many cases it is cheaper to replace the armature, the field coils, or the whole motor.

After many months of exposure to laboratory fumes and dirt, switch points may become coated or corroded. Cleaning with switch cleaner and buffing with fine emery paper may save much annoyance.

DC motors. These are provided for some types of laboratory centrifuges. Although the wiring detail is somewhat different from that of the AC motor, the two are quite similar in most respects. Rectifiers and capacitors are used to convert 60-cycle alternating current to the required direct current. The notes concerning maintenance given above apply equally to this sort of motor.

TYPES OF CIRCUITS

In the preceding pages many of the components that are used in electric circuits have been discussed. These are the tools with which the instrument designer works to make electricity do what he wishes. Circuit design is technical, and it is not the purpose of this text to give any particular detail of this science. It is necessary, however, that the student understand what is involved in certain types of circuits and what functions they perform. The following terms are of importance in understanding instrumentation.

Rectifier circuits. The fact that a direct current can be converted to an alternating current by the use of a chopper has been mentioned. Such conversion may be necessary because most amplifiers will not amplify a DC signal without distortion. Once the alternating current has been amplified, we may want to change it back to a direct current again. Most readout devices, such as meters, must have direct current; there are also other reasons why we may want to change AC to DC.

Discussion of vacuum tube and semicon-

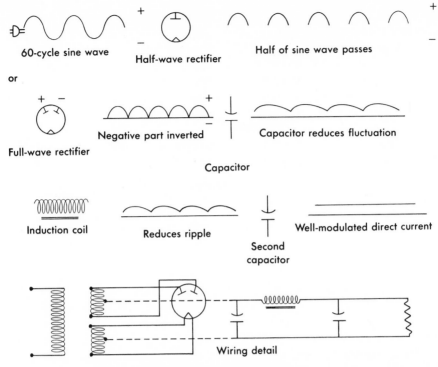

60-cycle sine wave

Half-wave rectifier

Half of sine wave passes

or

Full-wave rectifier

Negative part inverted

Capacitor

Capacitor reduces fluctuation

Induction coil

Reduces ripple

Second capacitor

Well-modulated direct current

Wiring detail

Fig. 2-22. Rectification process.

ductor rectifiers has shown that only the positive part of the AC sine wave is allowed to pass. We have also seen how two rectifiers can be used to convert both the positive and negative parts of the sine wave, producing a pulsating direct current. To use this signal effectively, however, we must convert it to a smooth, steady signal. (See Fig. 2-22.)

Alternating current is shown passing through a full-wave rectifier tube. Semiconductor or dry metal rectifiers could be used just as easily. The output signal is a pulsating current that all moves in a positive direction. If a capacitor is placed between the negative and positive sides of the circuit, the capacitor plate will store electric charge during the intervals of peak voltage and lose it during the period of low voltage. The process is similar to the storage of flood waters in marshes along the river and the subsequent drainage after the flood is passed.

After passing the capacitor, the DC current is more stable but still shows considerable fluctuation. If an induction coil is now placed in series in the circuit, the fluctuations will be further reduced because of the induction discussed earlier. Another capacitor can now be used, followed by another inductor, and the process repeated until the *ripple* arrives at an acceptable level. Thus alternating current is rectified and changed into a smooth, ripple-free direct current.

Amplifiers. We have seen that vacuum tubes and transistors can amplify a signal, and Fig. 2-18 shows three ways in which they can be arranged in a circuit to do this. When we refer to amplifiers in a broader sense, however, we think about all of the components necessary in a rather complex circuit to amplify and condition the signal. Thus the voltage of the amperage may be amplified, or both may be amplified. The amplifier circuit may have more than one amplifying tube or resistor and, if so, it is said to have more than one *stage* of amplification. DC amplifiers are made but are not used widely in laboratory instruments.

Linear-log converters. Discussion in the next chapter points out that the light absorbed by a solution is dependent on the concentration of the solute, if Beer's law applies. The relationship between absorbed light and concentration is not linear; if a graph is made by plotting one against the other, the curve will be logarithmic. It is possible to pass the photosignal, from a light detector, through a linear-log converter and produce an electric signal that is linear with concentration, thus allowing us to read the concentration of a solution directly on a meter or recorder. These converters will be further discussed in the appropriate chapters.

A to D converters. Whenever we measure the current from a photocell, a pH electrode, or other type of transducer, we get a signal that is analogous to the parameter being measured. We do not know what that electric signal means except in comparison to a similar one from a standard situation. The electric signal that is comparable or analogous to the parameter we are measuring is called an *analog signal*. If we wish to tell a computer, for example, what this signal means, we must convert it into numbers or digits. An *analog to digital* (A to D) converter is a circuit that performs this task.

Integrators. To understand what function an integrator performs, let us make a comparison to a totally unrelated subject. A restaurant serves no coffee at 10:30 A.M. but by 10:45 it is serving at the rate of two cups a minute. By 11:00 it is serving five cups a minute; and at 11:30, 8 cups a minute. This rate is continued until 12:45, when it drops off to 4 a minute; and by 1:30 the restaurant is no longer serving. With only these facts how could you determine how much coffee was served? The serving rates could be plotted and the points connected and (if you wanted to

work for many hours) you could estimate the quantity, minute by minute, and add it all up. Since the change in rate of serving was a variable, you could never arrive at a definite figure, however. If you could somehow figure the area under the curve of the graph you drew, you would have a total that would be fairly valid. If your minute-by-minute figures were accurate, you could have a very accurate answer. An integrator perfoms this type of function—one we can define as continuously summing the product of time versus rate to give a cumulative total. Since many of the phenomena we wish to measure are variables, this is an important device. Integration is accomplished electronically by a battery of capacitors that digitize a variable electric signal into units that can be counted. In the chapter on electrophoresis, integrators are discussed as they relate to densitometers.

Discriminators. Whenever a cell counter senses a blood cell or a gamma detector senses an emission, the detection may be thought of as an electrical event that produces a signal or pulse of some sort. To determine the size of the cell or the energy of the pulse, we must measure the amplitude of the pulsation and, if we are looking for a specific size of cell or one isotope, we must screen out all impulses that do not meet the criteria we have set. For example, the pulse from a white blood cell will be considerably larger than that of a red blood cell. We discriminate between them by measuring their electrical pulses, using a discriminator circuit. A capacitor may be set up in the circuit in such a way that only impulses exceeding a predetermined level will pass. All smaller pulses are shorted out to ground. This arrangement would be called a *lower* or *threshold discriminator*.

Another capacitor arrangement may be set up to short to ground all signals that exceed a given level. This would be called an *upper discriminator*. Both of these may be used in a circuit, leaving only signals that exceed a given level but are less than a predetermined maximum. This would leave a *window* through which pass only pulses from a red blood cell, for example.

If a large number of signals are being processed in a brief time period, there will be times when two signals occur at exactly the same instant and will appear to be one signal that is twice as large. This coincidence can be anticipated if we know the duration of the impulse and the approximate number occurring each second. Obviously the larger the number per second, the larger the number of coincidences will be. It is possible, mathematically, to calculate coincidence probability and, electronically, to make a correction for the error involved. Hence an *anticoincidence circuit* may be added to a discriminator.

Counting circuits. Having discriminated between pulses in the manner described above, we may now wish to count the blood cells or gamma emissions that the pulses represent. For this we use a counting circuit of some sort. The pulses we have selected may be occurring so rapidly that it is difficult to count them accurately. For this reason we may add a *scaler,* which selects only a representative number of pulses for counting. Two types are common. The *binary scaler* may be set to select first every second pulse, then every second one of these, and every second again, so that we may count one out of two, four, eight, sixteen, thirty-two, etc. The *decade scaler* will count every tenth impulse, then every tenth of these, etc.; the progression is 1, 10, 100, 1000, 10,000, etc.

Having selected the sampling ratio of pulses we will count, we may now send the pulse to a relay that mechanically causes a counter, such as a Veeder-Root tally, to turn and advance numbers on a dial. These devices are used less commonly now, however. A profusion of devices such as *glow tubes, Nixie tubes, bar tubes,* and *light-emitting diodes* are available, which will indicate the number of pulses coming to them. Readout instruments using such devices are generally referred to as *electronic displays.* This explanation is obviously an oversimplification of a fairly technical subject but should give some idea of the rationale behind these devices.

Current-summing devices. These circuits generally make use of capacitors to store all of the current involved in an operation, such as the counting of impulses of a given size, during a selected interval. This electric total can then be used for further operations such as averaging or integration.

Feedback circuits. When a part of the output of an amplifier is returned to the input side, to achieve some desirable effect, it is termed a *feedback circuit. Negative feedback* is often used in amplifiers, to stabilize the gain of the amplifier. Feedback information can also be used to inform the instrument of changes in conditions and hence cause it to modify its performance. At times amplifiers may inadvertently develop resonance from unwanted *positive feedback* causing oscillation and distortion.

Readers who are genuinely interested in the study of electricity are referred to the many fine texts and courses of study that are available. It is hoped that the foregoing may, by its simplicity, have clarified some concepts and awakened an awareness and interest in the subject.

REVIEW QUESTIONS

1. What are two ways in which capacitors can be used?
2. What does an integrator do?
3. How does a CRT produce a sine wave?
4. What sort of function does a Zener diode perform?
5. If a 300 μf capacitor has an applied voltage of 1 v, how many coulombs are present on the plate?
6. If a transformer is labeled "Input 115 V, AC—Output 115 V, AC," what is its function?
7. What is usually the function of the grid in a vacuum tube?
8. What is a thermistor and how does it perform its function?
9. The color bands on a resistor are red, blue, red, and gold. What are its value and its tolerance?
10. What do discriminators do?
11. What causes a relay to open or close?
12. What is a commutator?

3
Light and its measurement

A great many of the instruments to be discussed here will be devices that measure light in some way. Before we approach the actual instrumentation, let us think about light as a form of energy. An understanding of its nature, origin, and behavior will help us later as we consider its emission, absorption, and quantitation in laboratory instruments.

You will recall from the first few pages of this book, that the electrons of an atom possess most of the energy of the atom. When these electrons move from one orbital position to another, there is always some energy absorbed or given up. When an element is heated in a flame, certain valence electrons will move from their normal position, which is usually referred to as *ground state,* to a new characteristic orbital position. This means that the atom has absorbed a certain, definable amount of heat energy. When the atom cools, this energy is released as light energy. This very specific amount of energy will correspond to an exact color or wavelength of light.

Each electron of each element has a characteristic amount of energy that is required to perform this transition. This energy corresponds to a specific color of light that is emitted. Some electrons may have more than one discrete and definable new orbital position to which it will move; and consequently, when such an electron returns to ground state, it may conceivably emit more than one wavelength of light. Each wavelength given off, however, will

be characteristic of that electron position for that particular element. Also, more than one electron may be involved in transition at one time. Hence, several colors or wavelengths may be emitted simultaneously. (See Fig. 3-1.)

The human eye is not able to differentiate several colors at the same time; therefore, when presented with several wavelengths, the eye will see a composite, with the most intense color predominating. This helps to explain the variety of hues and colors that we see in a paint store. When all wavelengths of light are present at the same time, we sense the combination as white light. When there are none present, the eye does not respond, and we say that "it is black."

The light from the sun is normally considered to be pure white light because sunlight contains all wavelengths. The large number of elements in the sun and the very intense heat energy to which they are subjected make it a near certainty that all wavelengths are produced. When white light, such as that from the sun, hits a prism, a rainbow or *spectrum* of colors is produced. As we shall presently see, this is because the different wavelengths are diffracted (or bent) to different extents and each color comes out separately.

You may recall that the colors of the rainbow or spectrum go from violet, at one end, through blue, green, yellow, orange, to red, at the other end. If you observe these colors closely, you will notice that each color is not discrete but gradually blends into the next; thus it is impossible to say at what point one becomes another. Every shading of color represents a wavelength, and the spectrum actually represents a span of constantly decreasing wavelengths, which may be called a continuum of energy. On each end of this span are more wavelengths that are invis-

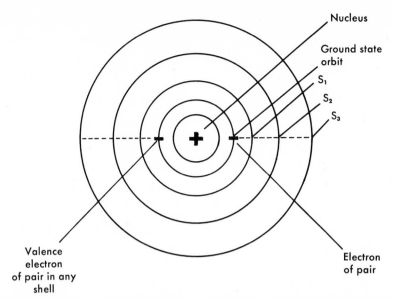

Fig. 3-1. Hypothetical atom to show transition of electron. Heat or light energy is generally required, to move an electron from ground state to a new orbital position—S_1, S_2, or higher. As the electron returns to ground state, light is emitted; its wavelength will be determined by the energy given up. Remember, violet is of higher energy than red.

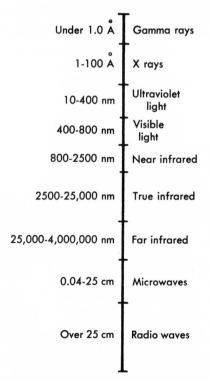

Under 1.0 Å	Gamma rays
1-100 Å	X rays
10-400 nm	Ultraviolet light
400-800 nm	Visible light
800-2500 nm	Near infrared
2500-25,000 nm	True infrared
25,000-4,000,000 nm	Far infrared
0.04-25 cm	Microwaves
Over 25 cm	Radio waves

Fig. 3-2. Continuum of electromagnetic energy, showing the wavelength span of each segment.

ible to the human eye. These "colors" that we cannot see can be characterized as infrared (IR) (beyond the red end of the visible span) or ultraviolet (past the violet color). Fig. 3-2 shows the entire span of wavelengths and the name we have given to each particular grouping. You will notice that visible light is a small segment of this entire *electromagnetic spectrum*. Let us look at some characteristics of this form of energy (Table 1), which we usually think of as "light."

Light or radiant energy is generally considered to travel in transverse waves. It has energy that is measurable in *photons*. Light waves have two characteristics that define them. First, they have *wavelength*, which is the distance from crest to crest of a wave. Wavelength is the factor that determines *color*. Second, they have *amplitude*, or wave height, which determines the *intensity* of the light. (See Fig. 3-3.)

In a vacuum all light travels at a constant speed, which is about 3×10^{10} cm, or 186,000 miles, per second. If we divide the distance light travels in 1 second by the length of 1 wave, the number of waves per second is determined. This is light's *frequency* per second. The energy of light depends on its frequency or wavelength. The higher the frequency (the shorter the wavelength), the higher is its energy (Fig. 3-4). Note that we can define light in terms of its wavelength, its frequency, or its energy. Physicists and engineers often express electromagnetic energy in terms of its fre-

Table 1. Electromagnetic energy

Types of radiation	Wavelengths
Gamma rays (isotopes)	Less than 0.1 nanometer (nm)
X rays and "soft" X rays	0.1 to 10 nm
Ultraviolet light	10 to 400 nm
Visible light	400 to 800 nm
Near infrared	800 to 2500 nm
True infrared	2500 to 25,000 nm
Far infrared	25,000 to 4,000,000 nm
Microwaves	0.04 to 25 cm
Radio waves	Over 25 cm

quency or *cycle per second* (cps). In discussing very short wavelengths such as gamma energy and X rays, it is more convenient to refer to the energy. Their energy is measured in thousands of electron volts (KEV) or millions of electron volts (MEV). When light is transmitted through matter, whether a liquid, a gas, or a solid, its *speed is somewhat slower* than in a vacuum but its *frequency is always constant*. The ratio of the speed of light in a vacuum to its speed in a substance is referred to as the *refractive index* of the substance. This varies slightly with the wavelength under consideration.

The energy of light may be calculated by the formula:

$$E = h v$$

in which E is the energy in photons, h is Planck's constant, or 6.6×10^{-27} erg-second, and v is the frequency. This is another way of saying that the energy increases as the frequency increases. The very high-

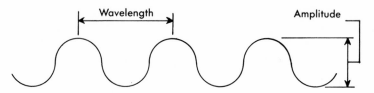

Fig. 3-3. Characteristics of light waves.

Violet light

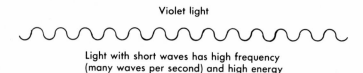

Light with short waves has high frequency (many waves per second) and high energy

Red light

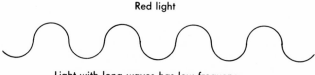

Light with long waves has low frequency (fewer waves per second) and low energy

Fig. 3-4. Short and long waves.

Table 2. Sources of electromagnetic energy

Wave-length	Common name	Source of energy	Fre-quency
Several meters to 25 cm	Radio waves	Electron-spin orientation	
	Microwaves (radar)	Molecular rotation	10^{11} cps
5,000,000 nm	Infrared	Molecular vibration	10^{12} cps
700 nm	Visible light	Valence electron transition	10^{15} cps
375 nm	Ultraviolet (soft X rays)		
5 nm	X rays	Inner-shell electron transition	
0.01 nm and lower	Gamma rays	Nuclear transition	10^{17} cps

Table 3. Units of length in measuring electromagnetic energy

$$
\begin{aligned}
1 \text{ meter} &= 100 \text{ cm} \\
1 \text{ cm} &= 10 \text{ mm} \\
&= 10,000 \ \mu \\
&= 10,000,000 \text{ nm} \\
&= 100,000,000 \text{ Å} \\
1 \text{ mm} &= 1000 \ \mu \\
&= 1,000,000 \text{ nm} \\
&= 10,000,000 \text{ Å} \\
1 \ \mu &= 1000 \text{ nm} \\
&= 10,000 \text{ Å} \\
1 \text{ m}\mu &= 10 \text{ Å}
\end{aligned}
$$

frequency gamma rays of radioactivity are quite dangerous, and we should exercise considerable caution in exposing ourselves to X ray. Even the lower frequencies of ultraviolet light (UV) can cause severe damage to the eye if we look directly into the source for more than a few seconds. The low-frequency rays of the infrared (IR) and the even longer radio waves may warm us or pass through us with no damage at all unless they are very intense.

We have noted that visible light is produced when a valence electron is involved in a transition. Other energy levels in the electromagnetic spectrum derive from other molecular energies. These are shown in Table 2. Gamma radiation, which is the most potent form of electromagnetic energy, derives from the transition of a proton from the very nucleus of the atom—a very fundamental change indeed.

You may recall, from earlier discussion, that the frequency of light remains constant regardless of the medium through which it travels. The speed, however may vary slightly and, as a consequence, the wavelength will also change. Also, the frequency may be expressed as cycles per second (cps), but wavelength is expressed in a confusing number of units—meters, centimeters, microns, millimicrons, angstrom units, etc. It is for these reasons that physicists like to refer to the *frequency* of electromagnetic energy. In biology and medicine we commonly use the *wavelength* as the term of reference. In practice, the change in wavelength in different media mentioned above is not significant for most purposes. Furthermore, the visible and near-visible light, with which we usually work, can be described in all cases in terms of millimicrons (or nanons). Hence the wavelength designation is adequate and is easier to visualize.

Table 3 may help you to remember the various units of length commonly employed in describing energy waves. The Greek letter *lambda* (λ) is used as a symbol for wavelength. The Greek letter *mu* (μ) is used for micron. One one-thousandth of a micron is called a nanometer (nm) or a *nanon*. The capital letter A or Å is used as a symbol for angstrom unit.

Early students of light used the intensity of a candle made in a specific way as a term of reference. The term *standard candle* is still used although it has since been more scientifically defined. *Illumination* is measured in *footcandles*. A footcandle is the illumination provided by 1 standard candle at a distance of 1 foot. Illumination varies *inversely* with the square of the distance.

The total amount of light hitting a surface at a given distance is called the *luminous flux*. A *lumen* is the luminous flux on 1 square foot of surface, all points of which are 1 foot from a light source of 1 candle.

$$\text{Total luminous flux} = \text{Candles} \times \frac{4\ R^2}{R^2}$$
$$= \text{Candles} \times 4$$

The surface of a sphere is equal to $4\ R^2$ and the flux decreases as the square of the distance (R = radius).

As the number of candles (or candlepower) of a light is increased, the intensity of the light obviously increases. If a photocell is placed 1 foot from a light source and the light intensity is steadily increased, the output of electricity from the cell increases; this increase in electricity is directly proportional to the light intensity. Note that this output depends on the *intensity* of the light source, not on the wavelength or the energy level.

If we keep the light intensity constant and locate the cell 1 inch from the light, then 2 inches, and later 3 inches, we will see that the output of the photocell varies *inversely with the square of the distance* from the light. This becomes a critical factor in the design of photometric instruments.

When light hits a surface that causes it to diffract, there is a tendency for the different wavelengths to bend at slightly different angles and form a spectrum. This happens because of the difference in refractive index of a substance for various wavelengths of light, mentioned above. The colors in the spectrum normally listed are violet-blue-green-yellow-orange-red. The blue, green, and red are, of course, the primary colors that stand out. The human eye can see green, at a wavelength of around 555 nm, better than any other color. The sensitivity of the eye falls off rather symmetrically in both directions, and one can-

not see much below 400 or above 700 nm.

Photosensitive devices are subject to the same sort of limitations as the eye, and most have an optimum range at which they are most sensitive. You will recall that the 100% T *(transmittance)* reading of a colorimeter must be reset each time the wavelength is changed. This is because of the difference in sensitivity of the photocell at different wavelengths. Scanning spectrophotometers may have a cam-driven slit or other device to regulate total light falling on the phototube, to compensate for this difference in sensitivity at different wavelengths.

Several devices are capable of breaking up white light to form a spectrum. Two that are commonly used in spectrophotometers are the *prism* and the *diffraction grating*. The prism is a piece of glass or quartz cut in such a way as to have interfaces at very precise angles. These can produce the fine quality of spectrum seen in some of the better instruments.

The diffraction grating is a highly polished surface into which a large number of parallel grooves have been cut. Such a surface is able to scatter light and produce a spectrum. The grating may either reflect light or transmit it. More detail will be given later on this subject.

Much of this book is devoted to the sensing or measuring of light by instruments used in the clinical laboratory. A surprising number of photometric devices are in use. In addition to colorimeters and spectrophotometers, there are flame photometers, fluorometers, atomic absorption photometers, isotope-counting equipment, some cell counters, some coagulation-measuring devices, and many other instruments that are either light sensing or light measuring. Some of these are important enough to merit individual chapters. They share many features with colorimetric absorption devices, which we usually refer to as *photometers*.

In the next chapter we shall consider

the "colorimeters" and "spectrophotometers" used in the clinical laboratory. Before we do, let us clarify our thinking about terms, many of which are often misused. *Photometry* is simply the measurement of light intensity, and the simplest photometer would be a light meter such as is used in photography. This is usually a photoemissive cell and a small meter to measure its electrical output. A *colorimeter* for people in the paint industry is a meter that will tell the color of paint by analyzing the light reflecting from its surface. (We, in the medical laboratory, mean something different, of course.) A *spectrometer* is a device designed to break down emitted, transmitted, or reflected light into its component colors. This information tells us something about the material that is emitting, transmitting, or reflecting the light. In other chapters you will find material about measuring light of fluorescence, flame emission, flame absorption, scintillation, and so forth, but devices for these functions can better be defined in the context of the chapter devoted to them.

The subject to be discussed in the next chapter is what we usually refer to as photometry or colorimetry. In reality it might better be called *absorptiometry*. After we have considered why, we can return to calling the instruments colorimeters and photometers; but first let us be definitive about the matter.

In chemistry we are concerned with measuring the ability of a solution to absorb light of a particular wavelength. The wavelength at which light is absorbed best may tell us a great deal about the nature of the material in solution. The degree to which the light is absorbed, under very closely defined conditions, tells us the concentration of the material in the solution. Therefore we shall want to produce a light that is *monochromatic,* or of one particular color. Next we shall want to identify an intensity of light as a norm (100% T) and then measure how much of the light is absorbed. This is, of course, a bit more complicated than simply measuring light. The identification of terms, establishment of standard conditions, refinement of mechanics, etc. pertinent to this subject will be considered in Chapter 4.

Any device for measuring the absorption of light by a solution will have certain basic components. The diagram in Fig. 3-5 shows these. A source of power of some sort is required for the exciter lamp, at least. An exciter lamp (*A*) provides light containing many colors or wavelengths (represented by many arrows at *B*). This light passes through a filter or other device (*C*) that allows one color of light (represented by the single arrow at *D*) to impinge on the sample (*E*). This light is called the *incident* light. Some of the incident light is transmitted through the sample and is

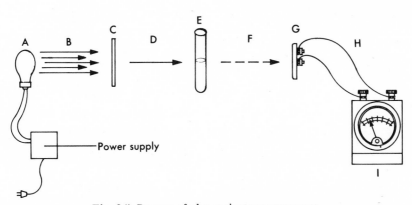

Fig. 3-5. Process of absorption measurement.

called *transmitted* light. The remainder of the light energy (remember that light is a form of energy) is absorbed by the molecules in the sample. This energy absorption represents energy used up in the displacement of valence electrons in the sample molecules. It is obvious that more energy would be used up if more molecules were in the path of the light. It would make little difference whether this increase in molecules were due to a longer light path through the solution or to the higher concentration of molecules in the solution.

The transmitted light, represented by the intermittent line (*F*), impinges on the photosensitive surface of the photocell (*G*), where it produces an electric current that is proportional to the amount of light. This current, called the *photocurrent* (*H*), flows through the meter circuit and causes the needle to move up scale on the meter (*I*).

Since absorptiometry is so important in the clinical laboratory, we need to thoroughly understand each step and each component. Let us go through this system again, considering possible additions and refinements.

BASIC ELEMENTS OF COLORIMETERS

When we speak of a colorimeter in the clinical laboratory, we generally mean an instrument for measuring light absorption in a liquid, using a light of a particular color. Furthermore, we are implying that colored glass filters are used to produce the incident light of the color desired. We may, however, use the term *colorimeter* in a generic sense, to include instruments of all types that measure light in this way. It is in this last sense that the word is used in the heading above.

Colorimeters (Fig. 3-5) all have essentially six parts. These are (1) power supply, (2) exciter lamp, (3) monochromator, (4) sample holder, (5) photodetector, and (6) readout. These parts may be very elementary or quite sophisticated.

Power supply. We might conceivably have an instrument with no power requirement other than the 110 v current almost universally available. The exciter lamp of most colorimeters requires a voltage of 6 to 8 v. A step-down transformer with a capacitor is often all that is required if a photoemissive cell is used and its output is not amplified. The light-measuring instrument may be much more sophisticated, however, and have many other power requirements, including some or all of the following:

1. Direct current plate voltage for amplifier tubes
2. 6.3 v alternating current for tube heaters
3. Ripple-free direct current supply for photoconductive cells
4. Well-regulated, high-voltage direct current for photomultipliers
5. High-voltage alternating current for firing mercury or hydrogen lamps
6. Direct current reference voltages
7. Alternating currents of various frequencies and wave forms for choppers, etc.

From this list, it is apparent that several power requirements may be present in one instrument. We may characterize these requirements for our purposes as alternating or direct current, regulated, low-ripple, etc. If we need alternating current, it is simple to pass 117 v house current through a step-up or step-down transformer, with the proper ratio of windings, to produce the voltage desired.

If we need direct current, we can use a full-wave rectifier as described in the second chapter, but we will have pulsating direct current. As shown in Fig. 2-22, this pulsation can be reduced to a ripple by the use of capacitors and induction coils or filters. The quality of a DC power supply depends on its regulation. A well-regulated power supply will have a ripple of less than 0.01%; that is to say, the rms value of the ripple is less than 0.01% of the total direct current.

Another significant feature of a well-regulated power supply is its ability to maintain a constant DC output when the AC input is varying. Also, as a heavier load is thrown on the power supply, the DC output is inclined to drop, and this variation must be controlled. Zener diodes and glow subes or ballast lamps may be used to control output voltage in these situations.

If alternating current is desired at some frequency other than that of house current (60 cps), the current is rectified and regulated and subsequently chopped at the frequency desired; the appropriate wave form may then be produced. (Production of various wave forms can be a little more complicated and is omitted here.)

In general, power supplies are very important to the stability and accuracy of a colorimetric instrument. Most of the newer power supplies are solid state, using semiconductors in place of vacuum tubes and printed circuits in place of wire connections. If large currents are rectified and regulated, a great deal of heat may be produced. Heavy grills or sets of metal vanes, called *heat sinks,* may be provided to protect delicate components by dissipating the heat and radiating it.

Exciter lamp. The exciter lamp must furnish an intense, reasonably cool, constant beam of light that can be easily collimated. The filament must be small and must provide an intense light; it must be of such a design that it can be exactly aligned when replaced; and it must be highly reproducible in all respects.

As any object changes temperature, it emits a somewhat different spectrum. This is apparent if one notices what happens when house lights dim during a power failure. Lamps take on a yellow color, and if the power surges back past its normal value, the light becomes whiter. If we could compare the spectra produced by the lamp in such cases, it would be immediately obvious that the same area of the spectrum does not give the same distribution of wavelengths. Hence, the temperature of the lamp is important. The quality and uniformity of construction of the exciter lamp are significant factors in the uniform performance of the spectrophotometric instrument.

For work in the visual and low infrared ranges, a tungsten lamp is a good source of radiant energy. Some light in the high ultraviolet region is emitted, but below about 360 nm this lamp is inadequate. If everything else about the system is optimal, a tungsten lamp may be used down to about 360 nm, but it is not recommended for routine use. Several other sources are available for UV work. The hydrogen lamp is probably one of the best choices. The mercury lamp has a much more uneven emission spectrum and is less desirable. A xenon lamp gives a brilliant light that is ideal for very narrow slit work but is almost too brilliant for routine application, since there is a large stray light problem with such an intense beam. The xenon lamp requires a high voltage to ignite or fire. Ozone is produced by ionization of oxygen around the lamp, in dangerous quantities, and must be dissipated in some way. At one time a mercury arc source was used in spectrophotometers because of its brilliance, but the spectral emission was erratic and the intensity was hard to control. Hydrogen, mercury and xenon lamps are all vapor lamps. In lamps of this sort a high voltage is applied through the envelope that contains the "vapor" of the element named. The molecules of gas are ionized and emit a characteristic light, which will contain the same wavelengths that would be seen if the element were burned in a hot flame. There is no filament in a vapor lamp. The high firing or ionization voltage is required only initially, after which a rather low voltage is adequate to maintain ionization and cause the lamp to glow.

For infrared spectrophotometers a silicon carbide rod heated to about 1200° C works very satisfactorily.

When the exciter lamp is changed in a

photometer, the calibration of the instrument should be rechecked. The calibration procedure is included in the discussion of calibration of spectrophotometers.

Most colorimetric instruments now use a *prefocused lamp*. This is a lamp having the characteristics discussed above and a flange around the base for alignment. There are three tear-shaped holes in the flange to accept and lock in three pins on the lamp socket. Since the lamp may be locked in only one position, any lamp of the same design will be positioned and centered in the identical way. The filament in each lamp is positioned in the same place in relation to the base. Even with the prefocused lamp there may be some slight, but important, error of alignment. As we shall see presently, the angle at which light strikes a diffraction grating determines the position of the spectrum and, hence, the color of light striking the sample. Recalibration is therefore necessary each time a lamp is changed.

Between the exciter lamp and the monochromator, collimating lenses are often inserted. These lenses collect the light rays and focus them in such a way that the light passing into the monochromator will be an organized beam of parallel light. A heat filter may also be placed in the light beam close to the exciter lamp to protect the monochromator from radiant heat. A heat filter is clear glass designed to absorb or reject heat-producing infrared rays while allowing visible light to pass.

Monochromator. A monochromator is a device for producing light of a single color from an impure source. The word *monochromatic* means "of one color." As we have noted earlier, it is difficult to identify the point at which one color begins and another ends. We identify monochromatic light specifically when we specify its wavelength. It is unlikely, however, that we will isolate a light of one uniform wavelength. We must, therefore, explain what range of wavelengths we are discussing. This range

is the *band pass*. A monochromatic light that appears to be grass green in color would have a wavelength of about 550 nanometers (nm), but wavelengths of 525 to 575 nm in length might also be present. The band pass would be from 525 to 575, or 50 nm wide.

The term "band pass" needs to be defined still more specifically. Consider the green light passing through a glass filter. All the light of 550 nm wavelength passes, but somewhat less blue-green light also passes. Blue light may pass in small amounts, and a trace of violet (400 nm) may pass. In the same way yellow-green, yellow, and orange (600 nm) may be present in decreasing amounts. If we were to plot transmitted light against wavelength, we would have a curve similar to that in Fig. 3-6. Since the outer edges of the curve extend more or less to infinity, the above explanation of band pass is quite vague. By definition, the band pass is the range of wavelengths *between the points at which transmittance is one half the peak transmittance.* (See Fig. 3-6.)

The simplest monochromator is a single *glass filter,* although we might question calling it a monochromator, since the band pass of a filter is very wide and the light that passes will include more than one color. Glass filters are made by suspending a coloring agent in molten glass. The thickness of the filter, molded from the mixture, determines how much light will be absorbed. The filter is identified by (1) peak transmittance, (2) band pass, and (3) thickness and/or opacity.

A narrower band pass may be obtained by cementing two glass filters of different colors together. Only the wavelengths that are passed in common by both filters will constitute the band pass for this compound filter. For special purposes such a compound filter may be designed to coincide exactly with the emission peak of a mercury lamp to produce true monochromatic light.

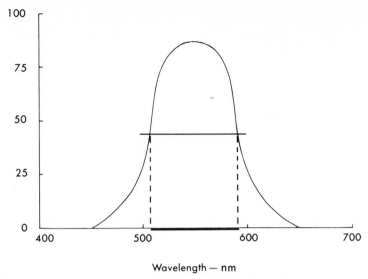

Fig. 3-6. Light transmitted through green filter. Shaded area at base indicates band pass.

Glass filters are only used for transmitting visible and near-visible light. Both UV-absorbing and IR-absorbing, visible light–transmitting filters are available, and near UV–transmitting, visible light–absorbing filters also exist.

For many purposes, filter colorimeters are quite adequate. A good filter colorimeter is sufficiently accurate and quite economical in a physician's office for doing such routine tests as hemoglobin and concentrations of BSP and PSP dye. Maintenance, calibration, and repair of these instruments are simple and foolproof. One does not need a cannon to kill a fly. Several general- and special-purpose filter colorimeters are discussed in detail in the discussion on some common photometric instruments.

Interference filters, made by placing semitransparent silver films on both sides of a thin transparent layer of magnesium fluoride, will give a narrow band pass. Side bands (harmonics) occur at other wavelengths, however, and may be blocked out by using appropriate glass filters. The band pass of interference filters is determined by the thickness and refractive index of

the magnesium fluoride and the angle at which the incident light strikes the filter. This type of filter may have an extremely narrow band pass.

The most widely used true monochromator is composed of an entrance slit, a prism or diffraction grating to disperse the light, and an exit slit to select the band pass (Fig. 3-7).

The *entrance slit* is generally fixed and limits the collimated light allowed to strike the prism or grating. Reflected light is reduced to a minimum. One measure of the quality of a monochromator is the amount of *stray light* it allows to pass. Usually this is expressed in terms of percent of total light. Less than 1% is acceptable for most routine purposes.

When it strikes a *prism,* white light is dispersed to form a spectrum. This occurs because of the fact that the angle of refraction of light at an interface (such as air and a glass prism) varies with the wavelength. Thus violet is refracted more than red and the spectrum is formed. The index of refraction determines the spread of the spectrum and the relative width of the color bands. Glass is the material of choice

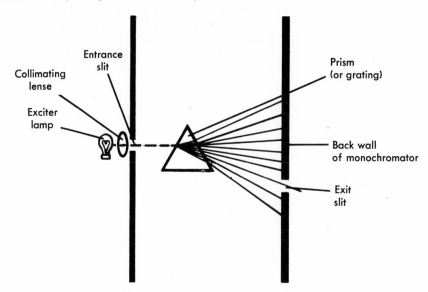

Fig. 3-7. Principal elements of a monochromator. Changing the position of the prism causes the spectrum to move up or down on the back wall of the monochromator so that another color passes through the exit slit.

for visible light; ultraviolet light is absorbed by glass. Quartz and fused silica are preferable for ultraviolet; but when they are used in the visible and IR regions, the color bands produced are two narrow for practical use. This is one reason it is hard to make one simple monochromator for UV, visible, and IR wavelengths.

In past years most high-quality spectrophotometers have used glass or quartz prisms in their monochromators. A very clean spectrum can be produced. The mechanics must be very precise, however; because high-quality diffraction gratings have become economically feasible, more spectrophotometers of good quality have appeared incorporating diffraction gratings.

Diffraction gratings are made by cutting tiny furrows into the aluminized face of a perfect, flat piece of crown glass. These furrows are cut at a very precise angle and at a very accurate distance from each other. Cutting is done with a diamond point, and there are usually from 1000 to 50,000 furrows to the inch. Needless to say, the engine, as it is called, that cuts these gratings is a very precise machine. Enormous weight

prevents any vibrations during the cutting. Original gratings cut in this way take many hours to produce and are very expensive. For this reason they are seldom used in spectrophotometers.

Original glass gratings are used as *master gratings* in the production of a molded product called a *replica grating*. In the process a parting compound is sprayed on the grating, after which a silvering layer is applied. Onto this a coating of epoxy is applied; and a carrier layer of plastic or glass, called an *optical flat,* is bonded to it. All this is done under vacuum. After it is cured, the replica is separated from the master.

Gratings may be of two types—a *transmittance* type, which passes the light, or a *reflectance* type, which acts as a mirror and reflects the spectra back in the general direction of the light.

As white light strikes the grating, it is diffracted to form several spectra (Fig. 3-8). Each of these is at a different angle from the grating. The brightest of these is called the *first-order spectrum*. It is generally used rather than the more diffuse, higher-order

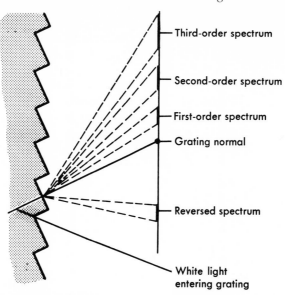

Fig. 3-8. Diffraction of light by a grating. Each ascending-order spectrum is more distorted and more diffuse than the preceding.

spectra. The angle at which the first-order spectrum is diffracted depends on the angle at which the white light hits the spectrum and on the blaze angle of the grating. The blaze angle is the angle at which the furrows are cut in the grating. (See Fig. 3-9.)

The spectrum, whether transmitted or reflected, falls onto the wall of the monochromator. A tiny exit slit in this wall allows a small portion of the spectrum to pass through and into the sample to be measured. The particular portion of the spectrum (wavelength) that passes the slit will be determined by the position of the spectrum, and this, in turn, is determined by the relative positions of the light, the grating, and the slit. Some spectrophotometers move the light (Coleman, Jr., for example), while others move the grating (Bausch & Lomb Spectronic 20) to select the light that passes through the exit slit.

The *band pass* of the monochromator depends on the width of the slit in relation to the length of the spectrum. A narrow band pass is generally desirable. (The discussion on spectral scanning explains

why this is true.) Hence a narrow slit is used. There is a practical limit to the size of the slit, however. For example, one fleck of dust in a very narrow slit may occlude it. Also, the amount of light energy passing a very narrow slit may not be adequate to measure accurately. If the monochromator wall and slit are moved farther from the prism, the spectrum becomes larger and a wider slit may be used. This may not help much, since light intensity decreases as the square of the distance traveled (as we have seen earlier) and the light energy of a narrow band pass is still not adequate. We shall see later that the best solution to this dilemma is the production of better detectors and amplifiers.

Many of the better monochromators have adjustable slits that allow the operator to determine the band pass. Some slits are adjustable in two directions, allowing adjustment of both the band pass and the total amount of light of those wavelengths that can pass.

In general, grating monochromators are capable of better *resolution* than are those

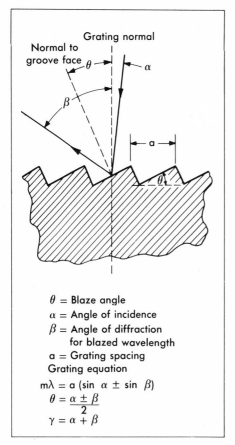

θ = Blaze angle
α = Angle of incidence
β = Angle of diffraction
for blazed wavelength
a = Grating spacing
Grating equation
$m\lambda = a (\sin \alpha \pm \sin \beta)$
$\theta = \dfrac{\alpha \pm \beta}{2}$
$\gamma = \alpha + \beta$

Fig. 3-9. Greatly magnified cross section of a diffraction grating. (Courtesy Bausch & Lomb.)

using prisms. Resolution is best in gratings with the most lines or furrows to the inch. Some stray light in grating monochromators is due to the first- and second-order spectra overlapping and reflecting light of other wave lengths through the slit. Sometimes a double monochromator is used to reduce the stray light. Gratings have the additional advantage of being practical for all wavelengths of light, in contrast to the glass or quartz prisms. In the UV region, only reflectance gratings are used, of course.

Transmittance gratings lose some light efficiency, since a certain amount of energy is lost in passage through the grating. Narrow–band pass instruments generally use reflectance gratings for this reason. Trans-mittance gratings probably allow simpler instrument design at the expense of increased stray light.

Replica gratings should never be handled, since fingerprints will seriously damage them. Dust or dirt on their surfaces is also quite deleterious. Laboratory fumes may cause damage to them in time. The condition of the grating can be checked by examining the light entering the sample compartment. If a small piece of white paper is inserted into the sample well, the incident light can be seen. The color should be reasonably monochromatic and clearcut. If the color is streaky or mixed, the grating may be in need of replacement. (*Note:* If the slits are adjustable, open them all the way before making the check.)

Sample holder. A few observations concerning *cells* or *cuvettes* used for samples may be pertinent. A square cuvette, which presents a flat surface to the incident light, has less light loss from reflection than does the round cell. This loss is more noticeable in an empty cuvette, since the difference in the index of refraction between air and glass is greater than between glass and a solvent. In routine work this loss is probably not significant, being fairly constant at about 4% for most round cuvettes.

It should be quite obvious that the cuvette must be thoroughly clean and free of fingerprints, etching, and clouding and that the sample and reference cells must be matched for transmittance. It should also be apparent that a longer light path will allow one to make more accurate readings in very dilute samples. Various types of horizontal cells and spacers are manufactured to provide long light paths for small samples. For routine work a light path of 1 cm has become fairly standard. Most definitions and values are expressed in this term of reference.

Ultraviolet light, as noted earlier, is absorbed strongly by lime glass. For this reason quartz or special-type glass cells must be used to hold the sample, in this range.

A very obvious but often ignored error is stray light entering from the top of the cuvette or elsewhere. A light shield over the cuvette well should be provided and used whenever a reading is being made.

When large numbers of readings are being made under favorable conditions, good chemists will often omit this precaution with impunity. A change in lighting may cause odd and mysterious errors and cause loss of accuracy and confusion unless this important potential error is kept in mind, however.

Many types of flow-through and flush-out cuvettes are available. These provide a constant light path and constant absorbance characteristics in addition to the obvious advantages of speed and facility of sample handling. In routine use care must be exercised not to allow them to become cloudy. Cells of this sort should be flushed very thoroughly between types of samples and should not be left in the instrument dry unless they have been rinsed several times with distilled water. Blanks should be run regularly.

Aside from the optical problems of the automatic sample-handling systems, there are often mechanical problems. These devices usually suffer from various annoying handicaps that render them awkward for routine use. Some are very slow, some rinse poorly or evacuate incompletely, and some are difficult to control. At any rate, the much more satisfactory mechanisms of totally automated chemistry systems are rapidly taking the place of these semiautomated sample handlers.

It is interesting to note that turbulence, even in a clear, bubble-free solution, will cause an increase in absorbance. This may be a problem in continuous-stream systems (such as the AutoAnalyzer) when the sample system is always in motion.

Photodetector. The simplest type of detector is the photoemissive cell. It is variously called *photocell,* Weston cell, selenide cell, barrier layer cell, photovoltaic cell, etc. Its construction may vary slightly, and different materials may be used; but it has the common characteristic of producing a small electric current when exposed to light. The selenide or oxide layer, which is the photosensitive part of the cell, emits electrons only when exposed to light. The number of electrons emitted (the amperage of the photocurrent) will be a function of the intensity of the light impinging on it.

The *spectral sensitivity* of this type of cell is similar to that of the eye. Peak response is obtained at a wavelength of about 555 nm, which is a grass green color. Sensitivity falls off in both directions for both the protocell and the eye. The cell is sensitive to shorter wavelengths and can detect near-ultraviolet fairly well. At the other end of the spectrum, however, the selenium cell is less sensitive than the eye.

Photoemissive cells are simple to use and are difficult to damage. Their output through the normal working range of simple filter colorimeters is reasonably linear with light intensity. There are a number of significant disadvantages to their use in more sophisticated systems, however. When light first strikes the cell, the photocurrent surges and gradually subsides to a reasonably stable output after several minutes. Hence these instruments should be turned on several minutes before they are to be used, and a blank should be read frequently to detect and correct drift. Also, temperature has considerable effect on output, and response will change as the instrument accumulates heat from the exciter lamp. At the extremes of illumination—very intense light or very faint light—this type of cell is not linear. Still another problem is the slow response of the photocurrent to fast changes in illumination. It is quite impossible to use a photoemissive cell with a light chopper, for example.

Photoconductive cell. Also called a *photoresistor,* this cell is similar to the photoemissive cell. A small electric potential is provided across the cell from an outside source. When no light is striking its surface, the cell acts as a resistor. When it is illuminated, its conductance is relative to the intensity of the light. The sulfides are good semiconductors for this type detector. The lead-sulfide cell is often used in the infrared region.

Since an external source of electricity is provided for the photoconductive cell, a larger current is available to operate a readout device. The stability of the output is somewhat better, also.

Phototube. A phototube acts very much like a photoconductive cell. It has a cathode of photosensitive material that has no free electrons when it is in the dark. When light energy strikes it, however, electrons are released, and under the influence of a plate voltage these flow to the plate to produce the photocurrent. The photocurrent is linear with the intensity of the light striking the cathode.

With a sizable plate voltage, there may be some slight seepage of electrons from the cathode to the plate, even in the dark. This very small current is called *dark current*. When amplified, it can produce an error in reading if it is not compensated. The dark current control on some instruments provides a variable resistance installed in such a way as to neutralize the effect of this small current.

Phototubes may be vacuum tubes or may be gas filled. In the gas-filled tube, the electrons flowing from the cathode collide with gas molecules, dislodging additional electrons, which are drawn along to the plate. These new electrons collide with other molecules, and the process is repeated. This process is called an *avalanche effect*. A relatively small plate voltage can produce a relatively large photocurrent. If too high a plate voltage is applied, the gas molecules are permanently ionized and the tube is destroyed.

The vacuum phototube does not have this limitation, and plate voltage may be

increased to its practical limit. Increasing the plate voltage obviously will increase the dark current, however.

Photomultipler tube. This detector is used in instruments designed to be extremely sensitive to a very low light level and to light flashes of very short duration. The considerable cost of the tube and its precise, high-voltage, power requirement render it impractical for use in moderately priced, routine instruments. The response time of the photomultiplier is in the microsecond range and the amplication factor may be over 2,000,000. The commonest use of these detectors, in routine laboratory work is in scintillation detectors, used for detecting gamma radiation.

Recently *photojunction diodes* and *phototransistors* have come into use in clinical laboratory photometers. Two types of semiconductors are generally considered in this class. (*Note:* Photoemissive cells and photoconductor cells make use of semiconductor materials but would not be thought of as transistors.) Point-contact phototransistors are PN-junction diodes especially arranged to measure light. A very thin slab of N-type material is mounted in a metal tube, which makes electrical contact with it. Behind the N-type wafer a tiny wire makes a point contact with it. A collimating lens in front of the N-type material focuses light on the junction. This diode is now biased backward; that is to say, the N region is positive and the wire contact negative so that almost no electrons will pass. When subjected to light, however, electrons are released from the covalent bonding and current flow is greatly increased. This point-contact transistor can be made very small. One of its commonest uses is in reading the bright light through the holes of a punch card in a computer-card reader. These transistors are also used, with increasing frequency, in laboratory equipment for sensing and measuring light.

The second type of phototransistors is called a *PN-junction* phototransistor. In this diode a P-type crystal and an N-type crystal are brought into contact and are reverse-biased. The light is focused on the junction. The entire unit is sealed in an evacuated plastic capsule. The two devices work in the same way. In both there is a dark current, since even in the absence of light a small current still flows. An early problem with both these devices was the lack of linearity. This problem has now been solved sufficiently to permit their use in many laboratory devices.

Readout. Not many years ago there were few options for a readout other than an ammeter and a null-balance galvanometer. Now there are many ways to retrieve the information conveyed by the photocurrent.

Historically, the first, commonest and most widely used device has been the microammeter. If a photoemissive cell is used as a detector, a 50 or 100 μamp meter does very admirably to measure its output. One or two pots are placed in the circuit to allow the cell output to be adjusted to exactly the value of the meter. Two pots, of 10 K ohms and 500 ohms, make meter adjustment easy. Meters of this sort are discussed in detail in Chapter 1. Recently taut-band meters, which are much more accurate and stable, have been introduced. Many companies now have such meters in mass production. They are more rugged than the pivot-and-jewel type of movement and may be more economical.

The string galvanometer has been discussed in Chapter 1. It is used in many photometric instruments in the same way that an ammeter is used. It is also frequently used as a null-balance device (Fig. 1-13). Instead of a reference cell, however, a second detector may serve as the balancing signal, as we shall see in the discussion on dual-beam instruments.

Recorders. These are now commonly used to record the output of detectors in easily readable form. There are many types of recorders and they are so ubiquitous in the laboratory that a separate discussion is provided elsewhere.

Digital voltmeters, such as those mentioned in Chapter 1, are finding considerable use now. It is much easier to read a number from a digital device than to read a pointer on a scale and interpolate a value. Although these devices are more expensive than ammeters, the time saved and the increased accuracy are probably well worth the cost. The same comments can be made about the *glow tubes Nixies,* and LEDs, which allow results to be read off as digits. It will be recalled that these devices work on a capacitance principle and, though expensive, are electronically fairly simple. As mentioned earlier, LED readout devices are becoming much cheaper as they are produced in greater numbers; they may soon be competitive in cost with ammeters.

REVIEW QUESTIONS

1. What is the source of most light?
2. What colors correspond to the following wavelengths: 400 nm, 550 nm, 610 nm, and 750 nm? Which has the most energy? Which has the least?
3. Discuss the relationship between slit width and band pass.
4. What are you actually doing when you calibrate a spectrophotometer?
5. Define ground state, didymium filter, electromagnetic spectrum, first-order spectrum, dark current.
6. What color does the human eye see best?
7. Discuss the relationship between percent transmittance and absorbance.
8. Explain Beer-Lambert's law.
9. What is the difference between spectroscopy and absorptiometry?
10. How does an interference filter differ from a glass filter?

4
Spectrophotometry

In Chapter 3 all the basic parts of an absorption colorimeter were considered. In practice, most instruments employ a great many modifications—to improve resolution, to make the instrument easier to use, to reduce the cost, or for some other reason. There are literally dozens of instruments on the market, and it becomes difficult to evaluate the various claimed advantages of brand A over brand X. The purpose of this chapter will be to discuss definitions and specifications, some of the details of spectrophotometer performance, and some actual instruments—with the goal of giving you a better basis for judgment.

DEFINITIONS

As stated earlier, a *photometer* is literally an instrument for measuring light intensity, but in the medical laboratory the term is usually used in its generic sense as *any* instrument that measures light. More often than not, the person using the term is referring to a filter absorptiometer. In the clinical laboratory a *colorimeter* is always an instrument for measuring the absorption of a colored light by a solution, and the colored light is nearly always produced by simple or compound glass filters. When we refer to a *spectrophotometer,* we mean an instrument that measures the absorption of monochromatic light, which has been defined by selecting a band from a spectrum produced by a monochromator. General usage of these terms has given them legitimacy in the laboratory; but we should think clearly about what we mean. Absorptiometry is not a commonly used term, but it better describes the functions that have been discussed.

Flame photometers measure the emission of an element burned in a flame. *Atomic absorption photometers* measure the light absorbed by certain atoms in a flame. *Fluorometers* measure the light, of a specific wavelength, that is emitted by a sample when it is excited by a light of a given energy or wavelength.

In work with absorbance spectrophotometry, there are a number of terms and rules that are commonly used. *Incident light* is the light that falls on the sample. We like to think that it is pure monochromatic light but in practice it will contain some *stray light,* of various wavelengths, that has somehow gotten to the sample. Usually the internal surfaces of a monochromator are painted black in an effort to make them *"ideal black body radiators,"* or surfaces able to absorb all wavelengths of light, but this is an ideal that is never completely effected. The *transmittance,* designated as T, of a sample is the percent of incident light that is transmitted through it. The *percent transmittance* or $\%T$ of a sample is its transmittance over the transmittance of its solvent alone. *Percent transmission* is a vulgarization of the correct term.

Absorbance is a measure of the monochromatic light that has been absorbed by the sample. One would suppose it would be the reciprocal of transmittance but, by general usage, it is expressed as the log to the base 10 of the reciprocal of the transmittance. Absorbance is designated by the capital letter "A." In laboratories the terms *optical density, OD, absorbancy,* and *extinction* are often used to denote absorbance. All of these terms are ambiguous and should be discouraged.

Absorptivity is a proper term and is designated by the small letter "a." Absorptivity is properly defined as the absorbance of 1 gram per liter of a substance, measured in a 1 cm light path at a specified wavelength. There are several other expressions of absorptivity in common use. For example, $\begin{smallmatrix}1\%\\-1\\520\end{smallmatrix}$ cm would mean the absorbance of a 1% solution in a 1 cm light path at 520 nm. *Molar absorptivity* is the absorptivity of a molar solution in a 1 cm light path at the expressed wavelength. Often the molar absorptivity may be a number (such as 4.6) that could not be read on most spectrophotometers. In practice a dilution of the molar solution is made, and the ab-

sorbance value is multiplied by the dilution factor. Molar absorptivity is a convenient expression but not usually practical for direct measurement. In the English literature absorptivity is often called *extinction coefficient.*

LAWS OF ABSORBANCE

Beer's law states that absorbance varies directly with the concentration of the solution in question. This means that, if a 1% solution of a substance has an absorbance of 0.1, then a 2% solution should read 0.2 A and a 3% one should read 0.3 A. Since most solutions obey Beer's law, it is obvious why absorbance is such a convenient expression. If we have only the %T

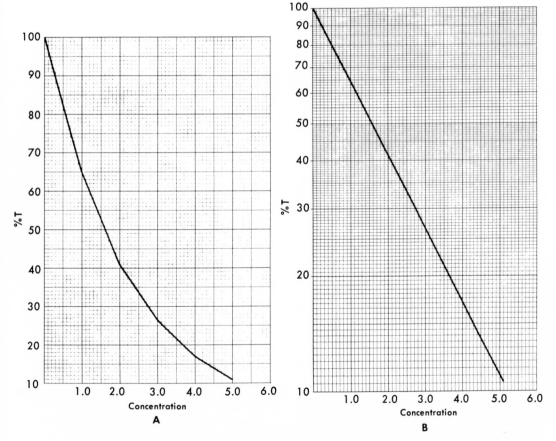

Fig. 4-1. Beer's law. If %T values are plotted against concentration on graph paper, the curve will resemble **A**. If semilog paper is used to plot the same information, the curve will be a straight line like **B**. Since absorbance units are log values, plotting them against concentration on ordinary graph paper will give a straight line exactly like **B**.

values, we can plot them against concentrations on semilog paper and obtain a straight line, all points of which should be true. See Fig. 4-1 to clarify your thinking about these values. Mathematically we would say A = log 1/T.

Lambert's law simply says that absorbance decreases exponentially with increases in the light path. In other words, the absorbance of a given solution in a 2 cm light path will be twice what it would be in a 1 cm light path. Since it is the number of individual molecules of the substance absorbing light that determines absorbance, it makes sense that increasing the concen-

tration of the substance *or* increasing the light path through the solution would have the same effect. It is for this reason that we often refer to *Beer-Lambert's law*, implying that the two expressions are saying the same thing.

It is obvious, from Lambert's law, that a small error in the light path through a cuvette may cause a significant error in reading.

SPECTRAL ABSORBANCE

It is not surprising that a blue solution transmits blue light almost perfectly. In fact, that is the reason it appears blue. It is

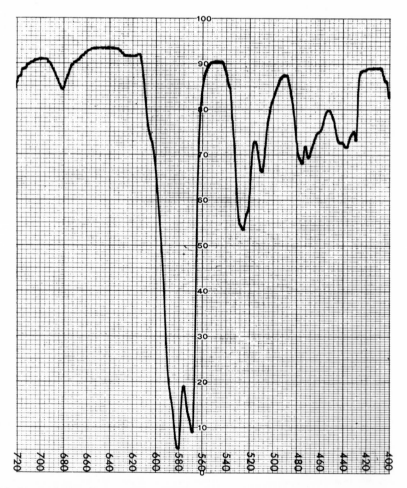

Fig. 4-2. Spectral absorbance curve of didymium, using the Beckman DB and the automatic wavelength adjustment option.

harder to say with certainty what colors the solution absorbs best. As mentioned earlier, the human eye sees only the principal component of light—blue in this case—but cannot evaluate what colors are present in lesser amounts. As a matter of fact, it is the absorbance of light at various wavelengths by a compound that provides us the most information about its identity.

Let us see how we arrive at this information. If we were to prepare a graph, using absorbance on the vertical axis and wavelengths from 400 to 750 nanometers (nm) on the horizontal axis, we could then plot the readings of a solution at each wavelength as we read it. From this *spectral absorbance* curve we would see that the solution transmitted (did not absorb) the color that it appeared to be, as in the example above. We would find some *absorbance maxima* or peaks where the solution absorbed strongly. These absorbance maxima are characteristic; indeed, the whole spectral absorbance curve is exactly characteristic of the substance being measured. (See Fig. 4-2.) In toxicology we often identify a

substance by its absorbance maxima and their relative heights when compared to each other. The absolute peak height—that is, the absorbance at a given wavelength—will depend on the concentration of the substance in the solution. When we set up a concentration curve (for blood sugar, for example), we are measuring the absorbance peak height at an optimum wavelength, which means at an absorbance maximum or peak.

When we set up our plot of the spectral absorbance curve above, it was necessary to take a number of individual absorbance readings to stake out the curve. If we had taken readings at 50 nm intervals only, we would have had a very poor curve that might have completely missed some of the absorbance peaks. If we had taken readings at every 25 nm, we would have had a much better curve. If we had used 10 nm intervals, it would have been even better. We can say that the peaks are better resolved, or identified, when more points are taken; that is to say that we have better resolution.

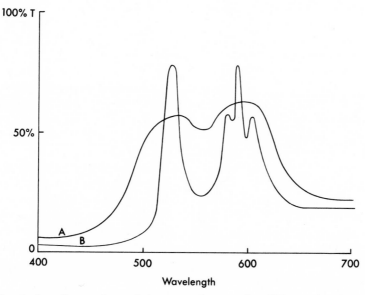

Fig. 4-3. Resolution. Comparison of the spectral scan using different band passes. *A* was made with a 35 nm band pass; *B* was made at 5 nm.

As we took the readings above, we were setting the spectrophotometer's monochrometer at given points. When we set the reading at 500 nm, we were using light that is nominally 500 nm but actually the band pass may have been from 490 to 510 nm. If the band pass was very wide (50 nm, for example), the *resolution* would have been very poor and we would not see many peaks. If a 2 nm band pass had been used, the resolution would have been excellent. Thus resolution depends on band pass. (See Fig. 4-3.)

CALIBRATION

Unfortunately, no one has ever developed a monochromator that is always true in all circumstances. If small changes are made in the light, the diffraction grating, the slit, etc., the geometry is changed and the band of color passing through the exit slit may be altered. Hence, when the wavelength dial says light at 520 nm is passing the slit, there may actually be light at 500 nm instead. We need to have a means of telling whether the monochromator is true or is properly *calibrated.*

It has been pointed out that absorbance maxima or peaks are highly characteristic. The result is that each solution of nickel sulfate, for example, will have a peak at exactly the same wavelength. We can use this information to calibrate monochromators. If we check absorbance values around this typical absorbance peak, the highest value should be found at the characteristic, defined wavelength. If this does not prove to be the case, we can adjust the position of the lamp or grating to correct the wavelength setting to correspond to true values.

It is possible to use, as a calibrating standard, almost any substance for which we have a spectral absorbance curve. If a solution is used, there is a risk that there are impurities or that a change in pH has changed the absorbance curve. If a pure crystalline substance is used, this is not a problem; in most cases the crystal will remain unchanged with time and conditions. The rare-earth crystal called *didymium* has a stable crystalline form and also happens to have some sharp characteristic peaks. It is, therefore, a good standard of reference. *Holmium oxide* is another crystalline compound with similarly good characteristics. Fig. 4-2 is a spectral absorbance curve of didymium. Fig. 4-4 shows curves of three commonly used solutions.

How an instrument is checked for wavelength calibration depends on the instrument itself and the type of scan it can produce. The first and most obvious means of checking is to identify a very characteristic, sharp absorption peak of a substance and see whether the spectrophotometer actually does show maximum absorption at this point. If methyl orange, for example, has an absorption maximum at 460 nm, we can simply put a sample of methyl orange in a cuvette, turn the wavelength selector knob slowly through the wavelengths from 440 to 480 nm, and observe whether the meter shows maximum absorbance at 460 nm.

This check presupposes, however, that (1) there is only one significant absorption peak in this general area; (2) the instrument has sufficient resolution to discern it as a sharp peak; (3) the absorbance value is on the scale (that is, readable at the concentration used); and (4) if one point of the spectral scan is correct, all others will be. These assumptions are not necessarily true or attainable in all cases. Let us take them, one by one, and examine the problems and their solutions.

Significant absorption peak. Many compounds have a great many peaks at close intervals, and it is hard to be sure whether the area of maximum absorbance is actually the wavelength sought. Three precautions may be taken. First, the scan of the substance should be examined to ascertain that the peak to be used is well separated from any other. Second, the color of the light should be consciously noted to

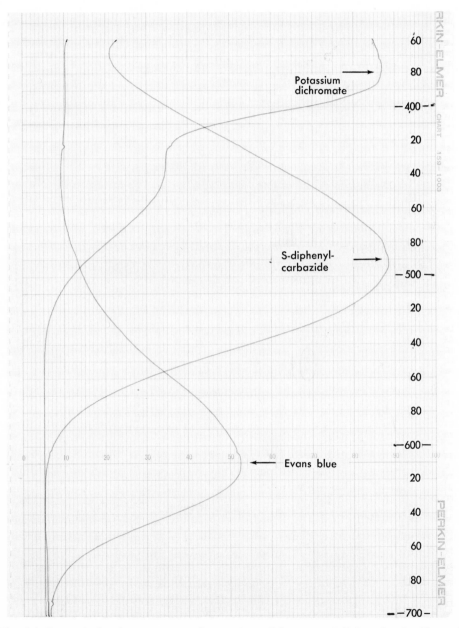

Fig. 4-4. Spectral absorbance curves of potassium dichromate, S-diphenyl-carbazide, and Evans blue dye.

verify that it is of the approximate wavelength under consideration. If the wavelength dial reads 650 and the color of light passing through the cuvette well is green, the instrument is badly out of calibration and the meter response is totally irrelevant. Third, the whole spectral scan should be followed to be certain that peaks are in proper relation to each other, in terms of both peak location and peak height.

Spectrophotometer resolution. The second problem—whether the spectrophotometer is capable of discerning the peak—can be better visualized if we look again at Fig. 4-3. Notice that the very broad absorbance bands in some areas of the spectrum are not truly peaks; it would be difficult to identify a point of maximum absorbance. This is, of course, true of all scans done at a very wide band pass. With wide–band pass instruments it is probably less important that calibration be absolutely correct, but every effort should be made to achieve the maximum that the system will allow. Calibration of these instruments is done on a somewhat different basis. If the spectral scan of didymium, for example (Fig. 4-2), is examined carefully, we can see that there is an abrupt change in absorbance between 580 and 620 nm. This characteristic can be used to calibrate roughly; if enough information is available, even a fairly close calibration can be attained. By turning the wavelength dial with didymium in the light path, it is fairly easy to locate the general area where absorbance drops off precipitously. Exactly what the absorbance reading will be at any one point, of course, depends on the band pass, grating characteristics, etc. If we are in possession of a didymium scan made on an instrument with the same band pass, grating, and other construction details, it is reasonable to assume that the trace can be duplicated and the absorbance of the instrument being calibrated will be the same at a test wavelength as that of the sample curve. This rationale is used to establish a calibration point for a broad–band pass instrument, and calibration performed in this way has proved to be quite adequate. This is the rationale of the calibration procedure for the Coleman, Jr.

Readable absorbance value. The next problem we might encounter in hunting for our test absorbance peak would be that it is off scale or that the peak is so small it is of little value for reference. When using a calibrating material in a strange instrument, we may find this is often the case; and if the material is a glass filter, no dilution or concentration of the sample can be done to solve the problem. What we can do if absorbance is too high or too low is change the absorbance by (1) using a brighter light (if the slit can be opened farther), (2) changing the attenuation of the detector by turning the control pots, or (3) using *neutral-density filters*. Neutral-density filters are filters that decrease the total light without selectively decreasing intensity at any given wavelength. Filters of this sort can be purchased in varying thicknesses. With a little experimentation, using neutral-density filters and the standard controls of the instrument, it is normally possible to get a usable scan on the commercially available calibration filters.

Reliability of readings. Our last problem is that the instrument may not be in calibration at all points throughout the spectrum if only one point has been calibrated. This is a major concern with some spectrophotometers, but only an occasional problem with others, because of the construction of the instrument. It is sound practice to check more than one calibration point occasionally on any instrument. When the instruction manual details it, several points should be checked routinely.

To understand the nature of the problem, let us consider an experiment with a diffraction grating. If we hold a transmittance diffraction grating in a beam of light, a spectrum will be formed on a sheet of white paper held in front of the grating.

The spectrum will not be directly in front of the path of light striking the grating but will be at an angle. At greater angles to the path of light, other, fainter spectra can be seen. The brightest of these spectra is called the *first-order spectrum.* The others are *second-order, third-order,* etc. The first-order spectrum has narrower bands of color and is more uniform in color distribution than are the higher orders. It is the first order that is used in spectrophotometers. Because of the very critical geometry of this system, it is quite difficult to keep the spectrum constant on the sheet of paper without having the light, the collimating lens, the grating, and the paper all held rigidly in position. If we devise a way of holding all these components in position, we can arrange them so that the spectrum is completely flat and all color bands are of essentially the same height and width. If a small window were cut in the paper where the spectrum falls, this would provide a "slit" through which a part of the spectrum could pass. The light that passed would be the "band pass." This arrangement is a monochromator.

If either the light or the grating is moved very slightly to the right or left, the spectrum will move, allowing a different band of color to pass. If properly done, the same proportion of the entire spectrum can still pass through the slit, but it will be a different color band. If we now move one end of the white paper a little distance, so that it is no longer parallel to the surface of the grating, we can see the spectrum distorted, with the blue portion very short, narrow, and bright and the red portion wider, longer, and more diffuse. If we now repeat the movement of the light or the grating, we can see the band pass in no longer the same proportion of the spectrum at the two ends of the scale. Also, the movement of the light that shifted the band pass from red to blue now moves it only from red to yellow or green. If we had calibrated on the red part of the spectrum both times, we would

have gotten totally erroneous results after moving the paper.

As it happens, the geometry of the monochromator is quite complicated and the movement of any of these components must be made very carefully if the spectrum is not to be distorted. In some instruments all these relationships are so rigidly positioned that only one element can be moved in one plane. In this case, barring major damage, a one-point calibration is probably adequate in all cases. In other instruments more than one element may be movable and calibration at several points is advisable.

Several techniques for checking additional points are available, and different filter materials can be purchased or prepared. Didymium is probably the commonest of the commercially available filter materials. The principal absorption peak is around 600 nm, and there are four maxima that are usable as calibration points. Didymium glass appears to be light lilac in color (Fig. 4-2).

Holmium oxide–glass is another specially prepared filter. The holmium oxide is mixed into the molten glass and molded to the thickness desired. This filter has about 10 sharp major maxima that can be used. Some of these are in the near ultraviolet, giving it some value for calibration in this area. Holmium oxide–glass is light yellow in color.

Cobalt chloride in solution is used as a calibrating agent. A 4.4% solution of $CoCl_2 \cdot 6H_2O$ in 1% hydrochloric acid should show a characteristic peak at about 512 nm (Fig. 4-5). Potassium chromate in a concentration of 4 mg per liter of 0.05 N KOH shows a good absorbance maximum at about 375 nm.

It should be apparent that almost any easily reproduced colored solution will have some characteristics that can be used in this way. For example, the green colored solution of nickel sulfate is often used.

Using any of these possible calibrating

Sample curve

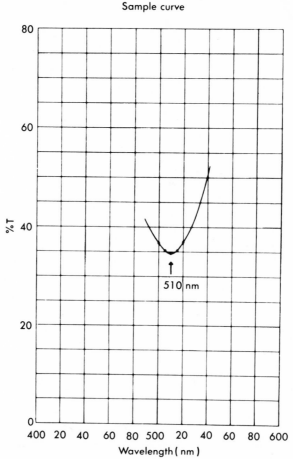

Fig. 4-5. Characteristic plot of percent transmittance versus wavelength using cobalt chloride as a standard with the B & L Spectronic 20. Details of this calibration check are given in the "Spec 20" instruction book. (Courtesy Bausch & Lomb.)

materials, it is fairly simple to dial through the length of the spectrum, observing the absorption peaks and comparing them to the available scans or printed values. Correction is then made by adjusting the light or grating according to the manufacturer's instructions.

Another calibration technique, which is excellent, uses a mercury lamp in place of the exciter lamp of the instrument. When mercury is heated, as in the mercury-vapor lamp, it emits a number of characteristic wavelengths. If this light is directed into the monochromator, these emission peaks will pass the slit as the grating is in the proper position and cause the meter needle to move upscale briskly. This calibration method is excellent for checking the entire optical system except, of course, that it does not tell anything about the positioning of the exciter lamp.

REFINEMENTS OF THE BASIC COLORIMETER

Up to this point we have been discussing *single-beam* colorimeters. In these instruments the light from the exciter lamp goes through the sample only and falls on one detector, from which the absorbance of the sample is calculated. There are a number of problems inherent in this sort of system, and various modifications have been made to solve them. Let us look at these design changes in relation to the problems they solve.

Problem A. When a heavy load is placed on an electric power system, lights dim and later brighten. If readings are being made on a photometer at this moment, results will be completely unreliable. If we take two photocells and position them at equal distances from the exciter lamp and attach both to the same meter so that they oppose each other, we can cancel this instability. Photocell no. 1 will drive the meter upscale and photocell no. 2 will drive it downscale. By the use of variable resistors we can locate the needle at 100% T (transmittance) with the blank in the cuvette well. If the two cells are balanced, a change in light intensity will not cause the needle to move, since both photocells will be affected equally. This is a very simple *dual-beam colorimeter.*

If we wish to make a *null-balance colorimeter* of this arrangement, we can locate the needle at midscale and, by means of a variable resistor, offset the absorbance of the sample with enough ohms of resistance to bring the needle back to exactly center scale. Ohms of resistance needed to balance the meter will be directly proportional to the absorbance of the sample.

Problem B. It is not quite true that the two photocells in our simple dual-beam photometer will balance each other. One beam is passing through a monochromator, and the photodetectors will not respond equally to the white light at the reference cell and the monochromatic light at the sample cell. We could use two monochromators to solve this problem. If we were using filters, this might be a workable idea and the cells would balance better.

Problem C. Using two grating monochromators to solve Problem B would be quite expensive, and the two monochromators might not be exactly correlated any-

way. It is quite easy to insert a beam splitter into the light path between the monochromator and the sample so that the light will go to both the sample and the reference detector. Beam splitters may be made in any of several ways. One of the simplest beam splitters is a half-silvered mirror, called a *dichroid mirror,* that allows half the light to pass through to the sample and the rest to be reflected to the reference cell. Other types of splitters will be discussed presently.

Problem D. Having two detectors can be expensive and, if phototubes or photomultipliers are used, the wiring detail and power supply become complicated. Also, the two detectors are costly and difficult to balance. We can use one phototube to read both the reference and the sample photocurrent. What we are really doing anyway is reading the net current when the two currents are presented to the meter biased against each other. If one detector output is 40 μamp and the other is 50, there will be a net current of 10 μamp if they are caused to oppose each other.

This signal comparison through one detector is accomplished by means of a photochopper, which may work in any of several ways. One common light chopper is a mirror that rotates very rapidly. At one moment it directs the light beam past the sample, then into a mirror, and into the phototube. At the next moment it directs the beam through the sample and into the phototube. Now refer to Fig. 4-6. When the beam is going directly to the phototube (position 1), 50 μamp of current flows. When the light passes through the sample (position 2), only 40 μamp of current flows. The output of the phototube is a square-wave current alternating between 40 and 50 μamp. If we now interpose enough resistance to consume 40 μamp, we have a current left that varies from 0 to 10 μamp. This can now be rectified to a direct current. (It will not be a 10 μamp direct current but will be proportional to any simi-

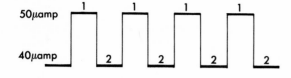

0μamp

Fig. 4-6. Square-wave signal from a phototube receiving "chopped" light, first from a reference cell, then from sample cell.

larly handled signal, and we assign it any meter value we wish.)

Problem E. We have to insert the blank solution in the sample beam, adjust to 100% T (transmittance), and substitute the sample to be read. With the sophisticated arrangement just described this is no longer necessary. All we need now is to provide a sample well for the reference, and we can compare the reference beam, with the blank in it, to the sample beam, with the sample in it. We can compare the two without changing tubes and can establish a ratio between them. If the output of the detector is fed to a recorder, we can call the system a *ratio-recording photometer*. This system is ideal for following a kinetic reaction in which the sample is changing absorbance as a function of time in response to enzyme activity, heat, or some other force.

Problem F. We would like to produce a spectral absorbance curve. This problem is rather easily solved. A drive motor is geared to the diffraction grating to turn it very slowly in the light path so that each color of the spectrum passes through the slit in succession. With the ratio-recording system we are continuously recording the relationship between the sample and the blank as different wavelengths pass through the sample. This geared motor attachment is called a *wavelength drive*. The recording which is

produced is called a *spectral scan* of the sample.

The spectral scan usually identifies a pure substance positively and hence is a very valuable tool. Concentration of the substance can also be calculated from known data, as will be explained later.

Problem G. The general outline of our spectral scan looks a little like a half-moon, and there is some difficulty in reading peak heights at 400 and 700 nm on the chart. As we have noted earlier, detectors have a spectral response similar to the human eye. At the center of the spectrum the response will be high, but at the ends the response will be considerably lower. This inconvenience can be eliminated by installing a variable slit in the light beam before it reaches the detector. This variable slit is operated by a cam or eccentric wheel whose shape is a function of the shape of the spectral response curve. The cam is turned by and coordinated with the wavelength drive motor so that the slit is widest at the ends of the spectrum and narrowest in the middle. Now the spectral scan will be true and the absorbance peaks in all wavelengths will be relative. This variable slit works at right angles to the band pass slit and controls the height of the beam but not the wavelength span.

Problem H. We cannot tell much about the spectral absorbance curve. There are only a couple of large humps that cover half the spectrum. Spectral scans have value only when there is good resolution; that is to say, we must be able to tell specifically what the absorbance at a specific wavelength is, compared to another wavelength 20 nm shorter or longer. To resolve absorbance peaks, the band pass must be short (Fig. 4-3). We might illustrate the relation of band pass to resolution by comparing rides in two cars, of long and short wheel base, respectively. A very long car evens out bumps and holes in the road, but a short car seems to climb every bump and go to the bottom of every hole. By the same token, the wide band pass levels out all the peaks and valleys of the spectral scan. We want to see every peak and valley, however. Often a very sharp, narrow peak may be the characteristic of a compound that positively identifies it. This would be completely missed if a wide band pass were used.

The peaks of an absorbance curve that show high absorbance are called *absorbance maxima,* and the points of lowest absorbance are the *absorbance minima.* Compounds may be identified in the literature by the exact wavelength of their principal absorbance maxima. Quantitation may be accomplished by comparing the peak height of the unknown with the peak height of a 1-molar solution at a given wavelength.

Problem I. Our spectral scan is not clear because of many jagged little peaks that are not in the same place the next time we scan. Some values change between scans. This sort of tracing is usually due to noise, and the change of values is due to amplifier drift. The output of a detector is usually not adequate to run a recorder pen or other type of readout, and an amplifier is needed to increase the signal. The photosignal from the detector usually is direct current. It happens that direct current is very hard to amplify without drift. Drift is a gradual change of value due to increasing or decreasing amplification. Direct current from a detector is generally put through an electronic chopper that produces alternating current of a given wave form. Sometimes the chopped signal from the detector, produced as a result of the photochopper's action (as in Problem D), may be amplified directly.

Electronic choppers may be of several types. One of the commonest is a simple vibrator or oscillator that opens and closes a circuit at a given frequency. Another system is the neon chopper described in Chapter 1. Recently *field-effect transistors* have been used to amplify a direct current without chopping. It is possible that the chop-

per may become unnecessary if the FET turns out to be as effective as present progress would indicate.

Noise in a recording is due to the amplification of various unwanted signal distortions. Ripple may be introduced at various stages and amplified. Static electricity and induction may introduce other artifacts. It is impossible to amplify a tiny signal without introducing some noise. The noise, however, must not be so great that it makes reading of the signal difficult. The *signal-to-noise ratio* is a measurement of the rms value of the noise compared to the rms value produced by a given input signal. The acceptable signal-to-noise ratio will depend on the nature of the measurement being made. A ratio of over 1:50 would be excessive in a spectral scan.

Problem J. We have a brand X recorder to attach to a brand Y spectrophotometer. The recorder pen goes off the paper when we hook it up. To hook up a recorder and a spectrophotometer, we must know the output of the spectrophotometer at the recorder leads and the sensitivity of the recorder in volts. This information is available from the instruction books but may be measured with a good multimeter. With this information we can apply the formula $R = E/I$:

$$\text{Resistance (ohms)} = \frac{\text{Recorder sensitivity (volts)}}{\text{Meter sensitivity (amps)}}$$

A resistor of this value placed in one of the recorder leads should cause full-scale deflection of the spectrophotometer meter to move the recorder pen full scale. Most of the better recorders now have multiple input possibilities. A span switch allows the operator to substitute various resistors by turning a knob on the recorder. For example, a variable resistor that allows use of half the spectrophotometer output to drive the pen full scale is built in.

We must also know whether the output of the spectrophotometer is DC or AC and, if it is alternating, we need to know its frequency. Recorders vary considerably in their capability to accept different frequencies. Some recorders also give full-scale response with a very small voltage change superimposed on a *common mode* voltage necessary to cause the recorder to operate. Because of these and related problems, it is usually wise, when purchasing new equipment, to get the recorder that was originally designed for the instrument in question. If this is not possible, it may save considerable time and effort to have a competent repairman work out the instrument coupling if problems are encountered.

SELECTION OF PHOTOMETRIC INSTRUMENTS

During the 4 years since the second edition of *Elementary Principles of Laboratory Instruments* was published there has been a revolution in the manner clinical laboratory work is performed. At that earlier time the performance of large numbers of profiles and large panels of laboratory tests was rarely done, and the automated equipment required in preparing such profiles and panels was found principally in the larger laboratories. By far the largest part of the laboratory's work load was performed by hand. There was a real need for ability to properly evaluate colorimeters and spectrophotometers, which were the workhorses of the clinical laboratory.

At the present time a large number of automated chemistry systems are in use in the United States, and many, many more very sophisticated systems are projected for delivery in the next year or so. The larger part of routine clinical chemistry is undoubtedly done by automated methods now, and the attention of those concerned with selecting new equipment is focused on automated systems.

For this reason new chapters applicable to automation (Chapters 9, 10, and 11) have been added, and the space devoted to the selection of the simpler spectrophotometric instruments has not been increased. To be

sure, there are still many laboratories that rely completely on these instruments, and there are still many methods that are not easily automated. There are also many laboratory workers who have well-founded doubts about the accuracy of automated methods and, in fact, question the whole concept of mass automation. For these reasons it is imperative that we give care and consideration to the selection of appropriate instruments.

The most important decision to be made is, "Exactly what function is this instrument to serve?" When an employee is being hired, it is of prime importance to have an accurate idea of the job description. By the same token, an instrument would be bought to fill a specific demand. Pathologists and technologists often overestimate the requirement of an instrument and buy something quite sophisticated to do a job that could better be done by a relatively simple device. On the other hand, it is being penny-wise to buy an instrument that is inadequate or one that takes valuable time away from important tasks.

Following are some considerations that need defining:

1. Who will operate the instrument? Be realistic.
2. What degree of accuracy is required? Be realistic.
3. How important is a narrow band pass?
4. Is scanning required?
5. What type of tests will be done?
   a. Repetitive tests done rapidly
   b. A few tests done at leisurely pace
   c. Painstaking procedures done in quantity
   d. Research-type activity
6. How important are economic factors?
7. Is ultraviolet required?
8. Does the instrument need to be a general-purpose tool?

Let us consider these questions in more detail. If you are a busy pathologist who needs a colorimeter to do hemoglobin determinations but who dreams of doing research with untrained helpers, do not buy a very sophisticated ratio recording spectrophotometer. It is foolish to buy an expensive or complicated spectrophotometer for most routine, repetitive-type tests. This is especially true if personnel are not trained in the use of such equipment. The large bulk of hospital and clinic laboratory work can be done adequately on a moderately priced spectrophotometer that is simple to use.

Instrument accuracy is probably overrated in most clinical situations. Most serious medical laboratory errors are errors in identification of patients, samples, reagents, wave lengths, or some similar parameter. Even an error of 5% in most reports would not be catastrophic. (This is not meant to discount the importance of care and accuracy.) Instrument errors are not usually of this magnitude, even with very poor ones. Simplicity, saving of time, and elimination of confusion are more important considerations for a routine instrument than is a narrow band pass.

Obviously, if spectral scanning for accurate quantitation of barbiturates, identification of carboxyhemoglobin and methemoglobin by scan, etc. are to be performed by this instrument, it must be able to scan and be capable of good resolution. In small hospital laboratories one instrument with these capabilities is sufficient.

If routine repetitive tests are to be done, it is wise to get an instrument that is easy to adjust, requires little maintenance, and accepts samples easily. If the load on the instrument is light, more latitude can be allowed for extras. If very careful work is demanded and the load is not heavy, a sophisticated instrument may save much irritation—especially if well-trained personnel are to use it.

In general, price is a minor consideration in buying instruments of this sort. Amortized over the lifetime of the equipment, the difference in cost is negligible if you get exactly what you need.

Service is an important consideration. Simple instruments require little service generally and can be repaired by relatively untrained people. The more sophisticated the equipment, the harder it is to get repair parts and service.

Multipurpose instruments that convert into several other instruments with the addition of gadgets are generally not satisfactory. The saving in money is not usually considerable. If the various devices are really needed, they are usually all needed at the same time. Adaptations are seldom as convenient or satisfactory as an instrument designed to solve the problem directly. In short, additional gadgets are a little like a Boy Scout knife designed as a mess kit and tool chest all in one. None of the functions are ideal.

Completely new and unproved instruments—even those produced by old companies—should be treated with some skepticism. Few instruments are trouble-free in their first production run. If you really want to experiment with a new gadget, admit it to yourself and buy the gadget with this in mind; but do not get into the embarrassing position of having to rely on your acquisition when it has to be recalled for "fine new improvements."

Most hospitals with over 150 beds should have at least three types of colorimetric instruments. The first would be a filter colorimeter or special-purpose instrument for hemoglobin determination. The second would be a general-purpose, moderately priced spectrophotometer. The third would be a wavelength-scanning spectrophotometer with thermostated sample compartment and ultraviolet capability.

Once the instrument is purchased, it should be studied carefully and properly maintained. Service personnel report that the majority of service calls occur because of failure to understand the equipment or failure to take reasonably simple maintenance steps or safety precautions. This situation is usually a result of either an overloaded work schedule or a mania for instant, trouble-free everything. The time required to avoid service pitfalls is usually time well spent, since service personnel are chronically swamped with work and beset by their own problems and repair may be delayed.

READING THE "SPEC" SHEETS

Advertising material about an instrument should always include a sheet or section listing the specifications of the instrument in factual terms (not the flowery prose sometimes used). These specifications are designed to set forth in scientifically accurate terms exactly what the equipment has and what it will do. In actual fact, many of these parameters are not quite as amenable to definition as we would like to think. For example, band pass is usually flatly stated in absolute terms even though the band pass generally varies at different points of the spectrum as previously mentioned. Most reputable manufacturers make a conscientious effort to be reasonably honest but often oversimplify the "specs" to make them more understandable.

Many details may be mentioned in these specifications, but the following are the commonest. In the interest of brevity, only a general idea of each is given here.

Light source. As mentioned earlier, tungsten is used in the visible range, and the vapor lamps such as mercury, hydrogen, deuterium, and xenon are used for UV. Both lamps are used if both the UV and the visible range are used. Quartz halide lamps are used in some newer instruments to cover both ranges.

Single beam or double beams. This distinction has already been adequately explained. We generally assume that wavelength scanning is not possible with a single-beam instrument. Gilford Instruments has produced scanning, single-beam instruments, Models 240 and 2400, in which the reference and the sample are moved in and out of the single light beam alternately several times per second. This approach has some advantages and some limitations.

Monochromator. Included here may be a glass filter, reflectance grating, transmittance grating, glass prism, quartz prism, interference wedge, etc. Technical details such as grating rulings per inch, blaze angle, and monochromator configuration are usually listed.

Detector. The major element may be identified as a photoemissive cell, phototube, photomultiplier, photodiode, etc. Often more technical explanation—such as catalog number, spectral range, or electrical characteristics—is given.

Readout options. Meter, printer, recorder, or BCD connection (for direct connection to computer) are included.

Wavelength drive. When available, the rates of scan provided are listed.

Sample-handling options. Automatic or manual sample changers, flow-through cuvettes, cuvette size options, etc. may be listed.

•   •   •

Several terms are used to define or characterize performance. *Wavelength range* tells the span through which the instrument is warranted to perform satisfactorily. *Band pass* is defined elsewhere and is, of course, a function of *slit width,* which is often stated. At times variable slits or multiple slits with different widths are available. *Resolution* is primarily a function of band pass but may be listed separately. *Stray light* is the portion of the total incident light that is not of the wavelength indicated by the monochromator. In grating instruments much of this comes from higher-order spectra overlapping the first order (unless eliminated by appropriate filters). Reflected light also adds some stray light. This is normally less than 1%, and on better instruments generally approaches 0.1%. *Base line drift*—results primarily from variations in the brilliance of the light source, sensitivity of the detector, and stability of the amplifier. *Noise* or *short-term stability* is a measure of the fluctuations in readings taken over a short time period. This is usually expressed as absorbance units variation per 15-minute period. *Drift* or *long-term stability* is essentially the same measurement but made over the period of an hour. *Wavelength calibration* should indicate the accuracy with which the wavelength scale reading may vary from actual wavelength when the instrument is in proper calibration. *Sensitivity* indicates the amount of light to which the instrument is accurately sensitive. This is indicated, in general terms, by the readout scale.

Most general laboratory spectrophotometers have scales that read from 0 to 1 A. If a higher sensitivity is indicated, the scale may go to 2 A or even to 3 A, suggesting that the instrument can read the very small amount of light that would be transmitted at this point of the scale. Sometimes an additional stage of signal amplification is added to provide greater sensitivity, and a separate scale may be used in this case. *Photometric accuracy* is a composite of several factors such as *meter accuracy* and *detector linearity*. *Photometric reproducibility* tells how closely repetitive readings will duplicate each other. Linearity tells us how faithfully Beer-Lambert's law would be enunciated with an ideal solution.

SOME COMMON PHOTOMETRIC INSTRUMENTS

Leitz Photometric Colorimeter (E. Leitz, Inc.). This is one of the most economical general purpose colorimeters on the market. It has stood the test of time with relatively little change in design. A transformer and capacitors provide and stabilize the 6 v current that the exciter lamp requires. This power supply is well insulated and rugged and almost never fails. It compensates fairly well for normal line voltage fluctuations but is inadequate to compensate for heavy surges and drops.

This instrument is typical of glass filter colorimeters. Having been on the market for about 40 years, this colorimeter has had many modifications and improvements added. It is simple, easy to understand, foolproof, and reliable. Like all glass filter instruments, it has a wide band pass and is severely limited in many characteristics but adequate for many situations.

Many manufacturers have introduced filter colorimeters. There are so many that they must have a gimmick to get any attention at all. There is space here to mention only a few examples of instruments in this class.

Unimeter (Bio-Dynamics, Inc.). The Unimeter attempts to use a single filter and a light level that is constant and is adjustable only with a screwdriver. All methods are performed at the same wavelength with prepackaged reagents. A separate dial face is provided for each method, and results are read directly in concentration. The attempt at simplification is to be applauded. The instrument, however, necessarily leaves much to be desired in terms of accuracy. I would not recommend it for hospital use.

Accu-Stat Blood Chemistry System (Clay-Adams, Division of Becton, Dickinson & Co.). In this filter colorimeter with prepackaged reagents, a dry heat block provides incubation at 37° and 100° C. Scale panels, calibrated in concentration, are provided for each method. As the panel is inserted into the colorimeter, the correct filter is automatically positioned. This is a fairly complicated small system that has found considerable use in doctors' offices.

Serometer (Serosonic Laboratories, Inc.). The Serometer has similar capabilities in a slightly neater package. A digital readout is provided, which can be caused to read out the temperature of the two dry bath blocks. This instrument, too, is primarily limited to doctors' offices.

Eppendorf Photometer (Brinkman Instruments, Inc.). The Eppendorf Photometer is quite a different instrument. This is possibly the most sophisticated filter colorimeter made. Very precise monochromatic light is produced by using mercury and cadmium lamps in combination with glass filters that eliminate all but the desired emission peaks of the lamp in use. High-quality components and workmanship along with good engineering have made this a quality instrument. Unfortunately it has not been widely accepted in medical laboratories in the United States—probably because its unique capabilities have never been properly mated to the needs of the clinical laboratory.

Bio-Tech Absorbance Spectrophotometer (Bio-Technology Instrument Corp.). This device, in a slightly different class, is a sort of continuously variable filter strip mounted in such a way that it can be moved in front of the light source to provide the desired wavelength. Since a gear track is solidly attached to the filter strip and the ends are locked into place, it is quite impossible for the wavelength to get out of calibration unless the filter deteriorates. Band pass is 8 nm through the range from 400 to 700 nm. This unique instrument provides a number of innovations and several options. A dry bath is provided, and the sample compartment is controlled at 37° C. Aside from the wavelength selector, one control knob does everything. It would seem to be possible to use ordinary test tubes, rather than selected cuvettes. The electronic factors seem quite well designed, with virtually all components on one easy-to-change circuit board. A 7½-inch meter, readable to two absorbance units, is available. A linear-log converter is incorporated in the instrument to provide linear concentration readout. A Nixie readout module is also available, which easily attaches in place of the meter. There are a number of other innovations incorporated. This appears to be an extremely well-conceived and well-engineered spectrophotometer that has gained considerable acceptance in some areas.

Eskalab (Smith Kline Instrument Co.).

Another instrument that is somewhat different in principle is the Eskalab, a spectrophotometer that makes use of an interference filter wedge. An interference filter, as mentioned in an earlier chapter, will transmit light at a wavelength equal to the thickness of the transparent part of the filter. If this transparent material is wedge-shaped, different wavelengths will pass, depending on the thickness of the wedge at the point where the light passes. By moving the wedge up and down in the light path it is possible to select wavelengths throughout the 340 to 700 nm range. Since the harmonics of the selected wavelength will also pass, it is necessary to use glass filters to eliminate them. The Eskalab also has a number of other innovations. For example, light passes through the sample, strikes a mirror, and passes again through the sample before striking the detector. This doubles the light path through the solution and doubles the sensitivity. A 10-inch meter scale is used. The full scale length may be used for readings from 0 to 0.5, 0.5 to 1, or 1 to 1.5 A. Thus, in effect, a 30-inch scale is available. A linear log converter linearizes absorbance values. A separate 340 nm interference filter is provided for enzyme work.

A tungsten iodide lamp, which has good emission in the UV range, is used and quartz optics provide good characteristics in this range.

Like all new departures in instrumentation, the Eskalab has had some problems. Most of these have been solved, however, and it seems to function well. Smith Kline has designed an automated enzyme system around it.

• • •

A review of the dozens of single-beam utility-type grating spectrophotometers that are on the market is likely to confuse even the experienced chemist unless he is prepared to spend considerable time in reading and research. Several manufacturers have taken basic instruments and, with different controls, readout options, etc., presented them as different models. Thus we will now consider models 101, 44, 54, 30, 139, 300, 88, 700, 100, and 330—certainly a confusing situation. To cut through this chaos let us consider the various offerings of each manufacturer and examine the difference between models in each case.

Coleman, Jr., Spectrophotometer (Coleman Instruments Division, Perkin-Elmer Corp.). The Coleman, Perkin-Elmer, Hitachi group has produced more spectrophotometers for the medical laboratory than any other. Whereas the product lines have been kept fairly distinct, these companies all share common ownership. In past years the Coleman, Jr., Model 6 has been the commonest spectrophotometer in the clinical laboratory. Since there are still many of these instruments in use and since it is a good example of this type of instrument, let us consider it in some detail. This instrument has stood the test of time well. Its power supply is usually an external 6 v constant-voltage transformer although an electronic power supply is available. The electronic supply is capable of handling greater fluctuations in line voltage, but it is relatively expensive and bulky and has had its share of electrical problems. If excessive line fluctuations are not a problem, you would be wiser to use the transformer. These transformers are, in general, good but may shift in value eventually. When problems are encountered, check the transformer output, which should be 6 v, except for the Model 6D, which will be considered separately. It is necessary to have the instrument turned on when the output of the transformer is checked. The wiring arrangement is such that 117 v will be measured at the input adapter of the instrument until the switch is closed. The transformers may burn out, with smoke and strong odor, but this is quite uncommon. If some shorting has occurred and the transformer output has changed, the only practical recourse is to replace the transformer.

From the receptacle at the back of the instrument, one side of the power circuit is grounded to the frame on the exciter lamp arm. The other side of the circuit goes across the back of the instrument to the switch and then back through a capacitor to the exciter lamp and galvanometer lamp.

Light from the exciter lamp passes through a collimating lens to strike the transmittance-type diffraction grating, which is immediately behind the lens. The spectrum created is thrown onto the front wall of the black chamber located between the grating and the sample compartment. A small slit allows a 35 nm band of light to pass through the sample and onto the photocell. Changing the position of the exciter lamp (by turning the wavelength knob) shifts the spectrum to the right or left, causing a different color band to pass through the slit.

The photoelectric current, produced when light strikes the photocell, activates the galvanometer. One side of the circuit goes directly to the base of the galvanometer while the other side is passed, in series, through the two variable resistors marked "coarse" and "fine." These potentiometers modify the photocurrent so that the galvanometer can be set on 100% T.

The galvanometer lamp is focused on the galvanometer mirror, through a collimating lens with a hairline that is mounted in a tubular mounting close to this lamp. The mirror reflects this image onto a second mirror at the rear of the instrument, from which it is again reflected onto the scale panel. All these components and relationships can be seen on the schematic diagram in Fig. 4-7.

The Coleman, Jr., Spectrophotometer is probably the most widely used spectrophotometer in medical laboratories in the United States. The basic design has remained unchanged for about 25 years until the advent of the Coleman, Jr. II, which will be discussed later.

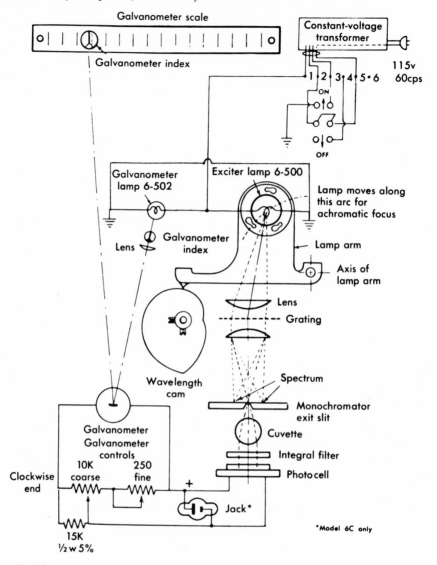

Fig. 4-7. Schematic diagram of Coleman, Jr., Spectrophotometer. (Courtesy Coleman Instruments Division, Perkin-Elmer Corp.)

The exciter lamp is designed to align exactly when properly installed. Removing the lamp may prove difficult if the mounting springs are strong; however, depressing these springs with a flat object will facilitate this operation. Be sure the holes in the lamp base are properly aligned with the lugs of the socket before forcing a new lamp into place. Care should be exercised not to bend the mounting arm. If the old

lamp appears cloudy or if it becomes impossible to set 100% T at 400 or 700 nm wavelengths, a new lamp should be used. Each time a lamp is changed or other internal changes are made, the calibration should be rechecked with the didymium filter. This procedure is outlined in the Coleman, Jr., manual and is further explained elsewhere.

As the instrument ages, the diffraction

grating (which is a replica grating) may deteriorate. The replica material may peel away from its base. If a strip of white paper is inserted in the sample compartment, the incident light can be seen by looking into the well. If the wavelength knob is then turned throughout its span, all areas of the spectrum can be inspected. Each area should present a clear-cut light of a single color. If more than one color can be seen at the same time or the light band appears uneven, the grating is probably defective and the instrument should be sent to a capable facility for repair. Replacement of the grating is not a difficult procedure, but it must be done by someone who understands the relationships. Proper positioning of the grating is the major consideration.

One of the commonest problems encountered in the operation of the instrument is the deterioration of the pots. Two simple checks can be made. (1) Turn each knob slowly and evenly throughout its span. The galvanometer light should move smoothly and evenly along the scale. If its movement is erratic, the pot is defective. (2) With the galvanometer index at various points along the scale, tap the coarse and fine control knobs solidly with the ball of the finger and observe whether the index jumps erratically. If so, the pot is in need of replacement.

The "coarse" control is a 10 K ohm pot, and the "fine" control may be 250 or 500 ohms. These may be obtained in any electrical supply house, but care should be exercised to replace with at least as good a quality component as was originally installed. The replacement can be accomplished quite easily by anyone reasonably proficient with a soldering iron; but, of course, care must be exercised to replace the leads in the same positions. A fixed resistor may be found between the two pots. This resistor is not critical. If damaged, it may be replaced by one of roughly the same value or even omitted completely.

Its function is to modify the effect of the smaller pot.

Occasionally the galvanometer lamp or its collimating lens gets out of line and the index light falls above or below the scale. This can be corrected by adjusting the position of the lens or the lamp. Sometimes the best way to do it is by slightly bending the brackets to bring the beam back into position. If the hairline of the index is not straight across the scale, it can be corrected by rotating the lens holder. Moving the lens holder forward or backward brings the index and hairline into sharp focus.

The photocell almost never fails unless physically damaged. Most of the eccentricities of instrument performance blamed on the photocell are caused elsewhere. The galvanometer is also quite reliable unless physically damaged. The grating, although not of particularly high quality, is satisfactory for this type of work.

In summary, the Coleman, Jr., models 6A, 6B, and 6C are single-beam, grating spectrophotometers with a band pass of about 35 nm. They are reasonably stable and rugged and have been proved by time. The band pass provided is adequate for most routine chemistry methods but is not usable for work involving high resolution. It is mechanically as trouble-free as any comparable laboratory instrument.

The model 6D is a modification designed to provide a 20 nm band pass without substantially changing the basic instrument. Few of these are currently in use.

Both models 6C and 6D are equipped with a jack in the back that allows the galvanometer to be used by another instrument, such as the Coleman Flame Photometer or the Coleman Photofluorometer. When the 6C or 6D is used in this way, the cuvette holder should be turned crosswise in the well to prevent exciter lamp light from falling on the photocell. The galvanometer thus provided is of good quality and is sufficiently sensitive for most purposes.

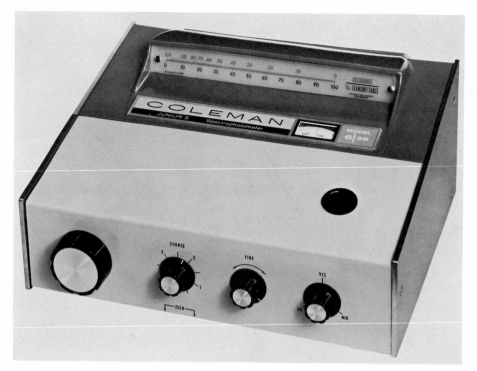

Fig. 4-8. Coleman, Jr. II. (Courtesy Coleman Instruments Division, Perkin-Elmer Corp.)

Coleman, Jr. II, Spectrophotometer (Coleman Instruments Division, Perkin-Elmer Corp.) (Fig. 4-8). This model has now superseded the Coleman, Jr., Model 6 series. An electronic power supply, built into the case, furnishes the 6.3 v current to the exciter lamp, and the signal from the photocell is amplified before presentation to the galvanometer. All circuitry is solid state. Meter response is faster and smoother. The grating seems to be unchanged although details are lacking in the published specifications. Both 35 and 20 nm band pass instruments are available. The exciter lamp is operated at the same voltage for both instruments; thus most of the objectionable features of the model 6D are eliminated from the 20 nm version. Access to the exciter lamp is still awkward.

Several design changes are worthy of note. A wavelength range from 325 to 825 nm is now claimed. The Coleman, Jr., Model 6 series was usable from 400 to 700 nm. This change is very welcome and worthwhile.

Three stray-light filters have been provided in conjunction with the wavelength-span expansion. Stray-light specifications have never been advertised for the Coleman, Jr., series, and in the earlier models they were something less than ideal. No stray-light figures are quoted in the Coleman, Jr. II, manual, but we may assume that these filters will improve the situation considerably. As explained earlier, higher-order spectra have a tendency to overlap slightly and also to allow some reflected light to pass the slit. Separate filters are provided for the 325 to 380 nm range, the 380 to 650 nm range, and the 650 to 825 nm range.

A receptacle that allows the instrument to be used with a recorder is provided. This option may be of value in recording reaction rates where time versus absorbance information is to be plotted, but it is unlikely that a recorder will appreciably increase the utility of this instrument in routine work areas, where it is already so outstanding. With the recorder and the UV range it is possible to perform some kinetic enzyme reactions.

The redesigned instrument has the knurled calibrating screw close to the back, where it is quite accessible. This is another welcome change.

Receptacles have been provided that allow the amplifier of the Coleman, Jr. II, to be used separately to amplify the signal from some other source. While this is quite interesting as an experimental device, we may wonder what practical value it is likely to have on this type of instrument. It is, of course, an inexpensive addition to make and may presage some instrument innovation by the company.

An interesting routine check procedure is recommended to detect power and amplifier error. Methyl orange is read at 460 nm in different serial dilutions to see whether absorbance is in the same ratio. This sounds like a very quick, easy way to detect amplifier linearity and other sources of erratic results. Details are as follows: Make up a stock solution of methyl orange consisting of 2 to 4 mg of the dye in 1 liter of 0.01 N potassium hydroxide. Serial dilutions of the stock are used. The solution should follow Beer's law and give a straight-line absorbance curve if amplification is linear.

The Coleman, Jr. II, has proved itself to be, after the tradition of the Coleman, Jr., a reliable and workworthy instrument. Like any new model (even automobiles), there have been some problems. Most of these have been with the power transistors and amplifiers. The power transistors are tightly seated in a heavy heat sink in the back access panel. They generate a great deal of heat, which may not be quite well enough dissipated. A few high-voltage shorts and component failures have developed in this area. Excessive heat has caused cracking of the plastic housing around the meter panel. It is interesting that the instruction manual suggests the instrument be turned off when not in relatively continuous use. As time goes along, however, problems are being solved, and the Coleman, Jr. II, is apparently on its way to becoming another "old reliable" of the clinical laboratory.

Figs. 4-8 and 4-9 show the exterior of the instrument and the rear interior view.

A modification of the Coleman, Jr. II, is the Jr. IIA. This instrument has a linear log converter built into the instrument, and the polarity of the output is reversed. When a selector knob is set on %T, the instrument functions in this mode as usual. When placed in the A or absorbance mode, zero absorbance is read at the left end of the scale and tenths of an absorbance unit are equally spaced along the scale. Since we can amplify the photosignal to whatever extent we wish, it is possible to standardize the instrument—that is, make a 5 mg standard read 0.5 on the scale, for example. Therefore we are able to read directly in concentration units on the scale.

A more recent Coleman Instruments entry has been the Model 44, which is essentially the same instrument as the Coleman, Jr. IIA, except that a 7-inch taut band meter is used in place of the galvanometer. With the development of sturdier and more accurate meter movements, some manufacturers are finding meters simpler to install and service. At the same time digital presentations of various types are becoming more common and much more economical, and these are gaining wide acceptance also as we shall see.

The Coleman **Model 101 Spectrophotometer** is a considerably more sophisticated instrument. It provides a 10 nm band pass and a range from 220 to 900 nm. To get this range both tungsten and deuterium lamps must be used and the lamps switched at about 375 nm. The detector that is used in this model is unique with Coleman. This phototube contains one cathode sen-

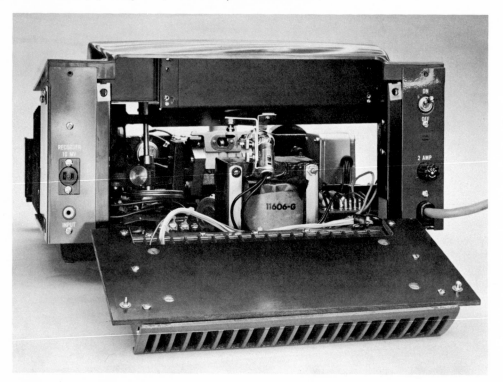

Fig. 4-9. Internal detail of the Coleman, Jr. II, as exposed with back cover open. (Courtesy Coleman Instruments Division, Perkin-Elmer Corp.)

sitive to the lower part of the spectrum and the other, to the high end. The two surfaces—antimony-cesium and silver-cesium—sense light energy, and the total output is compensated in such a way as to provide a smooth output throughout the spectrum instead of the abrupt shift that is noted with switching from one detector to another. This ingenious development considerably simplifies design and use. A three-stage amplifier gives the instrument good sensitivity and stability. The 6-inch meter allows readings to be made in %T and absorbance values from 0.04 to 2 A.

The Perkin-Elmer-Coleman Model 139 Spectrophotometer is capable of still higher performance. A grating ruled at 1440 lines/mm is used in place of the 600 lines/mm gratings used in the instruments just discussed. With the adjustable slits that are provided on this model, excellent resolution is possible. Stray light of less than

0.1% is claimed. Switching from tungsten to deuterium lamps is done by flipping a mirror lever to the new position. The dual-range phototube mentioned above is used here also. A photomultiplier is supplied as an option, if this is preferred, for higher sensitivity. The Model 139 is designed also to accept a number of accessories—to become a flame photometer, atomic absorption photometer, and fluorophotometer.

This presentation of the Coleman spectrophotometers is far from complete, but it should give some idea of what is available. It might be useful to mention two other Coleman single-beam spectrophotometers. The Model 295 is a small teaching instrument that has little to offer as an analytical tool but is nicely designed for student presentations. Another model worthy of special mention here is the Coleman Model 46 Digital Spectrophotometer. This model has all the excellent characteristics of the

Model 139 and adds a digital readout with inch-high neon numbers and a floating zero. The cell compartment can be easily temperature equilibrated. Controls are re-arranged and the presentation generally improved.

Spectronic 70 (Bausch & Lomb). Bausch & Lomb is another company having several number-designated spectrophotometer models on the market. The Spectronic 70 is their basic single-beam instrument. This instrument has a good grating, blazed with 1200 lines/mm at 300 nm. Its range is from 325 to 925 nm and the band pass is 8 nm. A tungsten lamp is used. A red and a blue phototube are used, and the interchange between them is automatic. The 8-inch scale is calibrated in %T and absorbance from 0 to 2 A. Stray light is less than 0.5%, which is satisfactory for this type of instrument.

Bausch & Lomb also have a Model 88 that is very similar to the Model 70 except that a linear log converter is provided, allowing readings to be made in %T, 0 to 1 A, 1 to 2 A, and in concentration.

The Model 100 by Bausch & Lomb is very similar to the Model 88 but has a Nixie read out display and a BCD connection for convenient computer hookup.

The Model 700 from Bausch & Lomb has additional capabilities. Both tungsten and deuterium lamps are provided with a simple switch-over procedure. The band pass is 2 nm, which should afford very good resolution. An 8-inch scale is provided on which %T, 0 to 1 A, 1 to 2 A, or concentration can be read. There is also an ex-panded scale capability that allows the op-erator to expand any portion of the scale by setting the low and high ends on what-ever values he chooses. This provides a very accurate readout capability. In the Model 700 again, we find a red and a blue photo-tube with automatic switch-over capability.

All of the Bausch & Lomb models are fairly recent entries into the field. They have not yet gained wide acceptance in most areas.

Turner Model 330 Spectrophotometer (G. K. Turner Associates) (Fig. 4-10). This is one of the more promising recent spectro-photometers, for routine heavy use. Its de-sign, both optically and electronically, ap-pears to be excellent, and a number of in-novations are included that seem to be very good.

It is a single-beam, grating instrument with a standard wavelength span of 335 to 710 nm that can be expanded to a range of 210 or 1000 nm with a deuterium lamp and IR accessory.

The band pass is 10 nm, which is excel-lent for a fixed-slit instrument of this sort. Stray light of less than 0.5% is claimed. This is a great deal better than most in-struments in this class.

The exciter lamp voltage supply is very carefully controlled. A feedback circuit ref-erence to a Zener diode maintains the volt-age to the lamp at a very accurate level.

The detector is a photodiode with an FET amplifier built into the photodiode socket. From the FET, the signal goes to the meter amplifier, where it is additionally amplified. Output terminals are provided for operating a recorder or other data-re-duction equipment.

The monochromator is of an excellent design, allowing a short band pass and very low stray light. Filters to reduce stray light from second-order spectra and other sources are provided. A digital wavelength dial to show wavelength setting is provided.

All electronics are solid state and appear to be excellently engineered. According to the instruction manual the instrument is designed to withstand vibration of the type it would receive if used on a van or trailer.

The operating and service manual is one of the most concise and straightforward in-struction books I have seen. All details are explained carefully and clearly and all pre-cautions are forcefully and clearly ex-pressed.

This is still a relatively new instrument and still not in wide use, but this situation

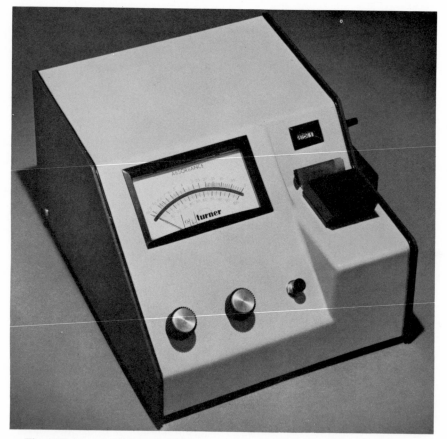

Fig. 4-10. Model 330 Spectrophotometer. (Courtesy G. K. Turner Associates.)

should change. From the information available, it seems to offer great promise. Its cost is low enough to place it in the routine-instrument class. See Fig. 4-11 for the schematic diagram of this instrument.

Micro-Sample Spectrophotometer 300-N (Gilford Instrument Laboratories, Inc.). This instrument was introduced several years ago and has gradually gained good acceptance in most areas. It is the only popular spectrophotometer designed primarily for micro samples. A 500 microliter sample allows a 1 cm light path. The spectral range is from 340 to 700 nm, with a band pass of 8 nm. A linear, digital voltmeter is used for the readout, allowing absorbance values from 0 to 2 to be read to 0.001 A. Concentration can also be read directly, of course. Adjustment of the 0 A

end of the scale is made by varying the intensity of the lamp. Lamp temperature is kept quite low so that lamp failure is unusual. Samples are drawn through a measuring cell by a vacuum pump that is outside the instrument. With practice, samples can be read at the rate of about one per minute. This instrument should be a particularly good choice for the laboratory performing many microanalyses. (See Fig. 4-12.)

Beckman Model DU Spectrophotometer (Beckman Instruments, Inc.) This instrument is a high-quality, medium-priced, single-beam spectrophotometer that has been widely accepted in laboratories of all kinds for many years.

The tungsten exciter lamp can be operated either from a 6 v storage battery or

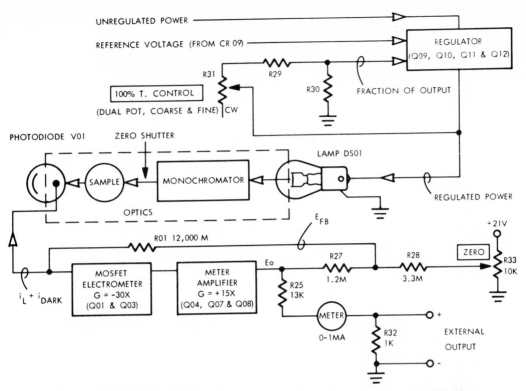

Fig. 4-11. Diagrammatic representation of the optical system of the Turner 330 Spectrophotometer. (Courtesy G. K. Turner Associates.)

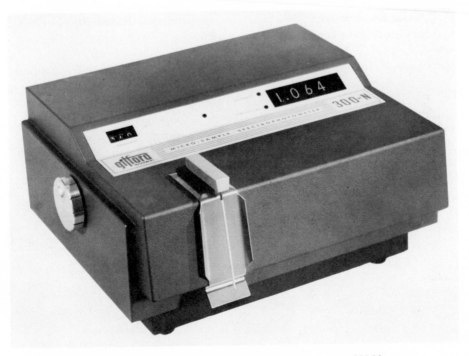

Fig. 4-12. Gilford Micro-Sample Spectrophotometer 300-N.

from an electronic power supply. The storage battery is an unreasonable inconvenience in most busy medical laboratories, and the electronic power supply has become more common. Light from the exciter lamp passes through a fairly elaborate series of collimating lenses and mirrors and is directed onto a reflective glass prism with a curved face. Rotation of the prism moves the spectrum to the right or left, determining which wavelengths will pass the exit slit. The monochromator is more elaborate and precise than those we have previously discussed. Resolution in the visible region is of the order of 1 nm and is somewhat better in the UV range. Output of the phototube is amplified, fed to a null-balance meter, and read against a reference current.

As with many Beckman instruments, modifications and additions to the basic system may be added. Changing of exciter lamps and detectors allows a range from 210 to 1000 nm. The use of a photomultiplier tube as a detector greatly enhances the sensitivity and accuracy of the instrument.

The DU is a fine, well-designed, and highly accurate instrument capable of high resolution and great accuracy. It is relatively expensive for a single-beam instrument and is not as easy to use as some of the newer, more versatile spectrophotometers. The cost and loss of convenience are not likely to be offset by its fine performance when used in the routine clinical laboratory, since this order of resolution and accuracy is seldom required in routine work.

In recent years the DU has found considerable use in enzyme work as a rate-recording instrument in conjunction with Gilford equipment. The very fine quality of the monochromator has made it particularly well adapted to this sort of application.

At one time the DU was a sort of status symbol in laboratories everywhere, since it had, beyond much doubt, the finest performance characteristics of a spectrophotometer in this price range. In recent years, however, spectral scanning has become more important; many advances that have allowed more convenience and speed with comparable accuracy have been made, and the DU has given way to such newer instruments as the Beckman models DB and DB-G.

All the instruments discussed up to this point have been classic single-beam instruments. The next instrument we shall consider serves as a sort of transitional one,

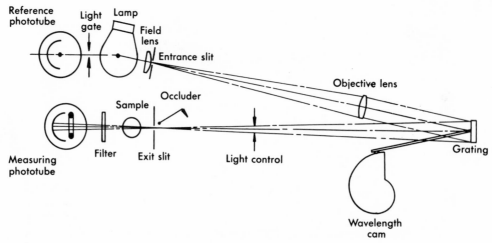

Fig. 4-13. Schematic diagram of the "Spec 20" optical detail. (Courtesy Bausch & Lomb.)

which is double-beam in the sense that it has a reference detector. It does not see a monochromatic light in its reference beam and it cannot monitor a reference solution simultaneously with the sample. Look at the optical detail of the "Spec 20" in Fig. 4-13.

Spectronic 20 (Bausch & Lomb) (Fig. 4-14). When this instrument was introduced in the early 1950s, it incorporated many new and promising features that had not been used in instruments of this class before. It was the first low-cost photometer to use a phototube as a detector. Printed circuit boards were also an innovation, as was electronic control of the power supply. The early models had many design problems that have been quite adequately resolved in newer models.

Three models of the "Spec 20" are available at present. These are a standard model, a regulated model, and a battery-operated instrument for field use.

The power supply for the exciter lamp is monitored and controlled by a feedback circuit from the phototube. Light is collimated through the entrance slit onto a reflectance-type replica grating of reason-ably good quality. Repositioning of the grating by a cam mechanism moves the spectrum to the left or right. The desired wavelengths thus pass through the exit slit, through the sample, and onto the phototube cathode. The optical system is shown schematically in Fig. 4-13. The fixed slits are arranged so as to provide a 20 nm band pass. The phototube used has suitable sensitivity through the range of 340 to 650 nm, above which a red phototube must be substituted to extend the range to 950 nm. This is an obvious disadvantage, and an accessory that allows use of the instrument through the visible range (from 400 to 700 nm) without changing phototubes has now been provided. A mechanical occluder blocks some of the incident light to allow for setting the meter at 100% T.

The photosignal is amplified through a bridge-type, Zener-stabilized amplifier circuit, which has worked quite well in the later models. The printed circuit boards have made the infrequent electronic repairs reasonably simple. Early models used vacuum tubes, which occasionally failed. Newer models are all solid state except for the detector.

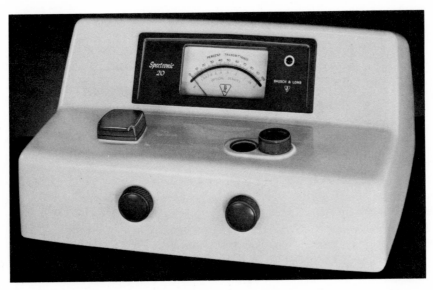

Fig. 4-14. Spectronic 20 Spectrophotometer. (Courtesy Bausch & Lomb.)

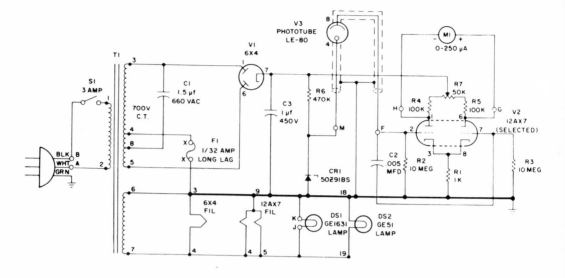

Fig. 4-15. Wiring diagram of the Spectronic 20 (standard model). A battery-operated model and a model with extra power regulation are also made. (Courtesy Bausch & Lomb.)

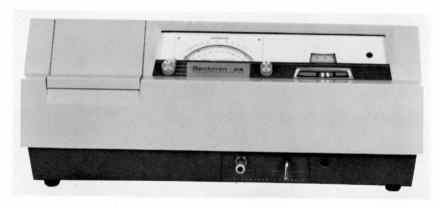

Fig. 4-16. Model DB Spectrophotometer. (Courtesy Beckman Instruments, Inc.)

The exciter lamps are easy to change. Changing of the phototube between the high (red) end of the scale and the low (blue) end is an annoyance but is not difficult. Power transformers fail occasionally but not excessively. Most other components have been reasonably trouble-free. Some instruments after heavy use have shown wear to the mechanical parts involved in positioning the grating, and this has caused instability when the wavelength knob or front panel is accidentally bumped.

In summary, the Spectronic 20 is a very economical, single-beam, amplified 20 nm band pass spectrophotometer that is well worth the price. Newer models have proved to be sensitive, convenient, and trouble-free. The wiring diagram (Fig. 4-15) is provided for further study.

Beckman Models DB and DB-G Spectro-

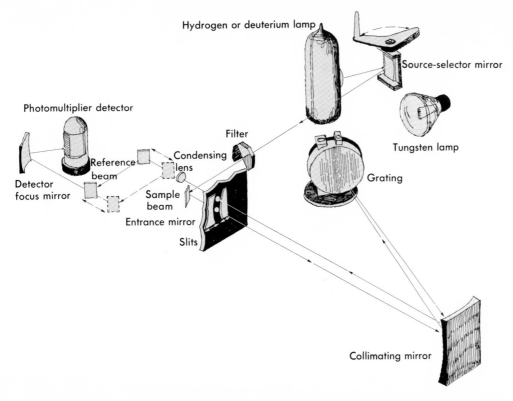

Fig. 4-17. Electro-optical system of the Beckman Model DB. (Courtesy Beckman Instruments, Inc.)

photometers (Fig. 4-16). These instruments are dual-beam and ratio-recording spectrophotometers capable of wavelength scanning. When equipped with an external power supply for the hydrogen lamp, they will cover the range from around 200 to 800 nm. They are capable of very high resolution for spectral scanning.

Fig. 4-17 shows the details of the electrooptical system. There are two exciter lamps—one an ordinary tungsten lamp, the other a hydrogen lamp for UV work (Fig. 4-17). The instrument's power supply provides a carefully modulated 6 v to the tungsten lamp. The UV power supply, external to the instrument, furnishes a higher voltage for firing and maintaining the hydrogen lamp. A mirror can be moved to the right or left to direct the beam from either lamp into the monochromator. Model DB has a

prism monochromator, but the newer DB-G uses a reflectance grating of high quality with a stray-light filter. The grating monochromator is rotated by means of a cam that can be mechanically driven through its entire wavelength span at either of two speeds. As the cam changes the attitudes of the grating monochromator in relation to the light, different areas of the spectrum are continuously presented to the slit; hence the term *spectral scanning*.

The band pass of light through the exit slit is directed to a mirror attached to a vibrating reed. At one instant the light is reflected by the mirror through the reference solution (blank), and at the next, the beam is reflected through the sample. At the other end of the vibrating assembly another mirror catches the transmitted light, first from the reference, then from the sample, and directs it to the phototube. This process causes the phototube to produce a square-wave alternating current, the high side of which is the reference photocurrent and the low side, the sample photocurrent. This new current is now amplified and presented to the meter and to a recorder (if so equipped). If such a record is made at a single wavelength, the optical changes of the sample may be recorded. If the recorder is running while the cam is rotating the monochromator, a spectral scan will be drawn, describing the absorbance of the sample at each wavelength of the spectrum. The narrower the band pass and the slower the scan speed, the better resolution is displayed in the spectral scan.

As mentioned earlier, detectors have a peak area of sensitivity, and sensitivity falls off toward both ends of the spectrum. Since this is true of the phototube of the DB Spectrophotometer, some compensatory mechanism needs to be made to take care of the greatly diminished output of the phototube in the violet and red areas. This is done by adjustable slits that open to accept more light at the high and low wavelengths. The slit adjustment is operated by the same motor that drives the wavelength cam, the opening being exactly proportional to the sensitivity of the phototube at any given wavelength.

The DB Spectrophotometer fills a definite need in the clinical laboratory. It is able to read the absorbance of a compound accurately and with fine resolution. It can monitor a chemical change in a solution by recording the change in absorbance. When plotted as a function of time, a rate of change that is especially useful in enzymology is established. This instrument can also do spectral scans and thus establish the identity and concentration of a substance in solution. All this capability has been provided in the instrument at a reasonable price and in good quality.

This is not to say that there are no problems with the Beckman DB Spectropho-

tometer or that it has no competition. The early models had many problems with components, and many people were discouraged with them before a workable system was developed. There have been problems with the automatic shutter assemblies, which have occasionally failed to operate correctly. Wear of the shutter parts has caused some problems. In the DB the small circuit board at the left rear of the instrument has generated too much heat and the 6973-6AK5 vacuum tube on this board has had to be replaced often. Unfortunately this replacement cannot be made without removal of the instrument cover, which is awkward and time-consuming.

The vibrating reeds are controlled by a neon chopper located directly below the sample well. The chop speed of approximately 35 cps is determined by an oscillator on the main power board. The rate of chop may be controlled by a pot located at the right end of the instrument and accessible through a hole in the cover. Variation in the rate of chop may cause serious meter instability when components fail or change values.

The DB-G is a newer instrument in which many of the troublesome features of the DB have been eliminated. The use of transistors has eliminated many problems of tube aging and failure, and redesigned circuitry has solved the overheating that was chronic on the amplifier board. A redesigned optical system incorporating an excellent reflectance diffraction grating and filter has improved the very good resolution to 0.5 nm, which is more than adequate for any routine medical laboratory work. Stray light is under 0.1% at 220 nm. Wavelength accuracy, which was a little erratic at times with the DB, is markedly improved.

The cell compartment is designed to allow its temperature to be accurately controlled. A water jacket surrounding the cells is fitted with ports so that hoses can be attached and water from a thermostated

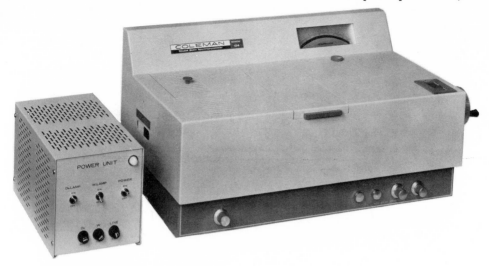

Fig. 4-18. Coleman Model 124 Double-Beam Spectrophotometer.

bath can be circulated through. This feature is essential for enzyme work, in which temperature is critical, and it is most useful for many other procedures.

Any piece of equipment as sophisticated as the DB and the DB-G is almost certain to have some mechanical and electronic problems if heavily used. These instruments are not exceptions, but the number and type of problems experienced with the model DB have not been excessive and its capabilities have far outweighed its shortcoming.

Coleman Model 124 Spectrophotometer (Perkin-Elmer Corp.) (Fig. 4-18). This is another double-beam instrument that has achieved considerable popularity in the past few years. In terms of general utility and price it is comparable to the Beckman DB. The Model 124 uses a tungsten and a deuterium lamp with a flip mirror to select between them. The UV power supply is external, as in the DB. There is a rotating mirror that directs light through reference and sample cuvettes alternately. In place of adjustable slits there are three slits that are easily selected by moving a lever. The respective band passes are 0.5, 1, and 2 nm. Readout may be in one of three modes: %T, linear absorbance from 0 to 2, and linear absorbance from 0 to 1. The linear absorbance scale can, of course, be used to read concentration. The wavelength range is from 200 to 800 nm. Scanning of the entire spectrum can be done in about $2\frac{1}{2}$ minutes with the 240 nm/min. speed. In addition, 30, 60, and 120 nm/min. speeds are available for better resolution. The reflectance grating is ruled at 1440 lines/mm and is blazed at 200 nm for good resolution in the UV region. Stray light is under 0.1% in the UV region, which is very good. The optical diagram is shown in Fig. 4-19. Stability, reproducibility, and accuracy are quite good. Temperature-equilibrating coils are not built in but must be added as an insert into the large sample compartment. With temperature control and with the automatic cell positioner that are available as accessories, four enzymes can be run simultaneously and recorded on any convenient recorder. The use of this sort of intermittent observation of enzyme rates will be considered in a section concerned with the automation of enzyme tests.

A newer model of the Coleman 124 is the 124D, which provides a digital readout with inch-high neon 7-bar numbers. Modes may be selected in the same manner as on the standard model. This newer model also has BCD output for computer or printer.

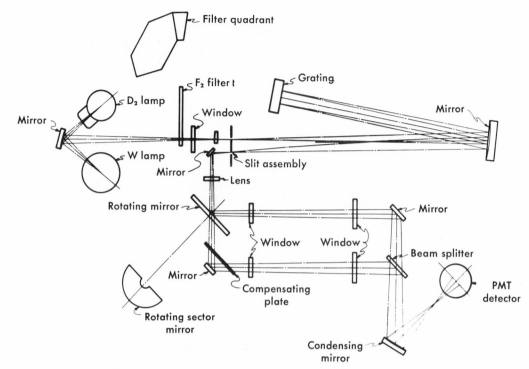

Fig. 4-19. Schematic representation for Coleman Model 124.

It is possible to set high and low limits for the tests being run. When these values are exceeded the printer (an optional accessory) will print results in red.

The 124 and 124D are good, stable, reliable utilitarian instruments that have been, for the most part, trouble-free. The infrequent repairs in my experience, have principally involved chopper mirror bearings and the UV power supply.

• • •

We have talked briefly about the Gilford Model 240 Spectrophotometer. You may remember that this is actually a single-beam spectrophotometer but behaves pretty much like a double-beam instrument. It can serve as a ratio-recording instrument or monitor a kinetic reaction by the device of moving the reference and unknown cuvettes alternately into and out of the light path. This is the only popular instrument operating in this way. There are ad-

vantages in simplicity of optics and electronics. At the same time, the mechanical movement of cuvettes adds moving parts, friction, and the possibility of turbulence in solutions. This instrument, using a fused silica prism, has a wavelength range from 180 to 800 nm, with maximum dispersion and highest energy in the UV region. The slits are adjustable from 0 to 2 mm, giving a claimed resolution of 0.25 nm when scanning at 30 nm/min. Either a tungsten or a deuterium lamp can be selected by a switch that operates both power supply and mirror. A unique photomultiplier circuit provides linear absorbance output, which is read on a 0 to 3 A digital indicator, in 0.001 A increments.

Performance characteristics such as resolution, stability, stray light, and accuracy are excellent. Time will tell how much maintenance the mechanical moving of cuvettes will entail. At the present time this innovative system looks quite good.

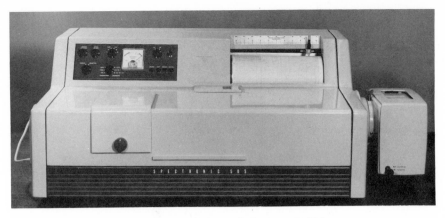

Fig. 4-20. Bausch & Lomb Spectronic 505.

The idea of moving samples alternately into a light beam, to record a gradual absorbance change in each (for kinetic enzyme tests), was an original idea with Gilford. In a discussion of the automation of enzyme tests the development of this idea will be traced and discussed in more detail.

Several years ago Bausch & Lomb brought out a large spectrophotometer called the Spectronic 505. Somewhat later the Spectronic 600 was introduced. Both of these instruments are quite similar in essential detail, so we shall consider them together and then note the differences. (See Fig. 4-20.)

Both instruments have a quartz-iodine lamp and a deuterium lamp as well as a mercury source for wavelength calibration, which is built into the quartz-iodine lamp housing. A 45-degree mirror is rotated to utilize the correct lamp. Two gratings are used in tandem to improve resolution and reduce stray light. The gratings are ruled at 1200 lines/mm and blazed at 300 nm. Two fixed band widths are provided. One is 0.5 nm and the other is 5 nm. The wavelength range is from 200 to 650 nm, but by changing photomultipliers the range can be extended to 800 nm. Readout is on a built-in 11-inch chart recorder. It is set up to record transmission. By changing gears, it can be made to record linear ab-

sorbance. An automatic gear-shifting accessory is available. Scale expansion is also available. Wavelength-scanning can be done from 10 to 300 nm/min. The chopper used in these instruments is somewhat different from the others we have seen. Details can be seen in the illustration provided (Fig. 4-21).

The Spectronic 600 has a combination tungsten and deuterium light source. A large high-contrast meter is provided, in place of the strip chart recorder on the 505. A chart recorder and a digital display are available as accessories, however.

These instruments have found wider acceptance in other scientific areas than in medical laboratories, apparently. Mechanically and optically they are rather complex. The performance characteristics are not appreciably better than those of the Perkin-Elmer 124 or the Beckman DB-G.

After this fairly detailed review of a number of routine working spectrophotometers, the mention of two instruments of especially high quality is included for completeness. These are expensive, versatile, and of the best quality. Their cost and complexity are such that they are not feasible for most routine clinical laboratory work. For the sake of brevity we shall cover only a few details.

The first of these is the Cary 15 Record-

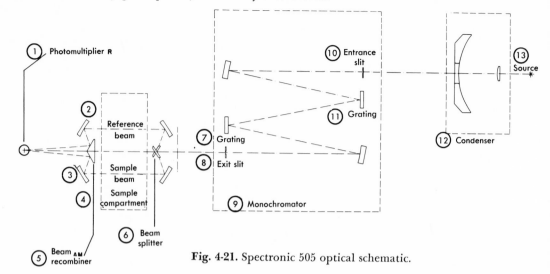

Fig. 4-21. Spectronic 505 optical schematic.

ing Spectrophotometer, which has resolving power down to 0.03 nm, reproducibility within 0.003 A, and excellent stability. With the built-in recorder, it offers a choice of many photometric ranges, scan speeds, pen responses, etc. Two prisms are used in tandem to improve resolution and other characteristics. The Cary 15 is a standard against which other high-quality instruments are measured.

For many years Beckman Instruments' DK series of instruments was accepted as among the best of the expensive, sophisticated spectrophotometers. This series has now been replaced by a newer series called the Acta Spectrophotometers. The Acta II, III, and V are all essentially the same except for readout details. All of this series have tungsten and deuterium lamps, selected by turning a knob. The wavelength range is from 160 to 1000 nm and the wavelength scale is graduated in 0.2 nm increments. Programmed or manual slits go from 0.01 to 7 mm, and a resolution of 0.2 nm is achievable. Readout on the Acta II uses a 4-digit neon glow indicator. Scanning speeds on this model are 5 and 100 nm/min., and BCD output is provided. The other two models are progressively more versatile. The Acta Spectrophotometers are

extremely fine, versatile, and convenient instruments but, of course, well out of the routine working spectrophotometer class.

INFRARED SPECTROPHOTOMETRY

Spectrophotometry in the infrared range, although not used to any great extent in clinical work at the present time, has great potential in analytical work. Energy at the wavelengths in the IR region is absorbed in vibrational and stretching modes within the molecule. These very specific absorbance maxima correspond with specific molecular bonds. It is thus possible to identify a compound with great accuracy on the basis of its component molecular structures. For this process to be used, it is necessary that the preparation be chemically pure or homogeneous. This eliminates its routine use for most clinical procedures.

One of the problems in IR spectrophotometry has to do with the fact that most cuvette materials such as glass and quartz do not transmit energy at these wavelengths. This is also a problem in optical design. For both the prism material and the sample container, crystalline sodium chloride, potassium bromide, and cesium iodide have been used. All optics are surface-reflectance type with aluminized surfaces.

A silicon carbide rod heated to about 1200° C is commonly used as an energy source. The range of wavelength usually employed in IR spectrophotometry is from 0.8 to 50 μ. Perkin-Elmer and Beckman Instruments have been active in the manufacture of instruments in this field and can provide more information to the student who is interested.

REVIEW QUESTIONS

1. Why is didymium a better calibration standard than a solution of potassium dichromate?
2. Why is 610 nm on the didymium filter scan used as the calibration point for the Coleman, Jr. II?
3. Why is a narrow band pass desirable?
4. Is the Bausch & Lomb Spec 20 a ratio-recording instrument?
5. What is an absorbance maxima?
6. On what does resolution depend?
7. What is a dichroid mirror?
8. What is the principal source of stray light in a diffraction grating spectrophotometer? How is it minimized?
9. Name two single-beam spectrophotometers. Name two double-beam spectrophotometers.
10. Can a single-beam instrument also be ratio-recording?
11. How does the Coleman, Jr. IIA, Spectrophotometer differ from the Jr. II?
12. Why are glass cuvettes not generally used in IR spectrophotometry?

5
Light emission and absorption measurement (photometry)

EMISSION FLAME PHOTOMETRY

When a metallic salt is burned in a flame, colors are produced. These colors are at very specific wavelengths that are characteristic of the ion being burned. The heat energy, which the ion absorbs, drives one or more electrons out of their usual orbital positions. As the ion cools, the absorbed energy is released in the form of light, the electrons returning to their normal positions (ground state). Any particular ion may have more than one electron that is excited. The heat energy absorbed and the light emitted on cooling are characteristic of the particular electron orbit involved as well as the ionic species. For this reason each metal, when heated, has its own emission spectrum, showing emission at various characteristic wavelengths. The number of emission bands may increase as the temperature of the flame is increased and more stable electrons in the ion are excited. If the temperature becomes high enough, the electrons may be thrown so far out of their orbits that the ion is destroyed and the electrons do not return to their proper positions with the characteristic emission of light. Electrons thrown out of position assume characteristic new orbits until they return to ground state. They may return to normal by drop-

ping to one or more intermediate new orbital positions before finally returning to ground. These partial energy releases also may cause the emission of light at other characteristic wavelengths.

Further confusing the picture is the fact that there are generally many different ionic species in a flame when a solution is burned; these ions may be present as free ions or parts of atoms, molecules, aggregates, or particles. Various areas of the flame will have different temperatures, and the introduction of water into the flame has a cooling effect. All these facts point up the difficulties involved in practical flame photometry. It is extremely important that conditions be duplicated exactly in all details and that exactly parallel standards be run if the results of flame photometry analyses are to be accurate.

The flame photometer is a device for burning solutions to be analyzed and for measuring the wavelength and intensity of their emissions. The design of the instrument is not complicated, but the details of construction must be quite precise. There are two major parts involved. The *atomizer-burner* assembly must introduce a constant amount of solution into the flame, which must burn at a constant temperature. The *colorimeter* portion of the instrument must measure the color and intensity of the light emitted by the flame. Since we are normally concerned with one element at a time, an interference filter for the wavelength of the brightest emission peak of the selected element is placed between the flame and the detector so that only this characteristic wavelength passes. There is then only the problem of reading the intensity of the light and comparing it to the intensity of a standard to establish the concentration of the element in the solution being burned.

The design of the atomizer-burner has

been the subject of a great deal of engineering research. A fuel gas such as propane, methane, or butane is brought together with an oxidizing agent such as oxygen or compressed air and burned to produce a flame of known heat. The choice of gases and the mixture of fuel and oxidant determine the temperature. The solution to be burned is pulled into the flame by *Venturi action* as the gases rush by the tip of a capillary tube whose other end is immersed in the test solution.

There are two general types of atomizer-burners in use. The first, called a *total-consumption burner,* draws the solution directly into the base of a small flame, where most of it is vaporized and burned. The second, called a *premix burner,* is designed in such a way that the gases rushing past the tip of the capillary nebulize the sample and spray it in a fine mist into a closed chamber beneath the flame. The larger droplets fall to the floor of the chamber and only the very fine droplets are carried upward into the flame by the flow of gas.

The total-consumption burner is a much simpler design. Concentric tubes around the capillary sweep the gases upward past the capillary tip and carry the droplets of fluid into the flame. Other factors being equal, it should be possible to work with smaller concentrations in this sort of system; but there are several rather serious disadvantages. The large droplets of water that are not dispersed cool the flame considerably. This is particularly bad, since small changes in viscosity, surface tension, and pressure may alter the size of the droplets and vary the flame temperature at any moment. Also a larger amount of solid material passes through the burner, and the part that is not burned tends to fall back to dry and cake around the burner orifice, causing further problems. The flame, because of the large droplets, has an uneven turbulent quality that causes erratic meter readings. For these reasons most of the newer flame photometers on the market are

of the premix atomizer-burner design with an atomizer chamber.

It should be apparent that the fuel content of the gas and the pressure and composition of the gas mixture are critical. Both gases should be accurately and consistently metered, and all gas lines and the burner should be clear and unobstructed. Moisture in compressed air, when such air is used, can be a serious problem, and a moisture trap and filter should be used. Where piped gas is used, care should be taken that the gas be relatively clean and consistent as to fuel content.

The total pressure of the gas mixture will determine the flame height, and it is important that the right portion of the flame be in front of the detector. In the base of the flame, where it is hottest, the element absorbs heat energy. As the element rises, it moves into the cooler part, where it gives off its light energy; it is in this area that the emission should be monitored.

Some instruments operate at a temperature that is barely adequate to achieve the desired emission. In most instruments fewer than 5% of the ions passing through the flame are energized. If the temperature falls slightly because of changes in gas pressure, fuel content, or water in the flame, the efficiency of the instrument may be seriously impaired. If this happens, there will be insufficient energy to activate the photometer properly and, when a precalibrated scale panel is used, it becomes impossible to set the high and low ends of the scale using the high and low standards.

The photometer part of the instrument must be designed to detect and measure a very small light signal. The light intensity of a flame is much less than that of an exciter lamp. Also, an interference filter with a very narrow band pass is generally used to isolate the specific energy peak (wavelength) that is characteristic of the element being measured. Hence the light reaching the detector is very weak. For this reason a phototube or photomultiplier is generally used and the output is amplified considerably before it is presented to the readout device.

Because of the many variables involved, it is expedient to use an internal standard whenever possible. An internal standard is a known concentration of an element with an emission peak appreciably different from the unknown so that the two can be readily differentiated. The internal standard is mixed with the test solution. A separate filter and photodetection system is provided. When the test solution with the standard is burned, the two photosignals are compared electronically. Since the standard and test will be affected similarly, variation in aspiration rate, atomization, or amplification will virtually be eliminated. To some extent, the effect of variation in flame temperature is also cancelled. Since the optimum emission temperature for the internal standard and the element being tested may not be quite the same, a disproportionate percentage of the two ionic species may be excited. In the case of sodium and potassium compared to lithium as a standard, this variation is minimal.

Calcium presents a special problem in that there are a number of emission maxima at wavelengths that overlap those of sodium. Since sodium is present in body tissues in concentrations up to 40 times that of calcium, the interference is very hard to completely eliminate. The problem is further complicated by the low percent ionization at low temperatures and the differences in the emission spectra at higher temperatures. An entirely adequate system for doing serum calcium determinations by emission flame photometry without previous chemical separation has not been developed.

For many years serum calcium determinations were done by flame photometry and normal standards were routinely found to read correctly, but many analysts complained that high or low values were not correct. Explanations were contrived, yet careful work revealed that the complaints were justified. Both sodium and protein seem to have contributed considerably to the error. These interferences could be eliminated by preparing a washed calcium oxalate precipitate of the calcium and redissolving in the solution to be aspirated. This procedure is rather pointless, however, since the calcium oxalate precipitate can as easily be titrated.

More recently attempts have been made to use a minor-emission peak, which is not influenced by sodium emission, and to amplify the photosignal as needed. At the present time this approach has not proved feasible. Spectral emission by calcium at some wavelengths is affected by small temperature changes, and this characteristic has rendered the problem still more difficult.

EMISSION FLAME PHOTOMETERS IN COMMON USE

Coleman Flame Photometer, Model 21 (Coleman Instruments Division, Perkin-Elmer Corp.). This was the first flame photometer to gain wide, general acceptance in medical laboratories and for many years was by far the commonest instrument in clinical use. At the time of its introduction in the mid-1950s it was the simplest and most trouble-free flame photometer available.

Oxygen and natural gas (or some similar fuel) are burned in a total-consumption burner. Interchangeable interference filters for potassium, sodium, and calcium are provided. Different dilutions of the sample must be made for sodium and potassium. The determination of calcium by this method is not generally accepted.

One of the principal problems with this instrument lies in the total-consumption burner, which has a tendency to get dirty, to clog, and to partially constrict the gas outlets. The result is poor sampling or a reduction in flame temperature. The temperature of the flame, considering the cooling effect of considerable water introduced by the total-consumption burner, is marginally adequate in most cases, and slight changes in the gas flow may lower the temperature enough to make it impossible to set the standards on the precalibrated meter scale. Strict attention to care of the burner is required and spare burners are a necessity. Also gas pressures and the gas mixture (regulated by a screw under an access plug on the top of the panel) must be watched carefully.

If the base of the instrument is removed, the photometer part of the instrument can be examined. Mounted on the baseplate is the power supply for the signal amplifier. Replacement of vacuum tubes and ballast lamps is a periodic service problem. If water gets into the base of the instrument (as can happen when laboratory accidents occur), the wiring may be short-circuited and the transformer, capacitors, resistors, or wiring may have to be replaced.

A cable connects the power supply on the baseplate to the amplifier box, which is attached to the underside of the instrument panel. If the cover of this black box is removed, the amplifier can be examined. At the front (toward the flame) there is a hole into the chimney housing. The interference filter is inserted in the chimney housing in front of this hole. As the filter is inserted, it depresses a blade that closes a microswitch, activating the amplifier circuit. Occasionally this blade may be bent so as to be inoperable. Just behind the hole is the phototube. This tube is quite durable and is seldom the cause of instrument malfunction. Behind the phototube and suspended in the air is a "peanut" tube (CK571AX), which is the amplifier tube for the photosignal. This tube occasionally fails. It is very hard to check and tedious to replace. In the manual for the instrument there is a check procedure for determining whether the amplifier circuit is properly functioning. If this procedure indicates that the circuit is not functioning

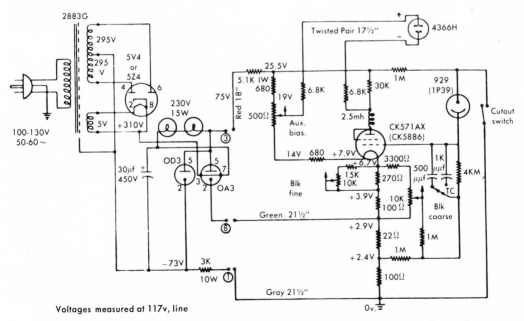

Fig. 5-1. Wiring diagram of the Coleman Flame Photometer. (Courtesy Coleman Instruments Division, Perkin-Elmer Corp.)

as it should, the instrument should be returned to a service facility that can make the necessary replacement or repair.

The amplified photosignal is relayed to a Coleman, Jr., Spectrophotometer or other suitable galvanometer by a small cable plugged into the backs of the two instruments. As mentioned before, the Coleman galvanometer is sturdy and trouble-free. The cable between the two instruments may, after considerable use, be broken or frayed. If this is suspected, the continuity of the cable may be checked with an ohmmeter.

A wiring diagram of a Coleman Flame Photometer is provided in Fig. 5-1. For practice in reading wiring diagrams, try to follow this rather simple one. If you do not recognize the component symbols, consult the Glossary.

The Coleman Model 21 Flame Photometer was undoubtedly the first truly practical flame photometer for the clinical laboratory, but instrumentation of this sort has evolved rapidly and today there are many flame photometers that are much better at prices only a little higher. Within the last year or so Perkin-Elmer has replaced this model with a newer, much improved instrument that admirably fills the need for an economical, simple flame photometer for the clinic or small hospital.

Coleman Model 51 Flame Photometer (Coleman Instruments Division, Perkin-Elmer Corp.). This Model 51 is the only widely accepted single-beam flame photometer on the market today. A hot-wire igniter has been provided that enables the operator to start the flame up without the adrenaline-stimulating process required with the old Model 21. All instructions for starting up and closing down the instrument are printed in logical sequence on the front of the instrument, with all the controls clearly labeled. This seems to be a most commendable step for any instrument. (See Fig. 5-2.)

The amplification factors for sodium,

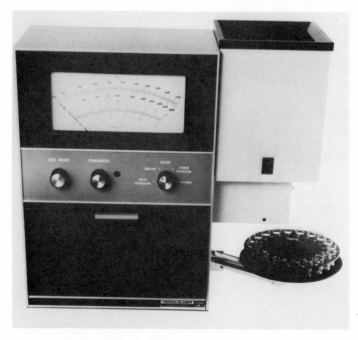

Fig. 5-2. Coleman Model 51 Flame Photometer.

lithium, and potassium have been adjusted so that, with a 1:200 dilution, the normal ranges for these elements in serum or urine may be read on the same 7-inch scale with good accuracy. A hand-operated rotary sample tray is provided for faster sampling. It is possible to attach a recorder and achieve a fair speed of reporting.

The atomizer has been redesigned, but a total-consumption burner is still used. I have not had routine experience with this improved version but the following points would seem obvious. The instrument is much more practical, since it is now possible to use the same dilution for sodium and potassium. Stability is obviously much improved and the igniter is a welcome addition. However, this is still a single-beam instrument, so that an internal standard cannot be used in the usual sense. Also,

the total-consumption burner would seem to be a drawback.

IL Model 143 Flame Photometer (Instrumentation Laboratory, Inc.) (Fig. 5-3). The IL Model 143 has been designed specifically for performing sodium and potassium determinations on serum and urine. It is a sophisticated instrument, well designed, with relatively few problems when used and maintained as recommended. Sodium and potassium values are recorded simultaneously within about 5 seconds on digital readout devices.

A plastic atomizer chamber attaches under the burner housing on this instrument. Compressed air entering the chamber through a small jet draws up the sample through a capillary and nebulizes it. The stream of air and propane sweeps the smaller droplets up into an open burner,

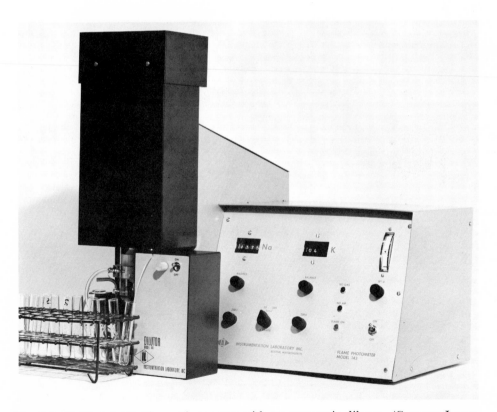

Fig. 5-3. IL Model 143 Flame Photometer with an automatic dilutor. (Courtesy Instrumentation Laboratory, Inc.)

where several small cones of flame burn and coalesce into a larger flame and emission occurs. The emission is monitored by three phototubes with interference filters for sodium, potassium, and lithium. The photosignal from each of these tubes is amplified. The sodium signal is then related to the lithium signal, and the difference is amplified and used to drive a sodium digital readout. The potassium signal is also related to the lithium signal, and this difference is amplified and used to drive a potassium digital readout. Meanwhile a portion of the lithium signal is fed to an edge meter, which serves to monitor the lithium concentration. Obviously, the lithium signal will be inadequate or unsteady if the flame is too high or low or if aspiration is poor. The electronics involved are all solid state and of high quality, giving negligible problems. Each function is on a separate circuit board to make checking and replacement easy.

In addition to the above-mentioned circuits, several convenience and safety checks and controls have been added. There is an automatic igniter that throws a high-voltage spark across the top of the burner when the machine is switched on. When the flame lights, a small indicator light, activated by a photocell close to the burner, indicates that the flame is on. If there is no gas pressure, a small pressure switch in the gas line closes a circuit to light a "no gas" indicator. A "no air" indicator works in the same way. If there is no air, a proportional mixing valve makes it impossible for the gas to flow, thus preventing a possible gas fire. When the machine is off, solenoid valves close both air supply and gas supply. Of course, for safety, the gas should be turned off at the tank also.

The propane gas comes in a small tank of the size used for hand welding torches. This tank is acceptable for use inside buildings without difficulty under almost all fire codes. Exchange of these tanks can be performed quickly and easily without

tools. Only a filtered grade of propane such as that sold by the company should be used with this instrument. Propane is a "dirty" gas normally, and industrial grades have debris that quickly clogs the built-in filter and causes considerable trouble. Even with the special propane provided, the filter gets quite dirty after a couple of years of use. A preheater, which is an aid to combustion, is provided on the gas line. The valve used on the propane tank is somewhat fragile and should not be forced closed and should be opened only about a half-turn. The small O rings on the valve stem are hard to find, and it is usually easier to replace the valve.

Most of the operational problems with this machine are the result of inadequate or irregular aspiration and clogging of the capillary of the aspirator. The ideal flow rate is slightly less than that required to get maximum deflection of the lithium meter. If the lithium meter is unsteady, the capillary may be partially occluded and should be cleaned or replaced. The newer models have an easily replaced capillary. Each time the capillary is replaced, however, the aspiration rate must be readjusted; this can be time-consuming.

Moisture in the air lines is a serious problem with this instrument. Compressor air may contain considerable moisture, and unless a moisture trap and filter are provided, difficulty will almost certainly follow. The moisture trap should be drained daily if any moisture is accumulating. The filter should be changed every 4 to 6 weeks. If air from piped compressed air lines is used, it should be dehumidified and filtered before it comes to the instrument. Piped air lines in moist climates can accumulate quantities of water, which must not reach the instrument.

The automatic striker on the IL Flame Photometer was one of the first built into this type of instrument. It is a real convenience and has been hailed as a most welcome innovation. Like most new ideas, it has had to go through a few design changes before problems were eliminated. The earliest models had a wire about 1 inch long positioned close to the flame. A high-voltage spark jumped from it to the metal burner and ignited the gas. The wire corroded badly and also got bent away from the flame area and would sometimes fail to ignite the gas. The next change was to have only a small unprotected tip of metal protruding from a ceramic insulator fixed firmly in place. This was a considerable improvement, but when corrosion of the igniter tip and buildup of material on the striker and burner occurred, the burned would fail to light and the high-voltage current short-circuited out through the buildup on the striker and burner. If the burner and striker surfaces were carefully cleaned, the instrument would work well again. A new striker housed in plastic is now in use. It has a replaceable electrode that can be discarded when it corrodes. It is easy to change and seems to work extremely well.

When the burner fails to light and air and gas are both available, the striker is usually the problem. You can easily check whether adequate current is getting to the striker. If the banana plug in the top of the Tesla coil (large black coil behind the flame compartment) is removed and the switch is turned on, a stream of sparks can be seen to jump from the plug to its receptacle. Absence of a spark indicates an electronic problem in the power amplifier. (Exercise care in making this check, for you are dealing with very high voltage.)

Just inside the case, below the burner, is a small valve that controls the flow of gas to the burner. Behind this valve is a proportioning valve that maintains a constant proportion of gas and air. Thus, although they enter the atomizer by separate lines, both propane and air are adjusted by turning the one gas-control valve. This setting is rather critical to good instrument performance, and, once the proper flame

height is set, the valve should not be readjusted. If the setting is far off, the instrument is hard to light.

An automatic dilutor with a peristaltic pump for attachment to this flame photometer is now available. The serum is picked up by a capillary sample line and drawn into the pump, where it is diluted with lithium diluent and fed into a pump line, from which it is aspirated in the usual manner. Both potassium and sodium results can be reported within about 15 seconds from the time the serum is available. This fantastic performance is not always without problems, however. The serum sample line and lithium diluent line of the pump are extremely narrow and stop up quite easily. Unfortunately the removal and clearing of these lines are awkward and time-consuming. Nevertheless, if many samples have to be diluted each day, it is well worth the trouble. Recent refinements of this dilutor have reduced earlier problems considerably.

More recently Instrumentation Laboratory has introduced an improved version called the Model 343. The old, sometimes troublesome, mechanical digital registers have been replaced by Nixie tube displays. The atomizer and burner assembly has been modified and improved from time to time, and all the improvements are used in this new model. A plug-in printed circuit board can be added to provide lithium analysis. With a new design and lighted push-button controls, the model 343 has more sex appeal, and, in fact, does have improved stability and ease of use. Fundamentally it is essentially the same as the Model 143 in most details.

In summary, the IL Flame Photometer system is sophisticated and efficient. In spite of problems that occasionally arise, it is superior to any similar equipment currently available. The company has done well since the introduction of the instrument with solving technical problems that have arisen. Replacement parts have

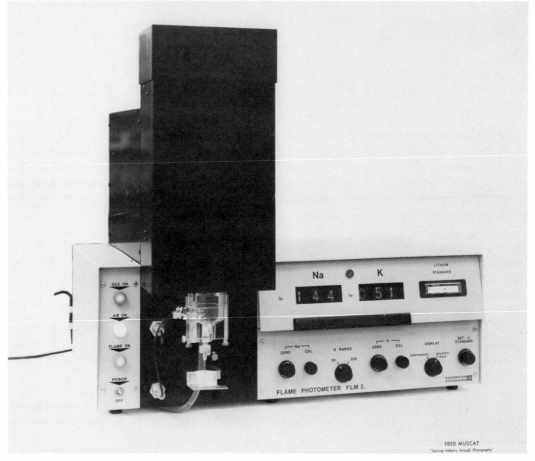

Fig. 5-4. Radiometer Model FLM 2 Flame Photometer. (Courtesy The London Co.)

seemed expensive, but, once parts are received, repair procedures are relatively simple and effective.

• • •

A Danish electronics firm, **Radiometer,** makes an instrument called the **FLM 2 Flame Photometer,** which is very similar to the IL Model 343. The principal differences are in the arrangement of controls and some electronic components. In terms of performance, the FLM 2 seems a little more stable and possibly a little slower. There are no truly remarkable differences. This instrument, as well as others manufactured by Radiometer, is distributed and

serviced by **The London Co.** The FLM 2 is shown in Fig. 5-4.

The **Yallen Model 101 Flame Photometer** is another instrument that is remarkably similar to the IL 143 in functional detail. In this model the electronics and digital readout are mounted in a cabinet separate from the atomizer and flame detector. This gives some increased flexibility. I have had no experience with this unit but it is reputed to be serviceable and comparable to the IL 143.

Turner Model 510 Flame Photometer (G. K. Turner Associates). This is a newer instrument that has received generally favorable comment. Its quiet, built-in compressor takes care of the air requirement, and one can switch very quickly from propane to natural gas in an emergency. Integrated circuits are used to make the unit quite compact while maintaining excellent stability. The sampler-atomizer is designed in such a way as to allow a reading to be made on 0.2 ml of diluted serum—representing 1 microliter of sample! The aspiration rate is from 20 to 40 sec/ml. The sampling area is arranged so that a rack with sample cups may be moved along under the atomizer and the tip may be lowered into each in turn. This arrangement and the fast response time make it possible to process fifty diluted samples in about 6 minutes. A constant-ratio dilutor is available as an accessory.

In general, the Turner Model 510 appears to be a good new instrument that would be especially useful in pediatric work. It seems to have advantages over the instruments that we have just discussed, which seem to all be copies of each other.

Klina Flame System (Beckman Instruments, Inc.). This is another flame photometer that is new since the last edition of this book. Beckman has had rather bad luck with clinical flame photometers in the past, but this unit seems very promising indeed and early reports on it are good.

There is an automatic ignition system, and in case of malfunction an automatic shutdown functions. The premix atomizer chamber is in the front, where it can be easily removed for cleaning. Dilution is performed automatically within the sampler-atomizer portion. A measured sample of serum and an aliquot of diluent are swirled together in a small cup from which the dilution is drawn into the atomizer. A vibrator aids mixing and the chamber is rinsed between samples. Three different dilution ratios may be selected with the flip of a switch.

There is a capability built in that allows one to switch over to reading sodium and lithium (rather than sodium and potas-

sium). When lithium is used as an internal standard, it is monitored and adjusted electronically. If the aspiration rate is incorrect or if certain other malfunctions occur, a system monitor reports the fact, thus reducing erroneous readings.

This system uses photomultiplier tubes, rather than phototubes, which makes possible a considerable improvement in precision and a reduction in background noise. Readout is by Nixie tubes, but a printer is available and BCD output is provided for computer connection.

If the Klina Flame System works as well as early reports seem to indicate, it should find wide acceptance in those laboratories that are not automating electrolyte procedures.

ATOMIC ABSORPTION PHOTOMETRY

In *emission flame photometry,* which has been discussed, a very specific amount of energy, in the form of heat, is absorbed by an atom. This energy causes certain valence electrons to move to new orbital positions more distant from the nucleus. We say the atom is *excited* or that it is in a higher energy state. Since this is an unstable state, the extra energy is given up in a very short time as the atom moves to a cooler part of the flame. This energy is released as light and the wavelength (energy level) is the precise energy involved in the electron transition.

In *atomic absorption* the process is essentially reversed. If we can dissociate the atom in question from its chemical bonds, we find that an un-ionized, unexcited atom will absorb light of a specific wavelength —that is to say, of a certain energy level. This is the exact energy required, in emission flame photometry, to excite the atom by moving certain valence electrons to new, defined orbital positions. In other words, the un-ionized atom will absorb light of the wavelength that it would emit if emission flame photometry were used.

The best way found, until now, to cause the atom to dissociate from its chemical bonds is to heat it in a flame. When heated, some of the atoms emit; but it is estimated that only about 1.5% do so, and all of them will absorb light energy. Thus the error is small and reasonably constant and can be compensated. The band that is absorbed is very narrow—in the order of 0.0001 nm— and at exactly the wavelength that would be emitted if the atom were excited.

These very fine emission lines of a metallic element are produced in the atomic absorption photometer by a *hollow cathode lamp*. This is a neon or argon lamp with a cathode composed of the metal in question. The lamp will emit only the spectrum of the gas plus that of the heated metal. If we direct this light into the flame containing the metal, the atoms of the metal in question will absorb the emission from the metal in the hollow cathode lamp. Absorption will follow Beer's law so that there is a logarithmic relationship between absorption and concentration of element in the light path, just as in spectrophotometry.

For this arrangement to work accurately, it is imperative that a very narrow emission peak of the hollow cathode lamp be measured and that all extraneous light be rejected. To accomplish this we must have a very good monochromator with a very narrow band pass.

Fig. 5-5 compares emission flame photometry with atomic absorption.

The atomic absorption flame photometer, then, in its simplest form, consists of a hollow cathode lamp, an atomizer-burner, a monochromator, a detector, and a read-out. You may be struck by the similarity to a spectrophotometer. The hollow cathode lamp acts as the exciter lamp and the flame acts as the cuvette. Fig. 5-6 may help you visualize the principle.

In actual practice most AA photometers include many additions, refinements, and details that are not described in this rather oversimplified summary. Let us consider some of these further.

A hollow cathode lamp is made for virtually every metallic element. Westinghouse and Perkin-Elmer, together, make almost all the hollow cathode lamps on the

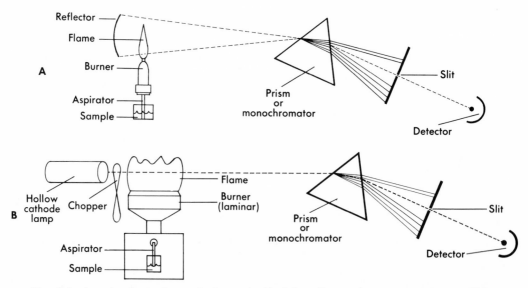

Fig. 5-5. Atomic absorption technique. **A,** Emission flame photometer measures light emitted by the flame. **B,** Atomic absorption photometer measures absorption of light, from the hollow cathode, by the flame. (Courtesy Beckman Instruments, Inc.)

market. Until recently the life of one of these lamps was about 100 hours of burning time. Since there was a rather long warm-up time for lamps of many elements, the actual use time was shorter. Recently lamps have been produced with a much longer life, and in some cases the warm-up time has been reduced. The price for these lamps is about $100 per lamp. More than one element has been inserted in one cathode in some cases so that one lamp can be used for two or more elements. This practice saves somewhat on initial cost; however, the lamp life is still the same. Also the multi element lamps may have interference between the elements.

The importance of lamp warm-up time has been somewhat controversial. The spectral emission of the lamps of certain elements fluctuates considerably during the first few minutes after the lamps are ignited. With some elements this instability has lasted for 30 to 45 minutes. In an effort to obviate the need for a long warm-up time, some companies have produced a double-beam instrument that works very much like a double-beam spectrophotometer. The emission from the hollow cathode lamp is directed to a beam splitter, which by one means or another routes half the light around the flame. Regardless of the variations of the cathode lamp output, the reference beam and the beam passing through the flame are now comparable. This modification is, in general, inclined to improve the stability of the instrument.

At least one company (Instrumentation Laboratory, Inc.) feels that this does not go far enough and that the double beam does not monitor variations in flame char-

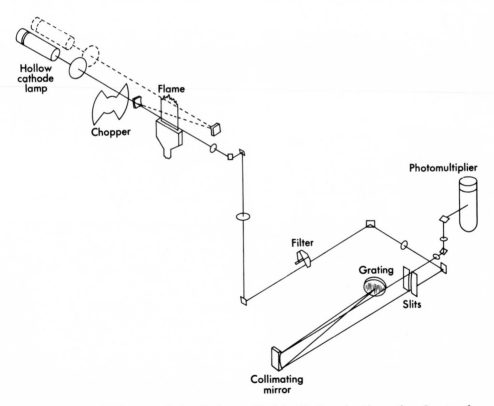

Fig. 5-6. Optical diagram of the Beckman Model 440 Atomic Absorption Spectrophotometer. It is a single-beam instrument with triple- and single-pass optics. (Courtesy Beckman Instruments, Inc.)

acteristics. It has inserted an internal standard (usually lithium) and has provided an additional hollow cathode lamp to continuously monitor the flame as the tests are performed.

Perkin-Elmer has a deuterium background corrector, which does essentially the same thing. Rather than use an additional hollow cathode lamp, such as lithium, this company uses a deuterium lamp with a broad band emission. Monitoring the deuterium lamp output gives the necessary corrective information.

As the flame burns the sample, a few atoms of the element to be tested are excited and give off light of the same wavelength as the hollow cathode lamp. Also some stray light from the room and the burner may coincide with the cathode lamp emission. In order to eliminate these sources of error, the beam from the hollow cathode lamp is chopped and only the chopped light reaching the detector is measured. As we have seen earlier, this is fairly easy to do. In the double-beam instruments, the chop may be the alternate viewing of the reference and sample beams.

Burner design has been the subject of much study during the past few years. Since absorbance varies directly with the optical path through the flame, it has seemed expedient to use a "curtain" or "fishtail" flame, with the hollow cathode beam passing through the length of the flame. Some instruments have the facility to turn the flame at an angle to shorten the path if this becomes desirable. The burner designed to give a curtain of flame is called a *laminar-flow burner*. Some burners have three slots in the head, which give the curtain of flame more width. A high-temperature, nitrous oxide burner is made for those refractory elements that will not atomize at lower flame temperatures.

It is important that the monochromator of the AA photometer be of very high quality, since the emission bands that are being measured are very narrow. A band pass of

about 0.2 nm is, on occasion, required for good resolution.

Atomic absorption is primarily used, in clinical laboratories, to measure trace metals of medical significance and to detect and quantitate metallic poisons. Zinc seems to be involved in the healing process, growth, appetite, and sexual drive. Copper is involved in porphyrin metabolism and is a constituent or activator of various enzymes. Many other metals such as cobalt, molybdenum, selenium, lithium, and tin are known or thought to be important to health—in very small amounts. Arsenic, lead, thallium, beryllium, and many other metals are poisonous, even in very small amounts. Increasing use of many of these in industry makes accidental poisoning more common.

Until recently many of these metals were very difficult to detect, and routine analyses of body fluids and tissues were seldom routinely checked. Food and water supplies could not possibly be monitored by the tedious chemical methods available. With the development of the atomic absorption spectrophotometer these analyses can be done quickly, economically, and quite accurately. This has allowed us to learn much more about these elements and this, in turn, has stimulated a heavy demand for many analyses. With the present emphasis on the environment, many more tests of this sort are being requested on industrial wastes and on water, air, and foods.

Although the use of these tests has become much more common, the measurement of atomic absorption is still restricted, in most cases, to the larger laboratories and hospitals or to specialized laboratories.

Several companies now have instruments that seem to be practical for clinical work. Some of these are presented here. The list is not exhaustive and only a cursory evaluation of each is made. Selection of a system such as an atomic absorption spectrophotometer involves many technical details and parameters, and space does not allow adequate consideration here. The serious student or prospective buyer should study carefully the claims for each, read all available literature on each, and talk with someone who has had experience with the instruments, if possible.

SOME COMMON ATOMIC ABSORPTION SPECTROPHOTOMETERS

There are probably more Perkin-Elmer atomic absorption spectrophotometers in use in clinical laboratories than any other. This company has produced instruments for study of atomic absorption since 1960. Perkin-Elmer scientists have published much material and conducted many fine workshops and training programs that have advanced the use of these instruments. There are two principal models in wide clinical use.

Perkin-Elmer's Model 290B and Model 303 (Perkin-Elmer Corp.). The 290B is a single-beam instrument designed with a readout in linear concentration units. The monochromator covers the range from 200 to 700 nm, using a grating ruled at 1800 lines/mm. Resolution of 0.2 nm is possible and a choice of 0.2, 0.7, or 2 nm band pass is available. Since some hollow cathode lamps require some warm-up time before their output is stable, a three-lamp warm-up supply accessory is available to save time. Where a large number of analyses are to be done on one element, the Model 290B is an excellent instrument. A scale expansion of $4.5\times$ is built into the instrument, which can be increased to $18\times$ by using an external 10 millivolt recorder.

Their Model 303, is a double-beam instrument. In this case the chopper is a rotating mirror that alternately directs the reference and the sample beam into the detector. The ratio is then read electrically. This process helps to offset drift in hollow cathode lamp output and detector sensi-

tivity. Lamp warm-up time can be virtually eliminated. With the Model 303 it is possible to use the deuterium background corrector, which emits a broad emission. Background in the flame absorbs both the deuterium and hollow cathode emission, whereas the element of interest absorbs only the hollow cathode's narrow band of emission, providing a basis for correcting for background effect. It is also possible to use the digital concentration readout accessory with the Model 303 to provide readout in units of concentration. See Fig. 5-7 and compare the light paths of Model 290B and Model 303.

The Model 303 is a sensitive, stable, and versatile instrument that is generally considered to be the leader among atomic absorption spectrophotometers in clinical use. This is not to say, of course, that competing companies do not have some extremely fine instruments and excellent points to make for their own developments and modifications. A wide choice of burners and other accessories is available.

Beckman Model 979 Atomic Absorption System (Beckman Instruments, Inc.). This system is designed to use the Beckman DB Spectrophotometer as its monochromator, detector, and readout. The system has two characteristics that are of special interest. First, it may be used as an emission-flame spectrophotometer. Second, since the spectral-scanning DB is used as the monochromator, the flame can be scanned for emission peaks. In practice, neither of these options is likely to be very heavily used, but both features add interesting dimensions. If you buy the entire system complete, it is obvious that you have also purchased a Beckman DB Spectrophotometer, which is a nice bonus.

This AA system is single-beam. Optics are arranged so that the beam may be passed through the flame three times before going to the monochromator. This has the obvious effect of tripling the light path through the flame and increasing sensitiv-

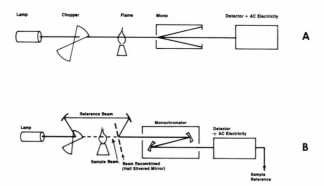

Fig. 5-7. Comparison of optical paths in single-beam and double-beam atomic absorption spectrophotometers. **A,** Single-beam AC system: in this system, light from the hollow cathode lamp is chopped, either mechanically or electronically, to differentiate it from unchopped light emission. The monochromator is tuned to select the resonance line of the element being determined. The chopped lamplight causes an alternating current flow in the photomultiplier detector—hence the name "AC system." The Model 290B uses this system. **B,** Double-beam AC system: in the Model 303, the chopper is a rotating sector mirror that divides the light from the hollow cathode lamp into two beams. The electronic output appears as the ratio of the sample and reference beams. The effects of changes in lamp emission and detector sensitivity are thereby eliminated. Compared to the single-beam system, double-beam gives better precision and detection limits. (Courtesy Perkin-Elmer Corp.)

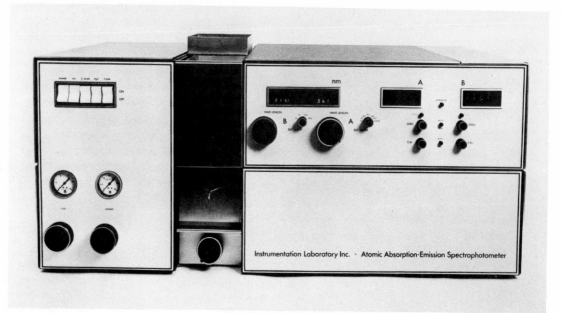

Fig. 5-8. IL Atomic Absorption–Emission Spectrophotometer, Model 453. (Courtesy Instrumentation Laboratory, Inc.)

ity considerably. The optical beam passing the flame is collimated to a very small diameter to avoid the outer turbulent edges of the flame as much as possible.

The Beckman laminar-flow burner has an interesting heating and cooling feature that is said to increase the concentration of the unknown in the vapor passing into the flame. The aspiration chamber is heated with infrared heaters to vaporize the sample as it passes. After leaving the atomizer chamber, the vaporized sample passes through a water-cooled baffle chamber, where solvent is condensed and removed. The company claims a significant increase in sensitivity with this burner. The laminar-flow burner is also available in a special construction for use with nitrous oxide.

The instrument does not have the advantages of dual-beam construction but seems to be sensitive, with good resolution.

IL Model 453 Atomic Absorption–Emission Spectrophotometer (Instrumentation Laboratory, Inc.) (Fig. 5-8). This instrument is by far the most sophisticated of those discussed here. It is, in effect, a double double-beam instrument; that is to say, the beams from two hollow cathode lamps are passing through the flame simultaneously, each with its own reference beam around the flame. The second cathode element may be used as an internal standard, or there is the option of performing tests for two elements simultaneously. This instrument also can be used as an emission-flame photometer. It is equipped with an automatic ignition as well as a number of monitoring functions.

There is a digital concentration readout, and scale expansion is possible. An ingenious correction circuit that permits linearization of nonlinear signals by means of a single adjustment is provided. Since atomic absorption is such a dynamic process, you would do well to check standards carefully at frequent intervals, however.

A great deal of thought has been given to safety in the design of this IL instrument. In addition to the automatic remote control of flame ignition and extinction, fail-safe devices that take over in certain circumstances have been built in. If air or gas pressure drops, all valves are immediately and automatically closed. If the flame becomes irregular or if it "lifts off" the burner, the fail-safe comes into play. If the wrong burner for the gas mixture being employed is installed, the ignition system is neutralized and cannot function.

Conversion to nitrous oxide may be effected by a control on the front panel and, when the N_2O flame is extinguished, air is injected into the system to prevent excessive soot formation and flashback explosions. If such a flashback does occur, a diaphragm ruptures gently away from the operator.

Another attractive feature of this unit that seems excellent is the built-in circuit-testing features. Using the controls on one panel, you can electrically check 20 different points without extensively dismantling the instrument.

The electronics are all solid state and superbly designed. The optical system seems very good. The band pass, of the Ebert-type (grating) monochromator, is 0.6 Å. Design of the gas-handling system, the fail-safe features, and the safety features appears to be excellent.

Many features that are provided as extra, optional accessories on other atomic absorbance units are built into this one. The digital readout, linearizer, electronic integrator, and built-in circuit-testing might be considered as extras. The price of the unit is comparable to the competitive units with these accessories.

An intriguing additional feature is a motorized wavelength scanning drive that permits scanning of the hollow cathode lamp's emission or the emission of the flame itself. This spectral scan may be recorded, of course.

The IL atomic absorption spectrophotometers have now established themselves as serious challengers and have had wide acceptance. Early arguments that the unit is overengineered seem, at least, to have been overstated, since its performance record seems good. There is possibly something to be said for the loss of sensitivity involved in the many optical surfaces of lenses, mirrors, and beam splitters. This loss seems to have been largely offset by good electronics.

Models AA-5 and AA-120 Atomic Absorption Spectrophotometers (Varian Techron). These instruments, from a company that has recently become active in the medical market with several instruments, are modular, single-beam instruments that are well built and convenient. The monochromator covers the range from 186 to 1000 nm and provides for automatic scanning of the entire spectrum in about 2 minutes. A lamp turret can power up to four lamps at the same time for fast switching between elements. In addition to atomic absorption, emission and atomic fluorescence can also be added. These models have been well accepted and have found wide use.

Almost all the better-known atomic absorption spectrophotometers now provide some flameless approach to deionization of the sample. Most of the methods consist of some device by which a small sample of material is dried and electrically heated at high temperature. Aspirating and atomizing the sample into the flame is not a particularly efficient process and only a small percentage of atoms are actually used. Also, they pass through the flame rather quickly. The various devices—carbon rod, carbon tube, tantalum boat, etc.—that are being used as substitutes for the flame, get maximum efficiency out of a very small sample and thus greatly improve sensitivity.

REVIEW QUESTIONS

1. How does a total-combustion burner differ from a premix burner?
2. What is the function of an internal standard?
3. What effect does water in the oxygen source have on flame photometry?
4. What is the principal argument for the double-beam approach to measurement of atomic absorption?
5. What is the source of monochromatic light in atomic absorption instruments?
6. Two methods were described for automatically diluting serum or urine samples for flame photometry. What were they?
7. Why would a glass filter probably not be used to produce monochromatic light for flame photometry?

Fluorescence and fluorometry

PHENOMENON OF FLUORESCENCE

When some types of molecules are exposed to light or other electromagnetic radiation, they absorb this energy and then re-emit it as light of another wavelength. The radiant energy displaces certain electrons from their customary orbital positions and moves them into characteristic orbital positions farther from the nucleus. In its natural condition the molecule is said to be in the *ground state*. When the electrons have absorbed energy in the above manner, the molecule is said to be in an *excited state* or a *higher-energy state*. Such electrons usually occur in balanced pairs. When one of the pair of electrons is raised to its first characteristic excited state, it is said to be in a *first singlet* or S_1 stage. If the electron absorbs still more energy, causing it to move into a more distant orbit, it may be placed in an S_2, S_3, S_4, etc. stage. A typical, highly reproducible amount of energy is required to place the electron in a particular orbit.

It was pointed out, in earlier chapters, that the wavelength or color of light determines its radiant energy. A specific color or wavelength of light will characteristically excite a molecule to a specific singlet stage by displacing an electron from its normal position.

At the same time other wavelengths of light, with different energy levels, from the same source may be displacing other electrons of the same molecule to new characteristic positions.

Excited molecules do not stay in this state very long. Within microseconds or even nanoseconds the displaced electron returns to its normal position, with the release of the absorbed energy. In the process, however, a little energy is lost and the *emitted* energy (light) is of a lower order (longer wavelength) than that of the *exciting* energy. Hence a molecule may absorb violet light and then emit red light. The energy that is "lost" in this process can probably be accounted for by vibration and by collisions. (See Fig. 6-1.)

This process is called *fluorescence*. The ability of a molecule to absorb light of a given wavelength and re-emit it at another, characteristic wavelength is such a specific and characteristic phenomenon that it can be used as a certain method of identifying a particular compound. Also the amount of light that will be re-emitted is a linear function of the concentration of the compound. These circumstances make *fluorometry* a very specific and sensitive testing procedure.

If energy is not released until a few milliseconds after excitation of the molecule, the process is called *phosphorescence*. The luminous dial of your watch provides an example of phosphorescence. For clarity we usually call it phosphorescence when a lapse of 10^{-4} second occurs before the light is re-emitted; much longer time lapses are, of course, very common.

When the electron is raised to the second or third singlet stage, it can lose its absorbed energy in two or more steps, thereby emitting more than one characteristic wavelength of light energy. Considering the possibility of electrons in different orbital positions, each re-emitting a characteristic wavelength of light, and further considering the possibility that some may lose their energy in several stages, we might predict that the fluorescent light

107

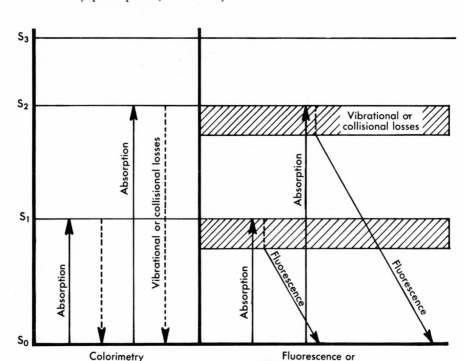

Fig. 6-1. Diagrammatic representation of the absorption and re-emission of energy in fluorescence or phosphorescence compared with the same process in normally non-fluorescing compounds.

emitted by a compound could contain a considerable number of characteristic emission peaks. This is, indeed, the case, and it is possible to identify a compound, in many cases, by the emission spectrum of that compound. If we wish to quantitate a compound by fluorescence, however, we select a specific characteristic wavelength *(an emission maximum)* at which we will measure the intensity of light emission relative to suitable standards.

Since some energy is always lost in the process of absorption and re-emission and since the re-emitted energy is generally visible light, it stands to reason that the exciting energy might often be in the ultraviolet or near ultraviolet region, where wavelengths are shorter and energy levels higher. The light source used to provide this energy in a fluorometer may be a *hydrogen lamp,* a *mercury arc,* a *xenon lamp,*

or another similar emission source. These sources require relatively high voltage to fire, and a high-voltage transformer is always a necessary part of a fluorometer. Fluorescent lighting such as that used in the home emits some energy in the near ultraviolet range and can be used in special situations.

It is interesting to note that the phenomenon of fluorescence is not limited to the UV and visible range. Some molecules may absorb energy from X rays and re-emit in the soft–X ray or far-UV range. Since it is more difficult to detect and resolve radiation of such short wavelengths, this region has never been used in routine analysis.

FLUOROMETRY

A very simple fluorometer would have a configuration similar to that in Fig. 6-2.

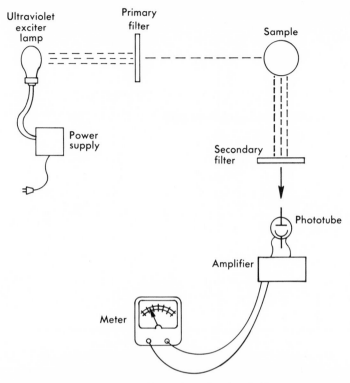

Fig. 6-2. Typical configuration of a simple fluorometer.

The power supply would need to be sufficiently stable to provide a constant voltage to the exciter lamp. The exciter lamp would have to have adequate emission at the specific wavelengths needed for whatever analyses were contemplated. The primary filter would provide the wavelength that would excite the solution under examination. The resolution required of the instrument would dictate the sort of monochromator to be used.

Since the entire sample in a fluorometer is saturated with light, the light does not have to be collimated into a sharply defined path through the sample. For the same reason, small blemishes and scratches on the cuvettes are of relatively less consequence as a source of error. If the material being tested is fluorescent, the entire content of the tube emits light and becomes, in effect, a light source, the brilliance of which we will measure with the detector. The detector is usually placed at a 90-degree angle to the beam of the exciting light so that only emitted (not transmitted) light is measured.

The secondary filter defines the specific emission peak that is to be used for analysis. Again, the quality of resolution required will dictate whether a filter or a more sophisticated monochromator is used.

A phototube or photomultiplier is usually used as a detector in fluorometers, since the total emitted light may possibly be much weaker than in photometry. Fig. 6-3 shows the optical path of a typical fluorometer.

As mentioned earlier, ultraviolet light is absorbed by ordinary glass, and the amount of this absorption is quite significant at the shorter wavelengths. Quartz or a special type of glass is used in the optics of better

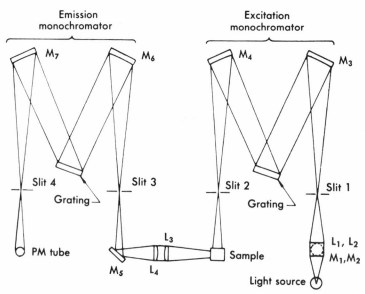

Fig. 6-3. Optical path of the SPF 125 Spectrofluorometer. (Courtesy American Instrument Co., Inc.)

fluorometers, and, in some cases, the use of quartz or infrasil cuvettes may be advantageous or necessary. Front-surfaced mirrors are also generally used.

The time required for fluorescent emission to occur after excitation may vary somewhat between orbital electron positions and between molecular species. This delay is usually in microseconds and is not significant when readings are taken reasonably soon after the specimen is exposed to light. If the specimen remains in the light path for a considerable time, however, this may result in a gradually increasing emission. A shutter is often supplied between the light source and the sample. The shutter is left closed until the reading is to be made, to prevent the sort of error just described.

As a general rule, the intensity of fluorescence is proportional to the concentration. When dealing with an unknown, one should plot a curve using known standards. In some cases a phenomenon known as "quenching" occurs, in which the fluorescence actually decreases as the concen-

tration of fluorophores exceeds an optimal value.

Fluorescent procedures should be followed exactly, since small changes in chemistry may make significant changes in fluorescence. Some fluorescing compounds are so sensitive to changes in pH that their emission can be used as a sensitive measure of pH change. In fact, there are several excellent fluorescent indicators for use in acid-base titrations.

It is interesting to note that the excitation wavelengths (those that excite a molecule and cause it to fluoresce) are the same as those at which the molecule will absorb light. The emission wavelengths are generally somewhat higher, but there may not be much resemblance between the total *excitation spectrum* and the emission spectrum. The term *quantum efficiency* is used to express the ratio of emitted light to absorbed light.

Fluorometry is a more specific means of measurement than absorptiometry. If we measure the light absorption of a solution at a given wavelength, we are measuring absorption by the material in question plus any other that might be present. In fluorometry, however, we are dealing only with the substance that absorbs at the specific wavelength *and* emits light at a second characteristic wavelength.

Fluorometry is extremely sensitive. It is estimated that it can detect materials in a concentration of one in ten billion. This is about 1000 times the sensitivity of absorptiometry. The material must naturally fluoresce or be made to fluoresce by some tagging technique, of course. This tagging technique can be accomplished with many materials, but it is often as easy and more expedient to detect and quantitate a substance by some other technique. Fluorescence for many substances, however, is the obvious technique of choice.

FLUOROMETERS IN COMMON USE

Coleman 12C Photofluorometer (Perkin-Elmer Corp.). This is a low-priced and simply designed filter fluorometer that has been available for many years. This instrument is a good one to use to demonstrate fluorescence, since all parts are easy to see and explain. A mercury vapor lamp is powered by an external transformer. There are a primary filter and shutter, a sample compartment, a secondary filter at right angles to the light path, a phototube, and a simple one-stage amplifier. The readout is an ammeter but an output plug in the back allows the unit to be connected to a Coleman, Jr., galvanometer by a short cable to improve sensitivity. All optics are glass. This instrument, of course, has limitations that would make it a poor choice for clinical work.

Model 203 Fluorescence Spectrophotometer (Perkin-Elmer Corp.). This more recent product is quite reasonably priced but can fill the needs of almost any clinical laboratory. This model uses a mercury vapor lamp. Xenon is also available. In place of the primary and secondary filters, monochromators are used. Both of these

use gratings, ruled at 600 lines/mm and providing a spectral range from 220 to 780 nm. The fixed exit slit gives a 10 nm band pass. Filters are provided to eliminate second-order interference. An R-212 photomultiplier is used as the standard detector. A twelve-step amplifier allows excellent sensitivity. Readout is on a 5¼-inch ammeter. Accessories are available for microcuvettes, solid samples, and recorder output.

Ratio Fluorometer (Beckman Instruments, Inc.). In this interesting instrument a patented double mercury vapor lamp is used. One half of the lamp lights, then goes off and then the second half lights. A light shield separates the two halves, and one side is used for the reference (standard) solution while the other is directed through the sample. Fluorescence excited by the two intermittent light signals, separated by a moment of darkness, is directed, through the secondary filter, to the photomultiplier. The ammeter is set at 100% using the reference and a blank. Thus the sample reading gives a percent of standard, or ratio, reading. The patented mercury lamp has a coated sleeve that, on rotation, selectively enhances the 310, 360, or 450 mercury peaks. In its normal mode it emits the mercury spectrum above 237 nm.

Turner Model 111 (G. K. Turner Associates). This instrument has become the standard for instruments in this category. Fig. 6-4 shows the optical configuration of its system. Light from the ultraviolet source strikes the sample, causing fluorescence that impinges on the photomultiplier. At the same time, light from the UV source is reflected from a diffuse screen and is reflected to the photomultiplier. A light interrupter (chopper) causes the photomultiplier to sense the fluorescent light from the sample at one instant and the reflected light from the diffuse screen the next. The forward light path, shown on the optical schematic, is a very small light signal that falls on the photomultiplier to

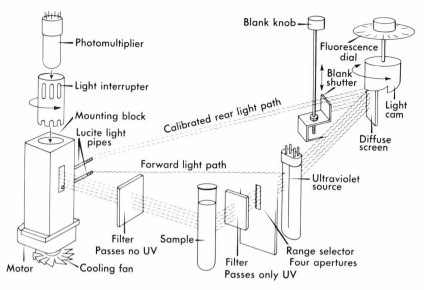

Fig. 6-4. Optical path of the Turner Model 111 Fluorometer. (Courtesy G. K. Turner Associates.)

produce a constant dark current to operate the servomechanism even when nonfluorescent blanks are used. The consequent photocurrent is an alternating current (square-wave) that can be amplified. This error signal is then fed back to a light cam that by a sort of servomechanism automatically adjusts the reflected light until the two light signals (sample and reference) are equal. The correction that has been made is indicated on the fluorescence dial. This correction is a linear function of fluorescence so the concentration of the sample may be accurately ascertained.

This sort of dual-beam arrangement, which Turner calls an *optical bridge,* eliminates the effect of variations in line voltage, light source, and detector sensitivity. As noted earlier, cuvette variations and light collimation are of minimal importance in fluorescence measurement; therefore the system has less chance for error than you would suppose.

As has been noted, glass absorbs ultraviolet rather strongly at lower wavelengths, so front-surfaced optics are used. The filters are glass. The secondary filters will not be in the UV range and the fact that the primary filter absorbs some UV light is not too significant, since this absorbance is constant for any particular filter.

A flow-through cuvette door is available, making possible the use of this instrument with the AutoAnalyzer for fluorescent methods. Also special doors are available for scanning fluorescence of filter paper strips, etc.

The electronics of this instrument are fairly complicated, and major repair should not be attempted by anyone but a factory-trained repairman. In use the Turner has had relatively few repair problems and has proved to be a very sensitive and reliable instrument.

G. K. Turner Associates has probably done more to advance the field of fluorescence measurement than has anyone else, both by its monumental design innovations and by its research and publication of fluorescence methods for clinical determinations. The company maintains an outstanding bibliography and reference service, which it has generously made available to Turner users and nonusers alike.

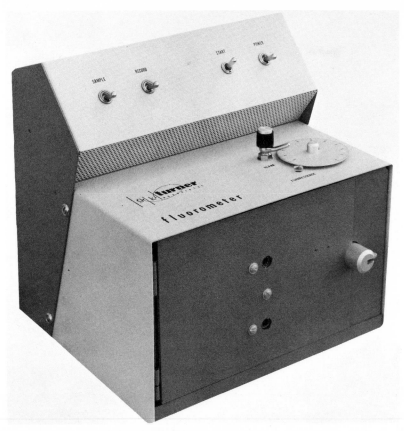

Fig. 6-5. Turner Model 111 Fluorometer. (Courtesy G. K. Turner Associates.)

The popular Turner Model 111 is shown in Fig. 6-5.

Spectrophotofluorometer (American Instrument Co., Inc.). This is a sophisticated and rather expensive instrument with more capability than the filter fluorometers we have discussed. In place of primary and secondary filters, this instrument uses grating monochromators.

A high-intensity xenon arc lamp is used. There is some danger from the buildup of ozone around the lamp, caused by ionization of oxygen. Ozone is normally considered healthful, but if present in excessive quantities, it may have deleterious effects. Such a buildup occurs only when the instrument is used continuously in quarters that are not well vented. Flushing the area around the lamp with nitrogen or ventilating the area is adequate protection. A high-

voltage DC power supply, required to fire the xenon lamp, is housed in a separate cabinet.

Several excitation and emission exit slits are provided to determine the band passes utilized. These slits are manually substituted in the instrument.

The high-quality monochromators are motor driven to provide automatic scanning. An X-Y plotter is available to correlate wavelength with emission regardless of scan speed or interruptions in the scan.

A photomultiplier tube is used as a detector. Even though this is a single-beam instrument, it has very good stability because of the high-quality electronic components employed in power supplies and amplifier circuits.

The output of the photomultiplier is amplified in the Fluoro-Microphotometer,

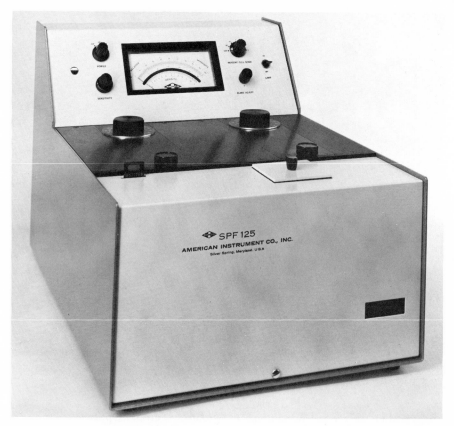

Fig. 6-6. SPF 125 Spectrofluorometer. (Courtesy American Instrument Co., Inc.)

which is housed in a separate case. This unit consists of amplifying and control circuits, chopper, amplifier, and a 6-inch ammeter. If it is used with the recorder and oscillograph, which may be attached, a total of five separate units are involved in the Aminco Spectrophotofluorometer system and at least 6 feet of bench space is required. It is an excellent research instrument with high resolution, good accuracy, and fine sensitivity but seems to be expensive and cumbersome for routine clinical use.

SPF 125 Spectrofluorometer (American Instrument Co., Inc.). In response to the obvious need for a smaller, more economical, and handier instrument, the American Instrument Company has introduced the SPF 125, which incorporates many of the features of the Spectrophotofluorometer in a much smaller unit and at a considerably lower price (Fig. 6-6). The instrument is all solid state (except for the detector, of course), and all components are housed in a single cabinet 15 × 22 inches deep (front to back) and 14 inches high. The X-Y plotter or printout accessories are not included in this cabinet but may be attached easily.

Resolution of the instrument is 1.5 nm, and sensitivity is very high. A larger thermostated cell compartment is available. Temperature control of the sample is important, since fluorescence, in general, increases with temperature; the heat build-up in this kind of instrument can be appreciable. Manual scanning is available if desired.

The fixed, substitutable slits are 0.1, 0.2,

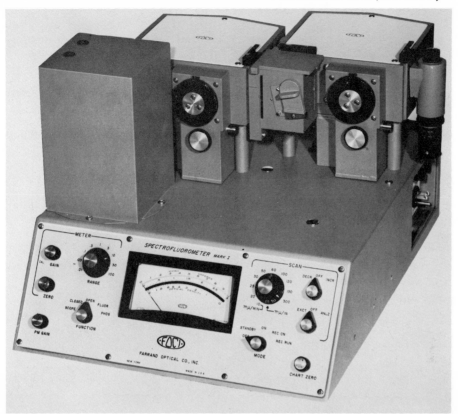

Fig. 6-7. Farrand Mark I Spectrofluorometer. (Courtesy Farrand Optical Co., Inc., Commercial Products Division.)

0.5, 1, 2, and 4 nm. These are mounted on a turret operated by selector knobs on the front panel.

The SPF 125 appears to be a great improvement over the excellent, but awkward, older Spectrophotofluorometer, which it is designed to replace. A flow cell and debubbler, as well as a strip scanner, are available and there are a number of other accessories. This instrument seems to be well adapted to clinical laboratory use and is of research quality.

Solid-State　Fluoro-Microphotometer (American Instrument Co., Inc.). American Instrument Co. also produces an economical filter fluorometer of good quality, called the Solid-State Fluoro-Microphotometer. This unit uses the company's very high-quality photomultiplier microphotometer as the amplifier and read-

out unit. Over the unit is coupled a saddle-type addition. One side of the saddle contains the power supply for the GE blacklight source, while the other side contains the sample well, primary and secondary filters, light source, and photomultiplier detector. The sample compartment is arranged to allow considerable versatility. Cuvettes up to 20 mm, temperature-controlled adapters, flow cells, or paper-strip scanners can be fitted into the provided space. Recorder jacks are on the back panel.

The Solid-State Fluoro-Microphotometer looks like a respectable challenge to the Turner Model 111.

Mark I Spectrofluorometer (Farrand Optical Co., Commercial Products Division) (Fig. 6-7). This company, which has been active in the development and manufacture of fluorescence equipment for many years, introduced the Mark I Spectrofluorometer, an instrument in the same general category as the American Instrument Co. SPF 125, to which it is similar in many ways. A xenon-arc lamp provides the excitation. Nearly identical monochromators are used for the excitation and emission beams. These are of highly quality and employ gratings manufactured by Farrand from the company's own master gratings. Interchangeable slits allow various band passes, which may be as short as 0.5 nm. The monochromators are driven by reversible stepper motors, allowing scanning in either direction, with synchronous plotting of fluorescence versus wavelength on an accessory X-Y plotter. The scan speeds are selectable by use of a panel selector knob. The X-Y plotter, oscilloscope, thin-layer scanner, paper scanner, phosphorescence accessories, etc. are available for the Farrand Mark I. This instrument is more sophisticated in many ways, and its controls are somewhat more complicated. The power supply is a separate unit.

The Mark I is technically excellent and provides high resolution, sensitivity, and linearity. With its optional accessories it would be well adapted to almost any sort of clinical research.

• • •

Other fluorometers that deserve mention include **G. K. Turner Associates'** excellent, moderate-priced **Model 430 Spectrofluorometer** as well as **Baird-Atomic Limited's** moderately priced **Floripoint** and their more expensive **Florispec, Model SF-100.**

The Turner instrument has a temperature-controlled sample compartment and provides a direct readout in concentration units but does not have automatic wavelength scanning. Both of the Baird-Atomic models scan automatically, and the more expensive Florispec has a complete line of accessories permitting paper strip scanning, automatic sample-changing, micro sampling as small as 4 microliters, recorder output, etc.

REVIEW QUESTIONS

1. How does the absorption spectrum of a solution compare with its excitation spectrum?
2. What can be said about the relationship between the emission spectrum and the excitation spectrum?
3. Why is quartz preferable to glass for fluorescence?
4. Do all substances naturally fluoresce?
5. Sketch the basic elements of a fluorometer.
6. What is phosphorescence?

7

Electrochemistry and measurement of pH

In a theoretical sense, nearly all chemistry is electrical in nature, since we are concerned with a movement of electrons, which can most often be measured. These phenomena in chemistry would include pH measurement, polarographic measurement of oxidation and reduction, electrophoresis, flame emission, and atomic absorption, etc. New techniques and devices are being developed constantly in the electrochemical area. For the purpose of this chapter we shall consider devices that are involved with the measurement of the movement of electrons in electrolytic solutions. These include pH meters and blood gas measuring devices, polarographs, ion-specific electrode systems, chloride titrators, and a few other miscellaneous devices. The logic of this grouping should become more apparent as we explore the rationale of these instruments.

Nearly all conductors of electricity are either metals or electrolytes. The carrier of current will be either electrons or ions. When current passes from metal to electrolyte or from electrolyte to metal, the type of carrier usually suddenly changes

and certain interesting phenomena occur. If a silver wire is immersed in a solution of silver chloride, ionization of the silver metal occurs with the formation of silver ions (Ag^+) and electrons. An electric potential now exists between the wire and the solution. To measure this potential we need a second electrode. We will find that the potential will depend on the concentration of silver ions in the solution and will be a logarithmic function of ion concentration.

If we use two *half-cells,* each with a silver wire or foil immersed in a different silver solution, and connect the two solutions through a meter, we can detect a difference in potential between them (Fig.

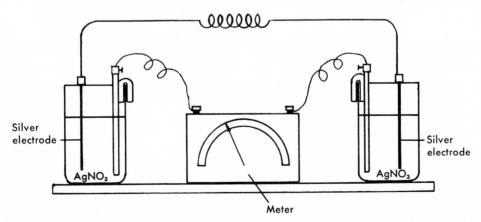

Fig. 7-1. Two silver half-cells connected through a meter. If we know the potential difference and the concentration of silver nitrate in one beaker, we can calculate the other.

7-1). Since the potential of each solution depends on the concentration of silver ions in it, we can predict the concentration of ions in one solution if we know the value for the other one and the difference in potential between them. A temperature difference between the two would affect the relationship, however, and there are other minor technical factors involved. In practice we can set up such a system and by calibrating it against known standards arrive at a very workable measuring system.

In the process above, it is not necessary that the two half-cells contain the same materials as long as two similar potentials are produced. In fact, it is possible to devise a reference half-cell that will give a very precise and reproducible potential. Using a reference half-cell with a highly reliable potential, it is possible to calibrate the system with known standards and measure the concentration of the ion in question on a precalibrated scale. Each half-cell is called an electrode.

ION-SPECIFIC ELECTRODE SYSTEMS

This is the rationale behind the electrode systems for specific ions. Reasonable and good electrodes have now been manufactured for chloride, sodium, potassium, bromine, ammonia, calcium, bivalent copper, fluorine, iodine, lead, silver, and a number of other ions. These electrodes measure activity and not necessarily concentration. There often are interfering substances also and methods must be chosen carefully. Orion Research, Inc., has published an *Analytical Methods Guide* to the techniques currently available using ion-selective electrodes. There are many quite usable methods and much progress is obviously being made. Perusal of the material reveals that only a very few methods have been developed for body fluids and that these have many problems.

The one outstanding exception is the **Model 417 system** manufactured by **Orion Research, Inc.,** for the measurement of the chloride content of sweat. This procedure is especially important in the diagnosis of cystic fibrosis in children. Using pilocarpine and an electric current, the child is caused to perspire profusely in a small area. The combination chloride-reference electrode is then touched down to this area and chloride concentration is read on a scale previously standardized with a standard chloride solution. This system is in fairly wide use in clinical laboratories. The absolute accuracy is probably not outstanding but, compared to the older methods of producing, collecting, and analyzing sweat, this is a very practical and clinically acceptable system.

Other companies, including Beckman Instruments and Radiometer Corporation, have produced chloride electrodes but there is no other widely used skin chloride electrode system.

pH MEASUREMENT

The concentration of hydrogen was originally measured by the same methods as described above. A hydrogen electrode was produced by coating a platinum electrode with lampblack (very fine carbon particles) and absorbing hydrogen gas onto the lampblack. This electrode was, of course, quite unstable and awkward to use. It is still the absolute standard for hydrogen electrodes but is not found in measuring systems routinely. In its place a glass measuring electrode is used. It has been found that an electric potential is developed on either side of a thin glass membrane when it is used to separate solutions of different hydrogen ion concentrations. This can be demonstrated only when the membrane is of a special type of glass. The glass electrode consists of a tube with a bulbous bottom made of this special type of glass. The bulb is filled with a solution having a known hydrogen ion concentration. When the bulb is then immersed in a solution containing hydrogen ions, the potential developed across the glass membrane of the bulb will depend on the concentration of hydrogen ions in the unknown solution.

If this hydrogen-measuring glass electrode is connected to a reference cell with a standard potential of its own, the difference between the potentials of the two can be measured and the hydrogen concentration calculated. Usually the reference used is a *calomel electrode,* containing mercury and mercuric chloride, which produces a reference potential that is constant and reliable.

When the glass measuring electrode and the calomel electrode are immersed in a solution containing hydrogen ions, the small potential difference between these two half-cells is measured on a very sensitive meter. When the instrument is calibrated against standards and adjusted for temperature effect, the concentration can be read very accurately. A very sophisticated, stable, and sensitive measuring train is of course required. This combination of parts is a *pH meter.*

The pH meter is designed to measure the *effective concentration* of hydrogen ions in a solution. In general terms three parameters are involved in the effective concentration. The first of these is the *actual molar concentration* of hydrogen. The second is the *dissociation constant* of the acid, or the pKa. The third is the *temperature.*

The *pH* is defined as the negative log of the hydrogen ion activity. Water at 25° C has 0.0000007 mole of hydrogen per liter. This may be expressed as approximately 10^{-7}; that is to say, the log of the hydrogen ion concentration is -7, and the negative log would be 7. Therefore the pH of water at 25° C is 7. An acid would have a higher concentration of hydrogen ions (as, for example, 0.08 mole per liter), which would represent a pH of about 2. A strong alkali solution such as sodium hydroxide would have a higher concentration of hydroxyl ions and a lower concentration of hydrogen ions. Such a solution might easily have

0.0000000000006 mole per liter of free hydrogen ions and would be said to have a pH of 13. The stronger the acid, the lower is the pH. We may also refer to the pOH or the negative log of the hydroxyl ion concentration. The sum of the pH and the pOH is always 14. Very strongly acid solutions, such as some pure acids that are highly ionized, may have a pH of -1. The pOH of such a solution is 15.

Buffer solutions have the ability of maintaining their pH when acid or base is added. Buffers are usually made up of weak acids and their conjugated base. The excess hydrogen ions are rendered inactive as they become part of the conjugated base radical and hence un-ionized and inactive.

Buffers have three properties of primary significance. First is their buffer value, which is indicated by the Greek letter *beta* and is also called the *Van Slyke buffer value.* The buffer value indicates the resistance of a buffer to pH change, on the addition of acid or base, and is defined as the amount of completely dissociated acid or base in gram equivalent per liter necessary to cause one unit of pH change. The second property of interest is the dilution value of the buffer, which is defined as the pH change of the buffer, on dilution with an equal quantity of pure water. The third property is the temperature stability or the magnitude of change in pH with a change in temperature. Obviously all these values vary with the pH under consideration. In selecting a buffer, the pKa of the buffer system should be close to the pH desired; this means that the pH should be close to the flat portion of the buffer titration curve.

This brief review of pH and buffers may be of some help in the discussion of the mechanics of measurement of pH by meters.

Since the early twentieth century, various workers have reported that a difference in electric potential could be measured between two solutions of different pH separated by a thin glass membrane. All the measuring devices available, however, had such a high internal resistance that the amplitude of the current produced could not be measured. Around 1930 an amplifier system was devised that allowed the pH meter, as we know it now, to develop.

In measuring the pH of a solution we are measuring the effect of hydrogen ions on the electrodes inserted into the solution. This is an *electrochemical* measurement in which chemical energy is converted to electrical energy in a quantitatively predictable manner. For the sake of simplicity, let us consider an electrochemical cell as consisting of two electrodes immersed in a solution. At the interface of each electrode a potential is established. When the two are connected through an external circuit, the electrons flow from one to the other, producing a measurable electric current. This sort of electrochemical system, composed of two *half-cells,* is called a *voltaic cell.*

Since the potential of this cell is a total of the potentials of two half-cells, one of the half-cells must be standardized so that measurement of the other is meaningful. This is done in pH measurement by the use of a reference cell whose potential is extremely constant. Reference cells such as the familiar calomel electrode (mercury–mercury chloride) or silver–silver chloride are commonly used in routine measurement. These cells remain stable for years when properly handled.

When such a reference electrode is used, the potential produced by hydrogen ions in this voltaic cell is quite constant, amounting to 59.15 millivolts (mv) per pH unit when measured at 25° C. As previously mentioned, temperature has considerable effect. Each degree of temperature increase raises the cell's output by about 0.2 mv.

The foregoing description of an electrochemical cell is considerably simpler than the actual situation in a pH-measuring train, but it should serve to clarify the nature of the system for the student.

The actual construction of the calomel reference electrode is somewhat complicated looking but depends on the constant potential produced where mercury comes into contact with a saturated solution of calomel in neutral potassium chloride of known concentration. Reference cells may be constructed in many ways. There is always some means of providing electrical contact between the inside of the electrode and the unknown solution. This may be a tightly packed asbestos plug, a fritted glass junction, or a ground glass sleeve separating the fluid inside the electrode from the solution being tested.

The glass electrode or measuring electrode is also complicated in appearance. The actual potential difference being measured occurs across a thin glass membrane, usually bulb shaped, at the tip of the electrode. The actual mechanism of electron flow across this membrane is poorly understood. Resistance across this glass barrier, however, is very high. Inside the glass bulb is an electrolyte solution with high buffering capacity that makes contact with an inner reference electrode. Fig. 7-2 shows some common glass electrode configurations.

For convenience both the glass measuring electrode and the reference electrode are sometimes built into a single glass housing and called a *combination electrode.* Combination electrodes are convenient to handle and can be used where a very small amount of fluid sample is available. No significant accuracy is lost.

It is immediately apparent that there are a number of interfaces in this total pH-measuring chain. We must assume that the potential at each of these interfaces is constant in all situations when we are making measurements.

To measure the flow of electrons between the two half-cells, a rather sophisticated electrometer had to be devised.

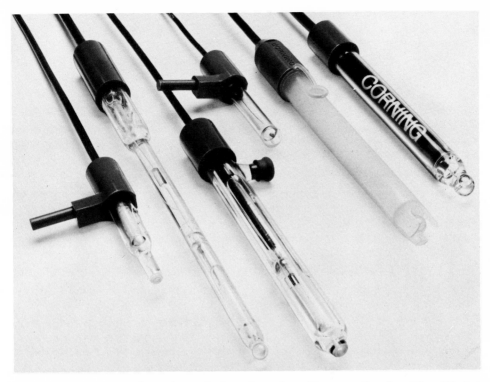

Fig. 7-2. Common configurations of glass electrodes. (Courtesy Corning Glass Works.)

If a difference in potential of 59.15 mv represents one pH unit, we must then have a device that can measure a voltage change of 1.2 mv to indicate a change of 0.02 pH unit. When we consider the many imponderables, such as the various junctions in our measuring train, the temperature effect on each of these, variables in electrical components, etc., we become aware of how complicated this process is.

Resistance of this circuit is between 500,000 and 200,000,000 ohms. The tiny potential we are discussing is extremely hard to measure. For this reason a device similar to a vacuum-tube voltmeter is used. Because of the high resistance of the electrode system, a circuit that will measure very high impedance is required.

GENERAL-PURPOSE pH METERS

Beckman Model G (Beckman Instruments, Inc.). One of the first pH meters

developed for laboratory use was the Beckman Model G. A few of these instruments are still in use. The meter was housed in a wooden case with an access door in the front of the cabinet to hold the electrodes. Reproducibility was not outstanding and sensitivity was not particularly high, but the meter was a pioneering, workable system.

A "battery" was used as a voltage reference for the Model G, a galvanometer was null-balanced by a slide wire as the reference, and the amplified unknown currents were compared. The resistance imposed by the slide wire, to null the two currents, was indicative of the pH, and calibration was established by use of standards. A resistance was introduced to compensate for temperature and a zero adjust was provided.

Although this sort of system might be considered somewhat primitive today, it was a landmark accomplishment at the time it was introduced. The system is still quite adequate if high accuracy is not needed.

Beckman Model 76 (Zeromatic) (Beckman Instruments, Inc.). In the currently popular Beckman Model 76 (Zeromatic) pH meter a feedback principle with a three-stage amplifier is used. The flow of current from the glass electrode is used to provide the grid current for the electrometer tube. The plate of this tube is connected directly to the grid of the second tube. The voltage at the cathode of the third stage is used to operate the meter. A temperature compensation and zero adjust are provided. A chopper converts the direct current signal to alternating current before amplification. This system, unlike the Model G, is a direct-reading system.

A scale expander that allows the whole scale width to represent 2 pH units is provided for this instrument; thus the reading accuracy is increased considerably. Switches of push-button type are used to switch from standby to read, from pH to millivolts, and from automatic to manual. The early meters of this type, like many new models, suffered from faulty components and "new model"–type defects. The instrument is quite well designed, however, and is an excellent general-purpose pH meter with good accuracy and reproducibility.

Model 601 pH Meter (Orion Research Inc.). This modern, compact, functional instrument is a good example of the recently introduced pH meters. Electronics are all solid state. The three-digit readout uses 7-segment planar display tubes. Only three controls are used on the front panel. These are a mode selector, temperature compensator, and calibration knob. An accuracy of 0.01 pH unit is obtained and drift is minimal. A BCD output connector is provided. The instrument is attractive, easy to use, conveniently small, and quite adequate for most laboratory pH work.

Digital Model 112 pH Meter (Corning Scientific Instruments). This is a highly accurate modern meter in a somewhat higher price class. The readout has a five-digit Nixie tube display with an automatically located zero. Accuracy is about 0.001 pH unit and stability is excellent. A pH range of 0 to 18 pH units is provided. Temperature compensation is automatic. Electronics are all solid state. This meter is of sufficient accuracy, reliability, stability, and convenience to be used as the meter for the blood gas system, which will presently be discussed.

Coleman Model 28C Metrion IV (Coleman Instruments Division, Perkin-Elmer Corp.). A very economical, general-purpose meter is Coleman Instruments' Model 28C Metrion IV pH Meter, which is shown in Fig. 7-3. This is a direct-reading system with a single stage of amplification, temperature compensation, the option of reading on the pH or millivolt scale, and very little else. It is an excellent example of a large group of small, economical, general-purpose pH meters that are commonly available. The versatility, ruggedness, stability, and accuracy of these meters are a contrast to the general-purpose instrument of a few years ago.

BLOOD pH AND BLOOD GAS INSTRUMENTS

During the past decade blood pH and the partial pressures of oxygen and carbon dioxide have become significant parameters in diagnosis and treatment. Many advances in the diagnosis and treatment of acidosis, electrolyte imbalance, emphysema, cardiovascular disease, etc. have been possible because of the improvement in instrumentation in this general area.

There is strong competition now among a few leading manufacturers of equipment. The leaders in the field at present (in alphabetical order) are Beckman, Corning, Instrumentation Laboratory, and Radiometer. All have systems for measuring the

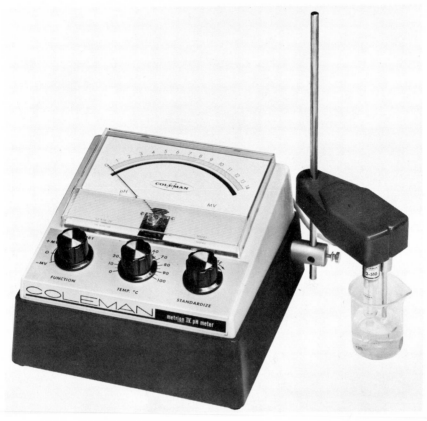

Fig. 7-3. Model 28C Metrion IV pH Meter. (Courtesy Coleman Instruments Division, Perkin-Elmer Corp.)

three parameters just mentioned. Some details of each system will be presented, although to discuss each one in detail is not feasible here.

Before discussion of the systems, however, a confusing expression that occasionally bothers students who are new to these techniques should be clarified. Reference is sometimes made to pH, P_{O_2}, and P_{CO_2} as if they were comparable terms of measurement. The term *pH* has been discussed earlier, and you will remember that it relates to the effective concentration (*puissance* or "force" in French) of hydrogen ions. The capital P of P_{CO_2} and P_{O_2} does not denote effective concentration but partial pressure.

Partial pressure simply refers to the part of the total gas pressure (atmospheric pressure, for example) that is contributed by the gas under consideration. To calculate the partial pressure of a known gas concentration, we take the following steps:

1. Determine ambient barometric pressure in millimeters of mercury (mm Hg).
2. Subtract the vapor pressure of water at the temperature of measurement. At 37° this is 47 mm.
3. Multiply the remainder by the percentage or decimal fraction of the gas under consideration. The product will be the partial pressure (P).

The technique of measuring pH has been previously discussed. Measurement of P_{CO_2} is accomplished in the same manner,

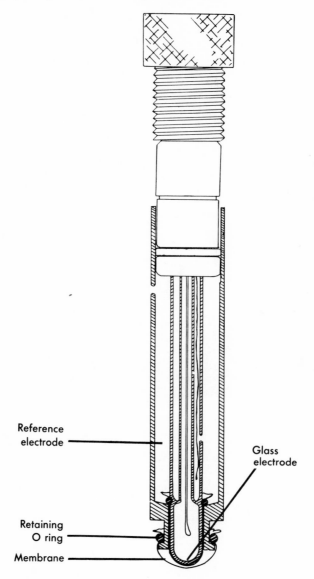

Fig. 7-4. Diagram of a Severinghaus P_{CO_2} electrode. (Courtesy Instrumentation Laboratory, Inc.)

but the details of the electrode require some explanation. The blood sample is separated from a combination pH electrode system by a membrane. CO_2 can pass through this membrane from the blood sample into an electrolyte solution, which perfuses the sensing tip of the electrode. As the CO_2 is absorbed by the electrolyte, carbonic acid is formed, altering the pH. This pH change is a linear function of the CO_2 content of the blood, and it can obviously be measured by the electronics of the pH meter on an appropriate scale. This arrangement is called a *Severinghaus electrode* (Fig. 7-4). The electrolyte solution perfusing its tip makes contact with both measuring and reference electrode elements.

Measurement of the partial pressure of oxygen requires a somewhat different approach. The P_{O_2} electrode works on a polarographic principle.

The fact that nearly all conductors are metallic or electrolytic in nature was mentioned earlier. When electricity passes from a metal to a solution of electrolyte or vice versa, the type of carrier changes abruptly, and either an oxidation or a reduction takes place. In the case of oxygen in solution, we find that oxygen is reduced, with the release of electrons, and the current increases as a direct function of the electrons released. Hence the change in current is an analog of the oxygen concentration in the solution.

This electrode consists of a platinum cathode with a tubular silver anode around it. The two are insulated from each other and make contact only through a drop of electrolyte at the electrode's tip. A gas-permeable membrane holds this drop at the tip of the electrode and separates it from the blood to be measured. Oxygen in the blood diffuses across the membrane into the electrolyte, where it is reduced and measured.

Measurement of the gain or loss of electrons in a chemical reaction, by electrical means as described above, is called *polarography*. Polarographic apparatus is widely used in analytical chemistry but is seldom applicable to medical laboratory situations. The very tiny change in current sensed by the P_{O_2} electrode is amplified and measured by a sensitive electrometer against a reference current provided by a reference cell or Zener source. The pH meter's ammeter can be used for actually reading out this signal on an appropriate scale. The polarographic electrode is the usual means of measuring P_{O_2} in the systems described here. Details of the electrode used by Instrumentation Laboratory, Inc., are shown in Fig. 7-5.

There are a number of instruments in use that rely on the *Astrup principle* for

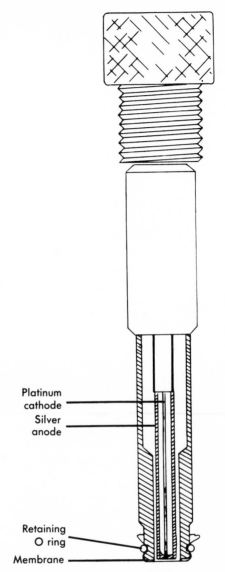

Platinum
cathode

Silver
anode

Retaining
O ring

Membrane

Fig. 7-5. Diagram of the polarographic oxygen electrode used by Instrumentation Laboratory in its blood gas system. Oxygen electrodes in all the systems discussed here are similar in principle. (Courtesy Instrumentation Laboratory, Inc.)

estimating the P_{CO_2} of blood. The pH of blood is measured before and after equilibration with two gas mixtures containing different concentrations of CO_2. A nomogram is then prepared, from which the estimated P_{CO_2} can be read. The instruments using this approach are primarily manufactured by a Danish Company, **Radiometer,** and the commonest of these was the **AME-1 Ultra-Micro pH and Gas Monitor System.** This instrument was well made but has been superseded by newer models. The CO_2 electrode method is more convenient and direct. This company now produces an instrument system using a CO_2 electrode as well.

At the present time nearly all of the systems for measuring blood pH and blood gas are produced by three major companies. These are, alphabetically, Corning Glass Works, Scientific Division; Instrumentation Laboratory, Inc.; and Radiometer A/S of Denmark. With the exception of the Astrup technique mentioned above, these systems all use essentially the same measuring system and their differences are primarily in refinements and quality of engineering and components.

IL Model 113 pH Blood Gas Analyzer (Instrumentation Laboratory, Inc.). This company was the first on the market to combine the pH electrode, the P_{O_2} electrode, and the Severinghaus-type P_{CO_2} electrode in one integrated system. This system, called the IL Model 113 pH Blood Gas Analyzer, has been in use for several years in a relatively unchanged form. Its popularity during this interval attests to its quality.

The Model 113 Blood Gas Analyzer is contained in two units. The meter, amplifier, chopper, etc. are in one unit while the thermostat, circulating water bath, and electrodes comprise the other. These two units are shown in Fig. 7-6.

The newer meters have eliminated the

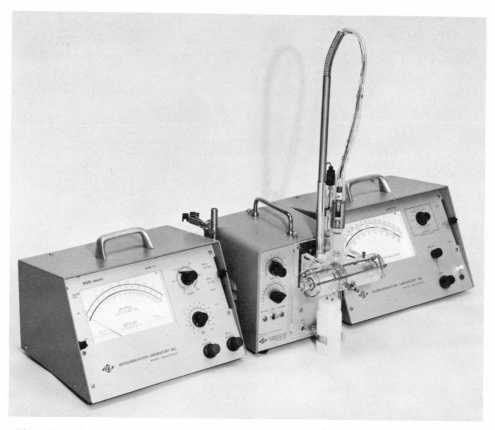

Fig. 7-6. Model 113 pH Blood Gas Analyzer. (Courtesy Instrumentation Laboratory, Inc.)

chopper and are now using FETs. See discussion of electrical components in Chapter 1. The use of direct-coupled amplifiers and other electronic innovations has provided a highly sensitive, stable, and trouble-free system. This instrument has fewer controls than any quality pH meter manufactured up to the time of its introduction. The meter portion of the Model 113 has been almost entirely trouble-free.

In the unit on the right in Fig. 7-6, a pump circulates water through the heating system and the plastic housings surrounding the electrodes. There is virtually no reservoir of water to be heated, and warm-up time is a few minutes when the unit is first plugged in. The circulating pump sends the water through the system by means of a whirling impeller rather than a positive-pressure pump. Unfortunately the impeller is rather easily air-locked and is sometimes time-consuming to restart. Also the rather ingenious wet seal around the drive shaft of the pump has been subject to considerable wear and leakage.

The water is temperature-equilibrated by means of a thermistor-controlled heat ring around the pump outlet. As we have seen in Chapter 1, a thermistor is a semiconductor that acts as a resistor whose resistance is a strong function of its temperature, this change in conductance being abrupt in a given temperature range. The thermistor is used here to allow (indirectly) just enough current to flow to the heater to maintain the desired temperature. A pilot light on the panel of this module glows brightly when the heater is heating to its full capacity and dims as the heater current diminishes. This heat-equilibrating system is extremely sensitive, fast, and largely trouble-free.

The pH-measuring system (Fig. 7-7) consists of the calomel reference electrode and a water-jacketed capillary glass electrode. The reference electrode stands in a plastic

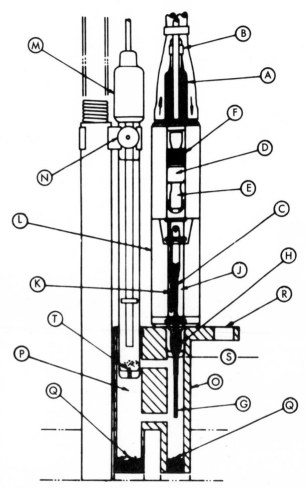

Fig. 7-7. pH-measuring electrode of the IL Model 113 pH Blood Gas Analyzer: *A,* glass electrode; *B,* coaxial UM electrode lead; *C,* active capillary glass; *D,* sample aspiration roller assembly; *E,* rubber tube; *F,* vacuum aspiration button; *G,* sample plastic tip; *H,* sample tip holder; *J,* electrolyte chamber; *K,* silver—silver chloride half-cell; *L,* water jacket; *M,* reference electrode; *N,* rubber cap; *O,* UM liquid junction assembly; *P,* saturated KCl; *Q,* undissolved crystals; *R,* support to hold pH electrode; *S,* filling height of KCl in liquid junction assembly; *T,* ceramic plug. (Courtesy Instrumentation Laboratory, Inc.)

well and makes contact with the glass electrode through a salt bridge.

The capillary glass electrode and its holder are more complicated, as can be seen by examining the right-hand side of the diagram in Fig. 7-7. The actual capillary glass electrode *(A)*, referred to by the company as the glass insert, is a cylindrical glass device provided with an electrical connection *(B)* at its top and a hub *(H)* at the bottom. When the electrode is properly positioned in its holder, blood can be drawn through the plastic tip at the hub end, through the sample tip *(G)*, and into the measuring capillary *(C)*. From here it may be drawn on out through the rubber hose *(E)* and exhaust port. (These details are perhaps difficult to visualize from the two-dimensional drawing but can be easily seen when the device is closely examined.) Water circulates through the jacket spaces *(L)* around the measuring electrode. The roller *(D)* can be released completely to allow the suction of the system to draw fluids through the electrode; or it can be moved upward with a peristaltic action to the hose, pulling a very small sample into the measuring capillary. The entire pH assembly is attached to a flexible support above the instrument. The hoses and electrical connections pass through the support to the unit. The electrode can thus be moved about to pick up samples as desired. When readings are being taken, the plastic sampling tip is inserted in the plastic holder, providing electrical contact through the salt bridge with the adjacent reference electrode.

A small vibrating diaphragm pump supplies the suction needed for loading and flushing the sampling electrode. A waste bottle is installed in the section line. If this bottle is not emptied when it is three quarters full, moisture will be pulled over into the suction pump, destroying its usefulness. Even spattered droplets of buffer drawn into the pump line can cause damage. The suction pump is quite easy to change, but

the inconvenience, down time, and expense are annoying.

The P_{CO_2} electrode is of Severinghaus type, consisting of a glass pH-measuring half-cell and a reference. Both these elements are enclosed in a single housing. As explained earlier, the carbon dioxide of the blood sample diffuses across a membrane into an electrolyte solution around the glass electrode tip. Dissolved in the electrolyte solution, the carbon dioxide forms carbonic acid, which alters the electrolyte pH.

The P_{O_2} electrode is a polarographic device. Oxygen passes through a membrane from the blood sample into an electrolyte solution in the electrode capillary. The oxygen is reduced, producing a flow of electrons, which is measured.

Both the P_{CO_2} and P_{O_2} electrodes are contained in a plastic, water-jacketed holder at the front of this module. An electrode is inserted into the plastic holder from each end. The tips of the electrodes are only a few millimeters apart, being separated by a sample compartment that is common to both electrodes.

The IL 113 system contains many innovations that have proved to be extremely useful. Such devices as FETs, thermistors, and integrated circuits are revolutionizing the medical laboratory–instrument field; and Instrumentation Laboratory, Inc., has been responsible, in some measure, for precipitating change. The introduction of the Model 113 was a monumental step forward in blood pH and blood gas measurement.

As with all new instrument systems, some problems developed at first with this system. As noted above, the circulating heating bath has leaked and has been subject to frequent air locks. The suction pump for the glass electrode has often been soaked by the overflow or spatter from the waste bottle, cables have been subject to breakage and interference, and membranes and glass electrodes have failed when exposed to air for long periods of time. Many of these problems have been brought about by poor technique and careless or inadequate maintenance. To alleviate these problems, the company has provided training classes and other in-service training programs. These have helped, but the ultimate solution to problems of this sort is designing problems out of the system. Instrumentation Laboratory has made large steps in this direction by the introduction of the Model 213 Blood Gas Analyzer.

IL Model 213 Blood Gas Analyzer (Instrumentation Laboratory, Inc.). This new system features an automatic flushing system that cleans electrodes at the end of the reading cycle to prevent damage to electrodes and membranes. The readout has been changed from the large ammeter of the Model 113 to three four-place electronic digital displays, one for each parameter. Electrode cables have been shortened and connectors improved to minimize electrostatic interference and fraying. Introduction of gas standards has been simplified and all operations are controlled by push button, eliminating many errors of technique. The bath system is simpler and more reliable and the sample suction system greatly improved. Monitor lights continuously check the membranes and the isolation of the glass electrode. About 20 microliters of blood is sufficient for pH measurement, and all three parameters can

be done on about 100 microliters. Values as close as 0.003 pH unit can, ideally, be obtained on repetitive samples. The chopper, which was somewhat failure-prone (as most choppers are), has been replaced by a field-effect transistor.

The introduction of the Model 213 modernized and made practical the measurement of blood pH and blood gases.

Recently the company has introduced a training series that they call "In Lab." Using bench-top projectors and tape cassettes, the series offers training in several techniques. This program can be utilized in the laboratory, saving time and expense of traveling to workshops or seminars. The idea is innovative, refreshing, and responsible. This idea for laboratory training seems to offer a solution to many problems of instrument maintenance and minor repair, and it is to be hoped that other manufacturers will follow the example.

Model 16 pH/Blood Gas System (Corning Scientific Instruments) (Fig. 7-8). This model has many similarities to the IL Model 213 and it will suffice to list a few features that differ. In this model, the glass and reference electrodes of the pH system are enclosed in a plastic housing along with the heater, thermistor, and indicator light involved in temperature equilibration. The fingertip, peristaltic sample control is also used on this uit. Originally the glass elec-

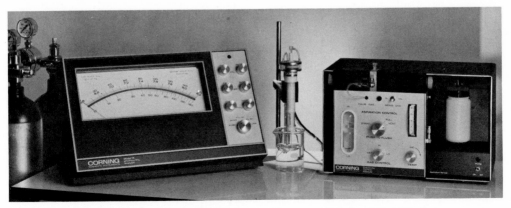

Fig. 7-8. Model 16 Blood Gas System. (Courtesy Corning Glass Works.)

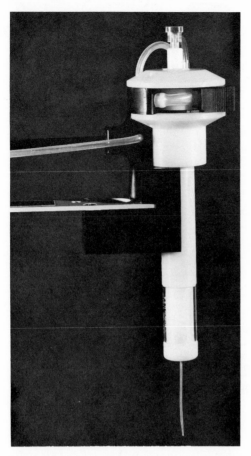

Fig. 7-9. Corning pH and reference electrode system. (Courtesy Corning Glass Works.)

the test, draws it off into a waste bottle and provides the suction for rinsing out the sample chamber. A rather simple but practical built-in feature is a pressure switch under the waste bottle that closes under the weight of a nearly full bottle to cut off the suction pump until the bottle is emptied. This feature prevents waste from being pulled into the pump system and causing damage. The same suction system and waste bottle serve both the pH electrode and the compartment between the P_{O_2} and P_{CO_2} electrodes. Also included in the electrode control module is a double bubble chamber in which the bubbles of gas, used for standardizing the electrodes, bubble up through water at a rate that is easy to monitor. A single gas valve makes it possible to switch between standardizing tanks quickly and easily.

Membranes for the P_{O_2} and P_{CO_2} electrodes are molded across one end of a plastic cylinder, forming a sort of thimble with the membrane providing the closed end. This thimble can be slipped over the end of the electrode with very little effort compared to the rather intricate task of installing the older-style film membrane.

The electronics of this system seem to be very good. Electronic drift is negligible due, in some measure, to the use of a photoconductive, solid-state chopper. Corning's advertising claims a repeatability of 0.002 pH unit. Corning electrodes are quite good, and the mechanical and electrical details of this system seem to be of high quality and well done.

Digital Model 165 pH/Blood Gas System (Corning Scientific Instruments) (Fig. 7-10). More recently Corning Scientific Instruments has introduced the Digital Model 165 pH/Blood Gas System. This modern, push-button system, pictured in Fig. 7-10, has eliminated many maintenance problems and greatly simplified operation. Each mode and the reading of each parameter are selected by push button. Total CO_2, bicarbonate, and base excess are calculated.

trode insert could be changed only in a repair facility but this feature has been modified. The whole unit has performed well, with very few problems. The combination of electrodes and supportive elements in one housing is pictured in Fig. 7-9.

The P_{O_2} and P_{CO_2} electrodes share a common sample chamber in a separate unit called the *electrode control module*. This chamber holds less than 100 λ and is temperature-equilibrated by a dry-bath heater with thermistor control similar to that used for the pH electrode. A vacuum system within the module aspirates the sample into the chamber and, on completion of

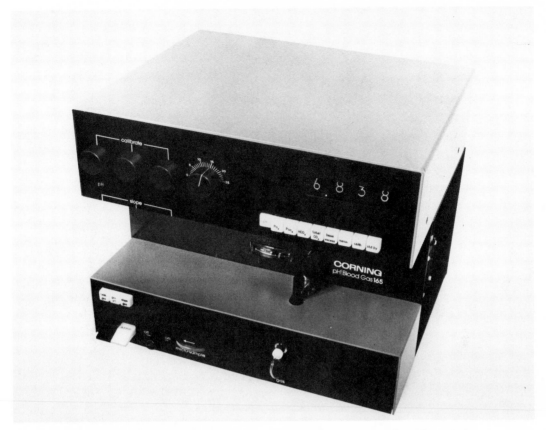

Fig. 7-10. Model 165 pH and Blood Gas System. (Courtesy Corning Glass Works.)

All six parameters are reported in 90 seconds, from 125 microliters of blood, injected into a single port. Electrodes and membranes are flushed by pressing one button. Calibration gases are available in disposable tanks.

• • •

The Danish company **Radiometer A/S** distributes in the United States exclusively through the **London Company.** As stated earlier, Radiometer has produced several instruments based on the Astrup technique. For a discussion of the theory behind these instruments the student should read "A Micro Method for Determination of pH, Carbon Dioxide Tension, Base Excess and Standard Bicarbonate in Capillary Blood" by Siggaard Andersen, Engle,

Jorgensen, and Astrup, published in *The Scandinavian Journal of Clinical and Laboratory Investigation.* This and other publications by the same authors may be obtained from the London Company. The work was careful and thorough and the approach is valid. This was, for some years, accepted as the best approach to the measurement of bicarbonate in blood. The method still has many adherents, in spite of the superior speed and convenience of P_{CO_2} electrodes.

Blood Micro System, Model BMS 2, produced by Radiometer is designed to measure blood pH with a microelectrode on samples as small as 30 microliters. A tonometer is provided to equilibrate the blood with gases of known CO_2 content. All components requiring temperature equilibra-

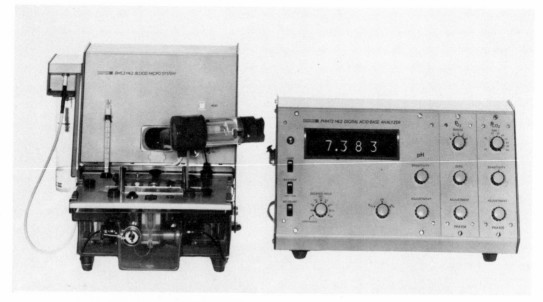

Fig. 7-11. BMS 3 Mark 2 pH and Blood Gas System from Radiometer. (Courtesy The London Co.)

tion are contained in a very accurately controlled water bath. This system is extremely well engineered and the very best components are used, making it excellent equipment. Controls are a little complicated for casual use, however.

Radiometer's newer instrument is the **BMS 3 Mark 2.** This system is a modern, compact measuring system incorporating the microelectrode for pH and the P_{CO_2} and P_{O_2} electrodes in the same excellent bath arrangement used for the BMS 2. Typical of the company, the unit is ruggedly constructed with excellent components and materials. This unit is shown in Fig. 7-11.

All three electrodes can be filled with a single sample insertion, after which the three parameters can be read out using either the Analyzer-Meter called the **PHM 71** or the **Digital Acid-Base Analyzer, PHM 72 Mark 2.** The combination of the BMS 3 and the digital PHM 72 makes an excellent measuring system for blood pH and blood gas—one that is hard to fault for quality. A little over 100 microliters is adequate for

all three parameters. Readability is 0.001 pH unit and stability is excellent.

Acid-Base Laboratory, Model ABL 1 (Radiometer A/S) (Fig. 7-12). A totally new system has been introduced by Radiometer. This piece of equipment automates the measurement of blood pH and blood gases except that sequential samples are not automatically presented to the analyzer. A built-in small computer does all calculations and calibrations and monitors the analysis. Pure CO_2 gas, from the only calibrating cylinder, passes through a gas-metering apparatus that mixes it with air to give 5.6% and 11.2% CO_2 and about 18.59% O_2. Electrical zero provides the O_2 zero concentration setting for the polarographic O_2 electrode. The gas mixtures are equilibrated with two buffer solutions. Barometric pressure will affect the resultant pH, but a built-in electric barometer provides the necessary barometric reading to allow the computer to calculate true values. The system automatically standardizes itself every 2 hours and will restandardize when a button is depressed. There are

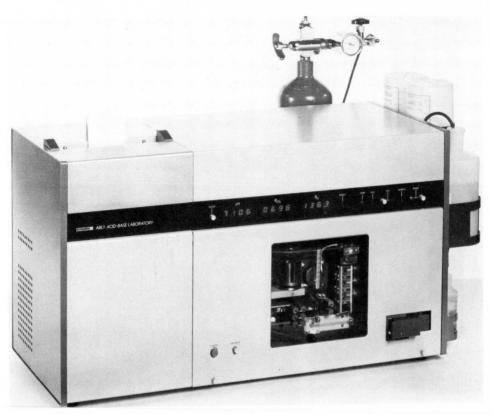

Fig. 7-12. New computer-managed acid-base Laboratory, Model ABL 1. (Courtesy The London Co.)

no calibrating knobs. Temperature is controlled by computer. Heat distribution is provided through heat sinks and a circulating fan. There is a flushing system that completely purges the sample from the system after results are reported out. If there is a power failure, the apparatus flushes itself using a discharge capacitor for power.

The apparatus measures pH, P_{CO_2}, P_{O_2}, and hemoglobin by conventional means and the computer then derives total CO_2, actual bicarbonate, standard bicarbonate, base excess, standard base excess, and oxygen saturation. All of the four measured and six derived values are obtained from the introduction of a single sample into the apparatus—without manual manipulation, calibration, or calculation. Results are printed out on a tape printer and the derived values

may also be read on a bar tube display. If a parameter is questioned by the computer, the printer places a question mark after the result. There is a bubble sensor at the sample entry port that allows rejection of results if bubbles are detected in the sample. The apparatus cycles in about 2 minutes, prints out all ten answers, and purges itself.

If this apparatus is as trouble-free as it seems to promise, it will eliminate a large part of the tedious technique involved in blood pH and blood gas measurement and provide faster and more reproducible answers. At this time it looks extremely good.

OTHER ELECTROCHEMICAL ANALYZERS

We have considered devices for the measurement of pH, P_{O_2}, and specific ions by

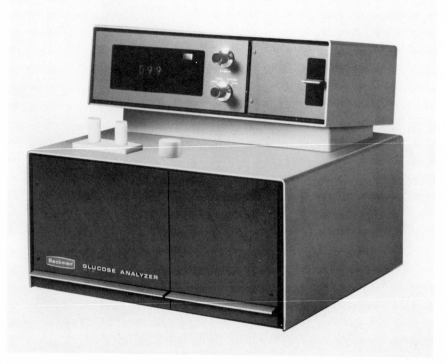

Fig. 7-13. Glucose Analyzer. (Courtesy Beckman Instruments, Inc.)

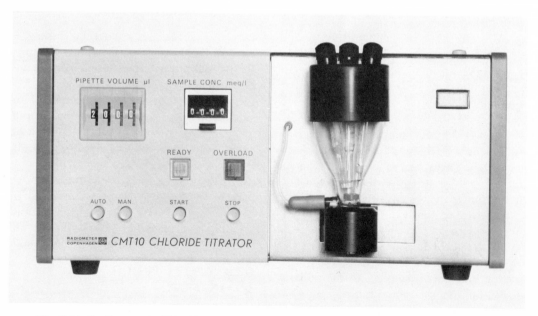

Fig. 7-14. Radiometer's Chloride Titrator, Model CMT 10. (Courtesy The London Co.)

electrode and polarographic devices in this chapter. Before going to our next topic, let us look briefly at the **Glucose Analyzer** produced by **Beckman Instruments.** This instrument has a P_{O_2} electrode as its detector. Serum or plasma is injected into a chamber containing glucose oxidase. As glucose is broken down to gluconic acid, oxygen in the solution is used to produce peroxide. The change in oxygen concentration is a linear function of the glucose. The analysis takes 10 seconds, and the glucose oxidase solution in the sample chamber will take care of many samples before it is replaced automatically. The method works well and this instrument has been well accepted, especially for stat blood sugar determinations. (See Fig. 7-13.)

Beckman has a similar system for blood urea nitrogen determinations. It is called the **BUN Analyzer.** Urease degrades urea to form ammonium and bicarbonate radicals which, being electrolytes, increase conductivity. The analyzer measures the rate of change of the conductivity. This instrument also works well.

Several companies manufacture *chloride titrators* that function on the coulometric principle. Chloride ions in the serum are precipitated as silver chloride as metallic silver is ionized, releasing silver ions into the titrating solution. As long as the chloride ions are free, they will conduct current freely. As soon as they are tied up in the insoluble salt, conduction effectively ceases. According to *Faraday's law,* the ionization produced when an electric current is passed from a metal into an electrolyte will depend only on the coulombs passing through the circuit. This is the same as saying that ionization will depend on the amperage multiplied by the time. If the amperage is constant, then the silver ions formed can be measured as a function of time.

The chloride titrator is a device that measures the time required for an abrupt change in conductivity to occur in a chloride solution to which silver ions are added at a known rate by electrolysis. This time can be read in terms of chloride ion concentration. Since chlorine ionizes so completely in the body and is so insoluble as the silver salt, this is a very good method. Additionally, the rate of ionization as given in Faraday's law is a precise, accurate, and easily controlled reaction.

Several excellent chloride titrators are on the market. Listed alphabetically, companies that produce instruments of this type include American Instrument Co., Inc.; Corning Scientific Instruments; Fiske Associates, Inc.; and Radiometer A/S. All of the instruments are remarkably similar in most details. The principle is the same in each case. All use good-quality solid-state electronics and similar mechanical counters. Titration vessels and electrode arrangements differ slightly. Most are offered with a dilutor of some sort and a printer, either as accessories or as integral parts of a specific model.

Radiometer Model CMT 10 Chloride Titrator (Radiometer A/S) (Fig. 7-14). This Radiometer instrument has a magnetic stirring device in the titration vessel and can routinely give reasonably consistent results on a 20-microliter sample. These characteristics and the high quality of components customarily found in Radiometer equipment recommend this model, but there is not a great deal of difference between the comparable models from the various better known companies. The Radiometer Chloride Titrator shown In Fig. 7-14 is the Model CMT 10.

REVIEW QUESTIONS

1. Sketch and explain a simple device for measuring the concentration of zinc chloride electrometrically, using known standards.
2. How does the Orion sweat chloride meter work?
3. What factors determine effective hydrogen ion concentration?
4. Define pH.
5. What is a combination electrode?

6. How does a Severinghaus electrode work?
7. On what does polarography depend?
8. How can blood sugar determinations be determined by polarography?

9. How is Faraday's law utilized in the chloride titrators?
10. What is a calomel electrode?

8
Chromatography and electrophoresis

THE GENERAL PRINCIPLE

Early in the twentieth century a Russian botanist by the name of Tswett worked at separating plant pigments and devised a system very similar to the paper chromatography that is in popular use today. Since he worked primarily with colored solutions, he suggested the name *chromatography,* and the term has persisted even though many of the separations commonly done today have nothing to do with color.

Chromatographic separation is accomplished by subjecting a mixture of components to two opposing forces. One of these forces tends to move particles in one direction while the other tends to restrain this movement or oppose it. Let us consider *ascending-paper chromatography,* for example. If a sheet of filter paper is suspended above a dish containing phenol so that the lower edge of the paper is in the solution, the paper will act as a wick and the phenol will gradually rise in the paper by capillary action. If a mixture of two components is placed on the paper slightly above the fluid level in the dish, the flow of phenol will have a tendency to wash the components upward while the texture of the paper tends to restrain them. The result is that the smaller molecules are washed along fairly easily while the larger molecules are held back. Over a period of time a definite separation occurs.

Components that have been separated in this manner can be identified with fair certainty by their R_F values, or the distance each has traveled relative to the moving front of the solvent used. In complex mixtures the R_F values of all the substances in the mixture are compared.

Recently a great many substitutes for paper have been introduced. *Cellulose nitrate, cellulose acetate, polyacetates, agarose,* and a host of patented film preparations are now in use. Most of these possess the advantage of having very even pore size. One of the problems in chromatography is that of *tailing,* in which some of the separated components migrate at a slower rate of speed, resulting in uneven separation. This is caused, in most cases, by variation in the size of the pores or open spaces in the support medium. Hence these newer materials allow migration to be much more regular and separations to be more discrete.

Thin-layer chromatography. This is a variant of chromatography that has made a large contribution to separation techniques during the past few years. A gel preparation is applied to a glass plate or film and allowed to dry. This very thin gel layer is used as the support medium for the separation of unknown materials. The technique is a valuable one, and there is a great deal of literature available on the subject. It is, however, outside the general scope of this book.

ELECTROPHORESIS

The technique of electrophoresis is similar in many ways to chromatography. In electrophoresis the *impelling force* is an *electric potential* that tends to move electrically charged particles toward the negative or the positive pole, depending on their electric charge. The difference in R_F value of various components depends principally on the difference in their electric charge and on their size. The *retarding force* is frictional in nature and is influenced by the porosity and general architecture of the absorbent material.

In electrophoresis a phenomenon known as *electroosmosis* occurs. When an electric current is conducted through a capillary filled with fluid, there is a tendency for the fluid to be displaced toward one of the electrodes. Other factors being equal, the larger the current imposed, the larger will be the flow of liquid toward the electrode. Porous material might be thought of as a collection of capillaries of various diameters, and the phenomenon of electroosmosis occurs in them also. This force may act to either impel or retard the migration of a material being separated, depending on the direction of the electroosmotic current relative to the direction of migration. It is a factor that has considerable influence in this type of separation.

Electrophoresis is especially practical for the separation of macromolecular substances such as proteins and lipids, although it is applicable to many other substances as well. In routine clinical testing the various protein substances in human serum are separated and quantitated, enzymes are separated and identified, and various hemoglobin fractions are identified. The isolation and quantitation of lipoproteins is also of practical value. Numerous other separations of biological materials are less often performed.

Recently *immunoelectrophoresis* has become an important diagnostic tool. In this variation, serum proteins are separated by electrophoresis. Specific antisera are spotted near to various zones in the gelatinous matrix, and the interactions of antisera and protein are observed. In this way specific protein fractions can be identified and roughly quantitated. The antisera may be placed in slits or small wells in the gel at a position and distance that have proved to be most advantageous. The technique is not difficult and may give very valuable diagnostic information.

The principal equipment for electrophoretic separation consists of a cell, in which the migration and separation occur, and a power supply that provides the electric charge to impel the particles to be separated.

Power supply. Typically the power supply must be able to convert line voltage into the required 100 to 500 v of direct current and provide 100 milliamperes or so, depending on the system. The current must be nearly ripple-free, and random variations of more than 0.1% would be quite undesirable. The components usually found in such a power supply are a step-up transformer, rectifier tubes or semiconductor diodes, capacitors, and chokes. Amplifier tubes and regulator tubes or their transistor equivalents are usually also present. Control of the voltage produced is usually by a potentiometer, and meters are used to indicate the voltage and measure the amperage. Many economical and adequate power supplies for this application are commercially available. The quality of the separation obtained depends on the quality of the current provided. Most newer power supplies are all solid state. These have proved to be trouble-free and convenient.

Some of the commoner problems with power supplies have been transformer failure, failing vacuum tubes, short-circuited capacitors, and resistors that have either short-circuited or opened. When a transformer fails, it usually short-circuits and overheats, with considerable smoke and odor. When the voltmeter needle vibrates rapidly, it may be that a capacitor has short-circuited. However, a capacitor may short-circuit without such a manifestation. Faulty resistors can sometimes be located by visual inspection. Potentiometers often become defective and cease to provide smooth control of voltage. Switches are always subject to failure. As with all electronic equipment, moisture is quite detrimental.

There has recently been a great deal of interest in *high-voltage electrophoresis*. Up to 50 v per centimeter or a 1000 v current has been used extensively, and some apparatus combinations have used much higher voltages. Obviously the power supply for such a system is, in general, more expensive and complicated. Much more heat is dissipated in the cell, and methods of cooling must be provided. With all power supplies, and particularly with these high-voltage sources, care should be exercised to shield all leads and to turn off the power supply when working with the cell.

Cell. There are many types of electrophoresis cells in use. Several requirements dictate their general design. The paper or membrane must conduct the current from one end to the other without contacting any conductor, which would shunt the current elsewhere or dissipate it. The membrane must be moist at all times, but fluid must not be allowed to pool or flow through it. The electrodes should not directly contact the paper or be too close to it, since breakdown products from the electrodes might contaminate the material being separated. Temperature should be relatively constant. Vibration and other physical disturbance should be minimal. If heat is generated in appreciable amounts, some system of cooling must be effected.

Obviously, better separation is obtained as migration distance is increased. The best arrangement from a theoretical point of view is to have the paper horizontal so that there is no gravitational effect on the liquid in the paper or membrane. Some cells have a flat surface on which the paper can lie. This encourages puddling of solution, with consequent shorts and eddy currents, but under ideal conditions it works fairly well. In cells of another type the paper is suspended between plastic or glass rods, but there is a tendency for the paper to sag and fluid to collect if the strips are very long. A center support is sometimes used to minimize this effect.

For several years paper has been the principal absorbent or support medium in general use. Whatman filter paper no. 1 and S & S no. 2043 are the most widely used types of paper. They both have a fairly high tensile strength when wet and are capable of absorbing a considerable quantity of solvent. They have reasonably small pore size, and the cellulose of the paper is chemically pure. In general the materials being migrated do not combine chemically with the paper and the paper is not soluble in the commonly used solvents. There is some tendency for components, notably proteins, to adhere to the fibers and produce an effect known as "tailing," in which the separation is not clearcut and some of the component lags behind the trailing edge of its zone. Also variation in the pore size of the paper does not permit the sharpness of separation that might be desired.

Several other support substances have been tried. *Agar gel* and *starch gel* have been used quite successfully. They have a tendency to melt as the temperature rises, and some cooling system may be necessary. Even with the best of equipment these are not as convenient as certain other materials.

With the advent of various membrane materials and the use of higher voltages, it has become possible to effect a clear separation within a very short migration. These materials and voltages have also allowed excellent separations with a very small sample. One of the best "micro" systems is Beckman's Microzone, illustrated in some detail in Fig. 8-1.

Recently a number of types of membranes for use in electrophoresis have become commercially available. *Cellulose acetate* is the commonest and most successful of these. Very sharp separations can be made if the material is handled properly. It is more brittle than paper, so it must

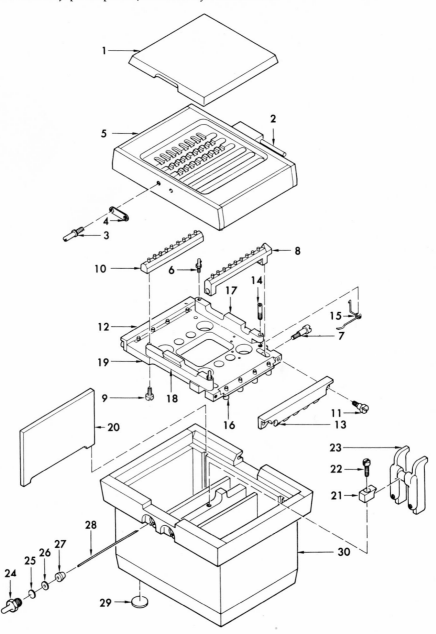

Fig. 8-1. Exploded view of the Microzone cell, showing minute detail. (Courtesy Beckman Instruments, Inc.)

be handled more carefully. It also readily absorbs contaminants from the fingers and other surfaces; therefore it should always be handled with forceps, and care should be taken to avoid contamination. Wetting of the membrane should be done carefully to avoid entrapment of bubbles of air in the fine porous structure. When these precautions are taken, very sharp zones can be obtained and tailing is almost nonexistent. Frequently materials that have migrated as a single zone on filter paper strips can be

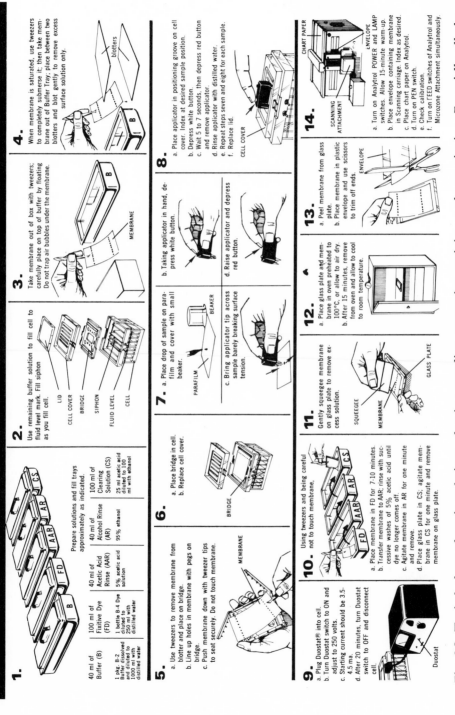

Fig. 8-2. Typical electrophoresis technique, showing sampling, separation, staining, and quantitation. Essentially all the systems in common use are similar in these details. (Courtesy Beckman Instruments, Inc.)

separated on cellulose acetate. The migration time may be reduced from about 15 hours to about 30 minutes. Other membranes now in use include *polyacrylamides, polyacetates, cellulose nitrate,* and *agarose film.*

The solvent used in the electrophoresis cell is of considerable importance. Changes in the pH of the system affect the mobility of charged particles by altering the actual electric charge. Ionic strength affects the electroosmotic current through the paper or membrane. Substances such as the *glycols* are added at times to reduce evaporation from the strips, especially when high voltages are used and there is evolution of considerable heat. *Urea* and other substances have been added to suppress formation of various complexes of the solute and the support material. Other materials have been added to reduce the amount of solvent that can be absorbed into the support material, in an effort to minimize the effect of electroosmosis.

In most cases the materials that are separated cannot be seen on the electrophoresis strips. Since the commonest means of recognition and quantitation utilize stained strips, the first step is proper preparation and staining. Techniques for staining will vary with the material in question and the choice of stain. Usually the protein materials are fixed by immersion in methyl alcohol. After the staining is performed, the strips are washed several times and dried. A typical electrophoresis routine for serum protein on cellulose acetate, as recommended by Beckman, is reproduced in Fig. 8-2, along with an explanation of the steps involved.

Quantitation of the stained material may be accomplished by *elution* and reading of the colored compound in a colorimeter if filter paper is used. The zones of material, identified by their R_F values, are cut out of the filter paper strips and placed in individual, marked test tubes. The stained protein or other material is then washed out in a measured amount of solvent and read on a colorimeter. A calibration curve can be prepared from the material in question or, in the case of serum protein, a measured quantity of albumin may be used to establish a curve on which all fractions can be read. This method is obviously slow and tedious, and better methods have been devised. With very small strips, such as those used in the Microzone system, it is quite impossible.

DENSITOMETERS

A densitometer is an appartus designed to measure the density of a deposit of material on a transparent or translucent electrophoresis strip. In effect, the instrument is built like a filter colorimeter in which a paper strip is used in place of a sample cuvette. Since electrophoretic separations are now done in large numbers in most laboratories, there has been a great deal of interest in the development of densitometers. Some of the types now available are listed below.

Beckman-Spinco Analytrol (Beckman Instruments, Inc.) (Fig. 8-3). This instrument was one of the first high-quality densitometers commonly used. Not many of them are still in routine clinical use, but there are a number used in teaching situations. It is a good teaching instrument, since it is rather easy to demonstrate and all essential parts are accessible and easy to understand. For this reason, considerable detail is included here. This densitometer is essentially a double-beam colorimeter. The exciter lamp is located about the center of the instrument. The sample beam is collimated and directed forward, where it passes through an interference filter before passing through a slit to strike the filter paper strip. The strip absorbs some of the light, and the transmitted light, which passes on through the paper, strikes the sample photocell located in the small black housing on the front of the instrument. At the same time, light from the exciter lamp passes through a similar interference filter toward the rear

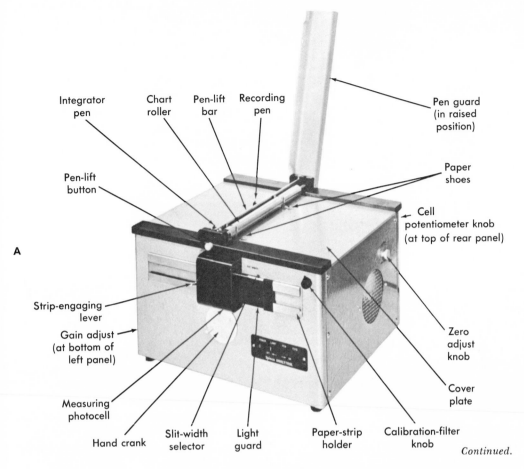

Fig. 8-3. **A,** Analytrol, showing all controls. **B,** Schematic diagram of internal details of the Analytrol. (Courtesy Beckman Instruments, Inc.)

of the instrument. This beam strikes the rear, or reference, photocell. The error signal from these two photocells is amplified and is used to drive the recording pen. An occluder is placed in the reference beam. By increasing or decreasing the amount of light that is allowed to strike the reference photocell, the cells can be balanced and the pen set at zero. Unfortunately the relation between the concentration of dye on the filter paper strip and the light that is transmitted through the paper is not a linear one. For this reason a cam is placed in the reference light beam in such a position that it will modify the amount of light allowed to strike the reference photocell, to compensate for the lack of linearity. Since the different stains

will absorb differently, various cams have been prepared for the dyes most commonly used. As the pen moves upscale, indicating an increase in absorbance, an attached drive assembly turns the cam to effect the modification of the light beam.

A single constant-speed motor performs three correlated functions by way of a set of drive mechanisms. First, the filter paper strip is fed through a channel between the exit slit and the photocell. Second, the recorder paper is fed through the recorder at a rate comparable to the movement of the filter paper strip. Third, the constant-speed disc of the integrator is turned at a speed relative to the other two functions.

A small wheel rolls on the surface of the constant-speed disc of the *integrator*. If it

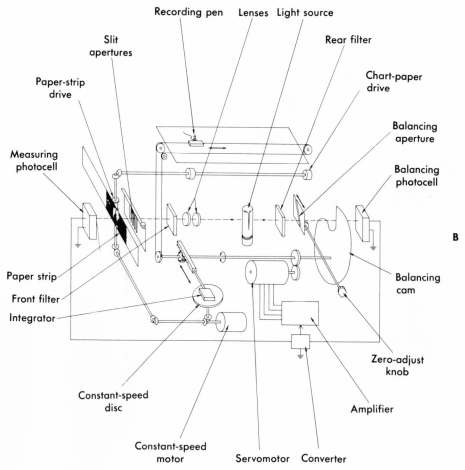

Recording pen   Lenses   Light source

Slit apertures

Paper-strip drive

Rear filter

Chart-paper drive

Balancing aperture

Measuring photocell

Balancing photocell

Paper strip

Front filter

Integrator

Balancing cam

B

Zero-adjust knob

Constant-speed disc

Amplifier

Constant-speed motor   Servomotor   Converter

Fig. 8-3, cont'd. For legend see p. 143.

is near the center of the disc, it turns slowly. As it moves out to the edge of the disc, it turns more rapidly. This might be compared to two cars on a racetrack. The outside car has to go faster than the inside car to make the same number of laps around the track. This small wheel is notched so that, with each rotation, five notches (in turn) cause a small rod to move up and down a total of five times. The small rod transmits these jiggles to an integrator pen at the bottom of the recorder paper. Since one of the notches on the wheel is larger than the rest, one of the blips of the integrator pen is larger than the others; thus it is easy to count total

turns of the wheel by counting the larger blips only. The small wheel, which drives the integrator pen in this fashion, is moved over the surface of the constant-speed disc by a gear drive attached to the recorder pen. As the recorder pen moves upward on the paper, indicating an increase in absorbance, the small wheel is pushed out to the edge of the constant-speed disc, where it is forced to run faster, thus making the integrator pen record more blips. This drive mechanism is accurately designed so that the number of blips indicates the relative area under the curve drawn by the recorder. The integrator may be operated as a planometer, to determine the area under

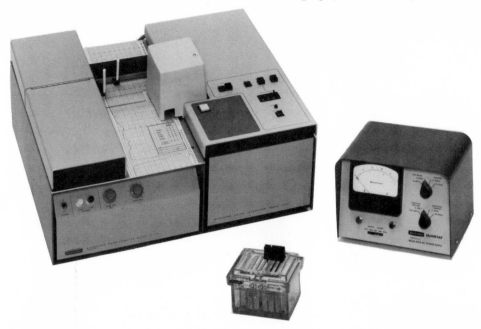

Fig. 8-4. Microzone densitometer Model R-110 with digital integrator Model R-111 and Duostat power supply. (Courtesy Beckman Instruments, Inc.)

a curve, by simply moving the pen along the curve with the controls as the recorder turns the constant-speed disc and feeds the chart paper through. This is a type of disc integrator.

The Analytrol was originally designed for fairly long paper strips that were migrated on a Durham cell (which has about disappeared from use). When the Microzone cell was designed, changes had to be made in the Analytrol to scan the very short and very narrow migration patterns. The total area of the membrane used is about 2 × 3 inches, and eight samples are migrated within this area. Obviously the bands of each sample are very small. The Analytrol was modified to scan these tiny bands; the slits were changed and a separate time control box was provided, which slowed down the membrane feed to make the pattern scan coincide with the length of the charting paper.

Beckman Model R-110 Densitometer (Beckman Instruments, Inc.) (Fig. 8-4). More recently Beckman introduced the

Model R-110 Densitometer, which was designed specifically with the very small Microzone membranes in mind. All eight patterns can be scanned in about 7 minutes. Interference filters varying from 450 to 700 nm (to allow use of any of the common stains) are available. Three neutral-density filters—0.4, 0.9, and 1.4 OD—are supplied in a turret wheel to allow a choice in energy attenuations if cloudy membranes or stain residues give difficulty. The integrator is electronic and seems to be more trouble-free than the mechanical device provided on the older model. Recently a digital integrator, capable of printing out results in grams percent or total counts, has been added to the system.

The combination of Microzone cell, power supply, sample applicator, and new densitometer is a very efficient system for performing large numbers of separations. The separations are sharp, and the traces are distinct, easy to read, and quickly made.

Schoeffel Spectrodensitometer, Model

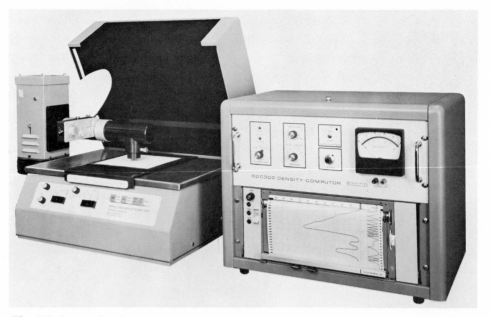

Fig. 8-5. Spectrodensitometer, Model SD3000, pictured here with the density computer. Note the flat scanning table for handling gels, columns, etc. (Courtesy Schoeffel Instrument Corp.)

SD3000 (Schoeffel Instrument Corp.) (Fig. 8-5). This is another densitometer that shows a great deal of promise. It does not use interference filters but has a high-quality quartz prism monochromator. It is a double-beam arrangement that can be coupled with a recorder to provide a continuous-scanning, ratio-recording system that can be used in many ways. The xenon light source and quartz optics make possible the scanning of protein fractions in the UV range, where they absorb reasonably well without staining. The monochromator has a range from 200 to 700 nm. The sample beam and the reference beam are located parallel to each other and a few millimeters apart. The reference beam scans the membrane, paper, gel, or other matrix as the sample beam is scanning the actual deposition of material. Each light signal is detected by its own phototube, and each photosignal is amplified separately. The two amplified signals are then fed to the ratio network and to the recorder. An accessory that will convert the transmission ratio to a concentration value is available. The entire system is solid state, except for the phototubes, of course.

The moving stage that carries the matrix between the monochromator and the detector is mounted on a flat tablelike surface that provides excellent versatility. Membranes, papers, gels, columns, and even capillary tubes can be read with good accuracy and reasonable convenience. The slits can be adjusted in both width and height, allowing adjustment of both band pass and area of observation.

The SD3000 Spectrodensitometer is an extremely well designed instrument with a high-quality monochromator. What it lacks in speed and convenience it more than makes up in quality and careful engineering.

Millipore PhoroSlide System and Phoro-Scope (Millipore Corp.) (Fig. 8-6). The arrangement of cells is quite flexible, allowing single samples to be run in small, economical cells; also larger cells to accommodate more samples are available. The

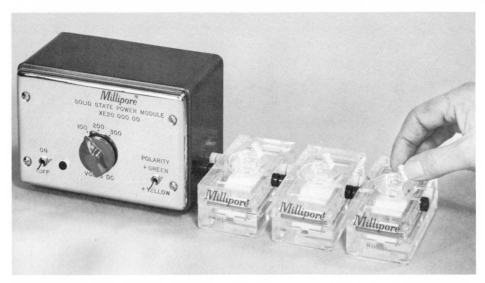

Fig. 8-6. Millipore system power supply and cells, showing chain arrangement of very small cells. (Courtesy Millipore Corp.)

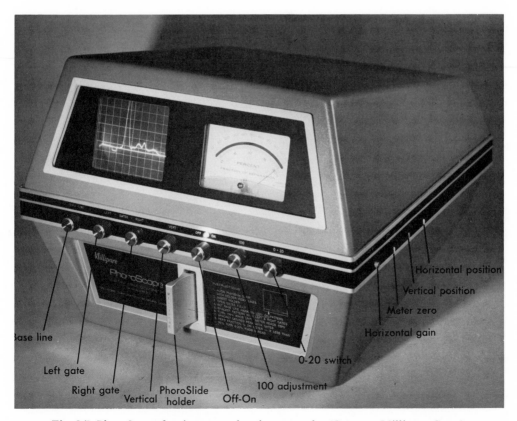

Fig. 8-7. PhoroScope densitometer, showing controls. (Courtesy Millipore Corp.)

power supply can carry several cells at the same time by interconnection with banana plugs. Membranes are of a resilient material and are simply placed in the cell in an arclike position, with either end immersed in solution. The preparation and insertion of the membranes are thus extremely simple. Each cell is 2 × 4 inches and 2 inches high, using about 11 ml of buffer.

The PhoroScope densitometer (Fig. 8-7) is the part of the system that seems the most revolutionary. A light beam passes through an interference filter and collimating lens into an oscillating mirror. The mirror directs the beam across the membrane from end to end in rapid sweeps. A condensing lens collects the transmitted light and directs it onto a silicon photocell that has a very rapid response time. The photocurrent is amplified and used to direct the vertical deflector plates of a CRT, producing a scan pattern on the screen. Within seconds the entire pattern is visible. An interesting system for interpreting the scan is also devised (Fig. 8-8). Gates at either

end of the scan pattern can establish the total current produced in each sweep. If the meter is set at 100% at this point and the gates are closed down to include only the peak to be considered, the meter will automatically indicate the percentage of the total represented by this peak. Thus each individual component can be quickly evaluated without the tedium of counting integrator peaks and calculating percentages. The whole process is fast and direct and provides a visual scan in seconds. A small recorder for generating a record is supplied, if one is desired. Each recording takes 3 minutes to make. The time required to work with each cell and membrane might be a bit longer than that required to produce the same result with Microzone membranes, but the instantly visible CRT pattern and rapid integration certainly seem to be desirable innovations. This system is interesting and innovative. However, the fast, accurate integrating and printing densitometers, like those described below, have proved to be more practical in many situations.

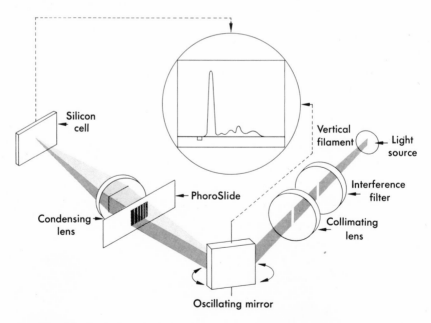

Fig. 8-8. Optical path of the PhoroScope. (Courtesy Millipore Corp.)

Densicomp Model 445 (Clifford Instruments, Inc.) (Fig. 8-9). This instrument is one of the most promising densitometers to be introduced recently. It is capable of scanning almost any type and size of material, including gels and thin-layer chromatography plates. With the addition of an accessory it can scan fluorescence in a migrated sample.

The completed strip is positioned in a holder. When activated, the strip is scanned in about 20 seconds. As the pen carriage of the recorder makes a fast sweep back across the paper, the printer prints the desired values on the recorder paper. If the total material value (for example, total protein) and sample number are dialed in, the printer may record (1) sample number, (2) total value, (3) area percentage to three digits, (4) grams percent of each peak, or (5) a digital count of the area of each peak. The recorder chart is 7 inches long, and various sample strip lengths can be accommodated to provide a full 7-inch trace. Full-scale response takes 0.3 second for the recorder pen.

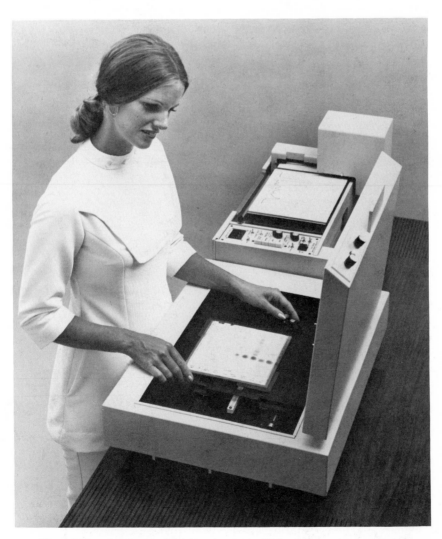

Fig. 8-9. Densicomp Model 445. (Courtesy Clifford Instruments, Inc.)

One may elect to choose the valley between fractions on the recorder chart or, with an accessory, to electronically sense the valley. The capability of choosing the valley becomes important in some cases where peaks overlap.

When a scan is completed, the sample strip holder automatically repositions for the next sample. An automatic zero accessory allows the system to zero itself. Uncleared strips can be read with good accuracy.

Wavelengths are chosen by changing the interference filters (2 × 2 inches). A number of filters are available for dyes, between 450 and 650 nm. The detector is a photodiode. BCD output is available.

The Densicomp 445 is a good, modern, and reliable instrument that has proved itself, in a very short time since its introduction.

Digiscreen (Gelman Instrument Co.). This is perhaps the most widely used of the newer generation of densitometers. When an eight-strip sample is positioned in the carrier, this instrument can automatically set zero and scan all eight channels in one minute. On a separate recorder module it provides a recorder chart with an integrator trace on each separation. To get the printout of grams percent of protein fractions, a "grams percent module" must be added. If more reporting sophistication is required, the recorder is replaced with a computer module.

Scanning is effected in much the same way as in the Clifford unit described above, with the membrane moving on a carrier between the tungsten light source and the photodetector. Interchangeable glass filters are used to optimize the light characteristics for each stain used.

Integration of peak areas is predicated on electronic valley sensing when the grams percent module or computer module is used. In most cases this is adequate but may occasionally be objectionable where there is overlapping of materials. As with most of the newer densitometers, a zero correction automatically makes allowances for the background opacity of the strip used.

This is a very practical, rapid, and accurate system for routine electrophoresis scanning. The basic unit apparently is primarily designed for conventional membranes and glass micro slides only. The manufacturer has opted for convenience and price advantages. Some workers may prefer the convenience and compactness of a single unit that provides all of the characteristics of Digiscreen's several modules. When all of the modules are considered, the total price of the system is comparable to that of other instruments providing the same functions. When everything is taken into consideration, the Digiscreen is probably an excellent choice for the medical laboratory performing routine electrophoretic separation.

RFT Scanning Densitometer (Transidyne General Corp.). This is a very sophisticated unit that is suitable for routine and research work. The letters RFT indicates the instrument's capability to scan reflected, fluoresced, and transmitted light, each mode being easily selected with the flip of a switch. Each scan requires 4 seconds. A monochromator of good quality provides wavelength selection from 190 to 720 nm with a 3 nm band width. Tungsten and deuterium lamps are both provided, and rapid switchover is possible. Detection is with a ten-stage photomultiplier. Almost any type of material can be scanned. The analog signal from the detector is reported out on a 4-inch recorder chart with an integrator trace. To get a digital printout, a computing integrator must be added. This unit, called the *PDQ Computing Integrator,* can print out in total percent, grams percent (when total is dialed in by the operator), and raw integral count.

Equipped with the computing integrator, the RFT is a high-quality, convenient, flexible, and expensive unit. Actually the

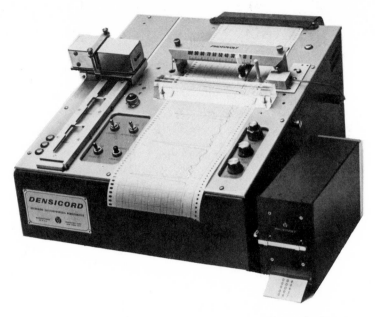

Fig. 8-10. Densicord densitometer. (Courtesy Photovolt Corp.)

price is not high in comparison to competing systems if the outstanding performance characteristics and overall quality of the system are considered. For the laboratory heavily involved in electrophoresis and chromatography and having a lively interest in developing new methods, this instrument would be an excellent choice.

• • •

Electrophoresis has become such a routine laboratory tool that nearly every medical laboratory has some capability in this area. For this reason, equipment manufacturers have become acutely aware of the potential market and much new equipment has been introduced. It is impossible to cover all of the good equipment available in the space of a few pages. In passing, a few other systems might be mentioned. *Photovolt* has a good densitometer called the *Densicord* (Fig. 8-10), which has good accuracy and a very wide field of application including paper, cellulose acetate, disc

gel columns, agar gel, fluorometry, UV and IR, etc. *Joyce-Loebl* has a high-quality densitometer called the *Chromoscan Densitometer* which is a double-beam, recording/integrating instrument for transmittance and reflectance through the UV and visible range. *Helena Laboratories,* thanks to many excellent contributions to methodologies, has become very active in this field. Their *Quick Scan Electrophoresis Densitometer* is economically priced, functional and convenient. It provides a trace and integration. The *Quick Quant Digital Computer* must be added to provide grams percent, percent, or raw integral digital printout. *Gilford Instrument Laboratories, Inc.,* provides a linear transport attachment for its photometer (discussed in an earlier chapter) to make possible scanning strips without a separate densitometer.

Passing mention should be made of the small, low-cost electrophoresis units especially designed for detection of Australian antigen and other hepatitis-associated antigens. These are usually gel systems using a specially prepared gel plate for the cell used. The patient's serum is placed in one well in the gel and the specific antibody is placed in a parallel well. Under the influence of the current, the antibody migrates in the direction of the serum well and globulin fractions of the serum travel toward the antibody well. If the antigen sought is present in the serum, a zone of precipitation occurs where the two come together after about 20 minutes of migration time.

B & L Spectrophor (Bausch & Lomb). This company has approached the problem of automating electrophoretic procedures from a somewhat different direction. The Spectrophor is a completely automated system for migrating proteins in a semi-solid medium and reading the fractions by absorption of UV light. The separation of protein fractions takes place in an eight-channel tray. The ends of the tray act as reservoirs and are overfilled so as to flood the flat quartz plateau between the reservoirs with a thin layer of medium. The medium used is an agarose-dextrin-buffer gel that is fluid but just viscid enough to prevent convection currents. The samples are applied to a cotton fiber immersed in the gel. A migration voltage causes the proteins to move along the sample channel and separate. The temperature of the migration tray is maintained at 25° C, ± 2°, by a refrigeration unit. Some heat is generated by the migration current, and the room temperature changes must be taken into account. At the end of about 20 minutes, the sample tray passes between the deuterium lamp and the photomultiplier detector, and the concentrations of the various samples are plotted by the recorder and integrator. A high-quality monochromator allows the operator to select any wavelength between 200 and 650 nm. Most methods utilize the natural absorptivity of protein for some ultraviolet wavelengths and no staining is required. The output of the photomulti-

plier operates the Y axis of the recorder.

The entire process is reasonably automatic once the samples are applied. The system has been improved and sixteen samples can now be completed in about 20 minutes. The Spectrophor is an expensive system and considerable training is required for its operation. It has not come into widespread use but it looks promising.

GAS CHROMATOGRAPHY

Gas chromatography is similar to column chromatography in many respects. In the simplest sort of system the material to be separated is in the form of a gas, and the substrate is porous material that is able to mechanically retard the advance of larger molecules in the material. The impelling force, pushing the sample forward, is flow of an inert gas through the column.

Although the basic idea of gas chromatography is quite simple, the devices that are in use may be complicated and may vary considerably in all details. The basic ingredients of a gas chromatograph are (1) a *carrier gas system* to carry the sample forward, (2) a *column* packed with some sort of material to selectively impede the forward movement of the sample, and (3) some means of sensing and measuring the sample as it passes a point in the system.

Many of the samples to be analyzed are in a liquid state. These may be volatilized by raising the temperature. In order to accomplish this, the column may be housed in an *oven* whose temperature can be accurately controlled. The signal from most types of detector is too small to measure conveniently without some amplification; therefore an *electrometer,* with some type of measuring device, is required. Let us consider these parts of the gas chromatograph in detail.

Carrier gas system. Any inert gas may be used to carry the sample forward. Technical considerations may determine which gas will be used. Helium is probably the most widely used although nitrogen is somewhat cheaper. Other gases in common use are argon and hydrogen. The flow of the gas must be extremely consistent, for any change in rate will vary the R_F values of the materials being separated and cause unstable and unreliable results. The flow of gas acts as a background value to the detectors, and a constant base line cannot be achieved if there is any fluctuation in the carrier gas. When the flow rate is increased, the material moves forward faster and the R_F value, measured in seconds or minutes, is shortened. When the flow rate is too high, the migration becomes ragged and the sample is presented to a detector as a less compact bolus, during a longer period. Thus the corresponding recorder peak is lower, wider, and less sharply defined. Usually a combination of at least two valves is used to control the carrier gas flow. A fairly common arrangement uses a two-stage regulator on the tank of gas and one or more needle valves. It is extremely important that the gas be very dry. It is usually passed through a filter of desiccant or a molecular sieve to remove moisture and other contaminants. On some systems several feet of stainless steel capillary tubing, before the column, serves as a resistance to reduce pressure and stabilize the flow rate. Metal and glass are generally used throughout, since rubber may be a source of contamination. Also, since helium is a very small molecule, it tends to pass through the walls of ordinary rubber tubing.

Column. Column technology has become an exact and complicated science. We shall discuss here only the principal considerations. The column may be made of stainless steel or glass and may vary considerably in length and diameter. A column of $\frac{1}{8}$-inch diameter is most widely used. However, when the system is to separate large quantities of material for commercial use or further study, a larger column may be desirable. Also a capillary column, which contains no packing material but a coating on the walls of the tube, may be used.

Materials with similar R_F values may require a long migration before they separate adequately, whereas easily separated materials may require only a short time. Most columns in routine clinical use are more than 18 inches and less than 10 feet in length.

The columns are generally packed with a porous material to help retard the progress of the sample. This material is called the *solid phase, stationary phase,* or *column support.* Crushed fire brick, diatomaceous earth, and molecular sieve are examples of commonly used solid-phase materials. There are many others. The size of the particles of material is spoken of as the *mesh.* Granular material that is 40 to 50 mesh will pass through a screen that has 40 wires per inch but will not pass through one with 50 wires to the inch. For various situations solid-phase packing of 60 to 120 mesh may be used. The smaller the particles, the more tightly the material will pack and the slower will be the passage of gas through it; also the more will be the retarding action on the migrating sample.

The material used as a solid phase is commonly coated with a viscid liquid to help retard the progress of the sample. This material must be stable at high temperatures and must be effective in the differential partitioning of the sample components. It must be a good solvent for the sample components and must not react with them or with the solid phase. Various glycols, silicone oils, paraffin oils, etc. have been employed.

After the solid material is coated with the liquid phase, the column must be conditioned by heating and flushing with inert gas. Excess liquid phase and various impurities are driven off, and the system is gradually stabilized. At high temperatures the column may continue to "bleed" or lose some volatilized liquid phase.

Columns are formed in U shapes or coils

so that they will fit easily into ovens of workable dimensions. The ends are attached to the carrier gas supply and to the detector by means of threaded Swagelok fittings or some similar easily connected device. Different analyses require columns of different length and composition, and it is desirable to be able to change them easily, even when they are hot.

The oven into which the columns are installed is designed to control the temperature within very narrow limits. Most modern systems include controls that enable the oven to heat up to a preset temperature quickly, to maintain that temperature very exactly, and to cool back to room temperature with a minimum of lost time. They are also programmed so that increases in temperature can be performed at a regular, even rate that can be controlled. A regular and even increase of 1° per minute or 20° per minute can be attained with ease and accuracy. This aids in the differentiation of compounds that volatilize at different temperatures.

There is usually a separate temperature control for the point in the system where the sample is injected into the column. This *injection port* is usually maintained at a slightly higher temperature than the column so that the material will be driven into the column immediately and not remain at the point of injection. There is also a separate temperature control for the area around the detector. This temperature is also maintained a little higher than that of the column to prevent the material from redistilling at the detector. The temperature at these points may be monitored by a system having a thermistor probe in each location, a switching arrangement, and a single meter.

Detector. There are many types of detector used with gas chromatography. The simplest of these is the *thermal-conductivity cell*—a type often referred to as a TC detector. A hot wire conducts electricity at a rate dependent on its temperature. Heat

is dissipated at a rate that is dependent on the type and concentration of gas passing the wire. The resulting change of temperature of the wire determines its resistance and hence the flow of electricity through it. Two such *hot wire detectors* may be used in conjunction. One of these monitors the stream of inert gas prior to injection of the sample, and the other monitors the effluent from the column. The difference in resistance between the two wires is then amplified and used to drive a recorder, meter, or digital readout. Many instruments actually use two hot-wire cells located before the column and two located after the column. This serves to average the signals in each case, minimizing errors caused by slight variations in gas pressure and hot wire temperature. A thermistor may be used in place of the hot wire. The thermistor works on the same principle as the hot wire. A semiconductor material that conducts much more readily at high temperatures than at low is enclosed in a small glass capsule and installed in the flow lines.

A second type of sensing mechanism is the *ionization detector*. As the material being separated is swept out of the end of the column, by the carrier gas, it is burned in a small but very hot hydrogen flame. The resulting breakup of molecular structures produces ion pairs. An electric field of high potential is set up in the area of the flame. The ion pairs contribute to the current in the field, and the increase is measured by a highly sensitive electrometer. For this system to function, the current passing across the detector must be very constant when at base line. Gases must be dry and the flow rate must be extremely steady. Impurities from the column must be minimal. Since the ionization current is very small, even slight variations in these factors can cause severe problems.

Since many of these conditions are hard to control with adequate precision, two columns, each with its own detector, are sometimes used. The second column and detector act as a reference system against the sample side. Hence the two must be parallel in every detail. The columns are the same length and contain the same packing. They pass through the same heating oven in proximity, and the injection-port heaters and detector heaters are at the same temperature. As the column temperature is raised, there is a tendency for the liquid phase to volatilize or bleed, causing some ionization at the flame. If dual columns and detectors are used, this bleed is compensated and the net effect is negligible.

Ionization detectors are most efficient for the detection of compounds with many electrons that are easily displaced. Organic compounds rich in carbon are easily detected, and the hydrogen-flame detector is best suited for these.

Another type of detector occasionally used is the *cross-sectional ionization detector*. The sample is ionized in a small cross-sectional area of the column by a stream of beta radiation from an isotope. The amount of ionization occurring is measured by a sensitive electrometer in the same manner as with the hydrogen flame.

The *argon detector* is a two-stage mechanism. A radioactive material ionizes argon gas molecules, which then collide with the molecules of the sample to be measured, causing ionization.

In the *electron-capture detector* the process is more or less reversed. Certain halogenated gases, peroxides, and metal organic compounds are able to capture and bind free or loosely bound electrons. As the sample reaches the end of the column, it is bombarded by beta radiation. The free electrons are captured by the electron-binding gas, thus decreasing the current flow.

There are several other types of detector available for specific analytical problems. The hot-wire and hydrogen-flame detectors just discussed are the commonest systems in medical applications.

It is possible, in the case of the hot-wire detector, to reclaim the entire sample fraction in its naturally occurring state. Various gas traps are provided to collect these fractions as they leave the detector and are flushed out of the column. In the case of the hydrogen-flame detector, a *stream splitter*, which allows a portion of the sample to pass into the flame while the rest goes on to the fraction collector, may be provided.

• • •

Some discussion of the various control devices, electrometers, etc. involved in gas chromatography should be made at this point. There are many instruments on the market, and they vary in detail enough to make such a discussion difficult at best. To the novice the total system may seem hopelessly complicated. Actually each of the components is reasonably simple if considered by itself. A brief discussion of some of these follows.

A power supply must be provided for the detector. For the thermal-conductivity detector, this is a low-voltage system whose chief requirement is stability. It is a fairly simple low-voltage, DC power supply. For the ionization detectors, a high-voltage supply is required. Voltages between 10 and 1000 v at a very low amperage are supplied to the electrodes. This current must be extremely stable and ripple-free. High-quality potentiometers are used to effect very precise control.

For the ionization detectors, an electrometer of very high quality is required, to amplify and measure the small change in current. Most of these are solid state at the present time. A series of very accurate resistances is built into the system to allow for attenuation of signals too large to be measured directly.

A recorder with an integrator must be provided since the area under the curve is the measure of the sample passing the detector. The information from the electrometer may be fed directly to a computer for analysis, but a recorder is still a rather necessary component, since visualization of the column output for monitoring is, at least, highly desirable.

Simply seeing a blip or peak on a recorder chart is not sufficient evidence of the identity of a compound, even if the R_F value of the compound is known. Conditions are very hard to duplicate from instrument to instrument and from day to day. It is therefore necessary to run standards in all cases and compare them with the unknown. The solvent (normally organic) used for the unknown sample and the standard will be detected as it passes through the detector, and there may be some problem of separating the solvent peak from the sample peak. This may be done by adjusting flow rates of gases, sample size, solvent/sample ratio, and choice of solvents.

Oven controls are usually located remote from the oven because of the amount of heat involved. The oven is heated with electric elements. Increased rates of heating may be provided by using additional elements or a higher voltage or both. Fast cooling is achieved by means of fans that blow the hot air out rapidly. Regulation of the rate of increase in temperature is accomplished by a timer that operates the voltage control.

As mentioned earlier, a temperature-monitoring system is provided. Thermistors are installed in each location where the temperature information is required. Each is supplied with a current, and the resistance to the current is relative to the thermistor's temperature. One meter is usually used for all the thermistors, and a switch is provided to monitor each as desired.

A very large amount of work has been done in the field of gas chromatography in the past years. These instruments are beginning to find use in the clinical laboratory. Gas chromatography shows promise in steroid chemistry, toxicology, and several other areas. It is reasonable to assume that workable methods for the routine analysis of many compounds of medical importance may be forthcoming in the next few years. As time goes on, however, it is becoming increasingly apparent that the very critical procedures of sample preparation will reduce the general utility of the method for routine work. It is possible to detect extremely small amounts of some compounds by this method with fantastic accuracy. Identification can be made with a high degree of certainty by comparison with standards. By the same token, very small traces of contaminating materials or small changes in structure may cause extreme difficulty.

Gas chromatography has become a fairly routine tool in toxicology, and there are a few practical techniques in routine clinical laboratory work. This is a rather specialized area, however, and the instruments are not common enough in routine clinical use to justify much discussion of individual instruments here. American Instrument Co., Antek Instruments, Inc., Perkin-Elmer Corp., and Varian Corp., among others, have good instruments and provide abundant technical information. The student who is especially interested in gas chromatography is referred to these sources and to texts on the subject.

REVIEW QUESTIONS

1. What is electroosmosis?
2. What does the R_F value tell us?
3. How does immunoelectrophoresis work?
4. What is the disadvantage of valley sensing?
5. What causes "tailing"?
6. How does an electronic integrator store information?
7. Most methods used by the Spectrophor system do not use a stain. Why is this possible?
8. What does the carrier gas do in gas chromatography? The liquid phase?
9. Why is the injection-port temperature usually kept higher than the oven temperature in gas chromatography?
10. What is the source of the analog signal in a hydrogen-flame gas chromatograph?
11. What is a TC detector?

9

Automation in hematology

As recently as 15 years ago the average medical technologist spent an appreciable part of every day counting red blood cells and white blood cells in ruled areas of a slide chamber to estimate the average number of red and white cells in a cubic millimeter of a patient's blood sample. In most laboratories a total of 30 counts a day for one technician was considered a heavy day's work.

In performing a red cell count, the technologist counted about 500 cells, out of a total of nearly 5,000,000 cells per cubic millimeter. The inescapable error due to random sampling, plus a multitude of dilution and preparation errors, glassware-calibration errors, and human errors of judgment and fatigue, could add up to a very large total error indeed. One of the most significant changes that have been made in laboratory equipment has been the introduction of devices for counting red and white blood cells quickly and accurately. These devices have arrived at a high state of mechanical efficiency and have become so trouble-free that the technician employing them may be totally unaware of their operating principle.

Before the advent of today's counting instruments a few attempts were made at estimating a cell population by various indirect methods. The Leitz Photrometer used the total absorbance of the suspended red cells in a simple dilution of blood as an indication of red cell population. This method assumed that all cells were equal in size, that the serum was essentially colorless, that no clumping existed, etc. In practice this method turned out to be useless except as a very rough screening method.

An instrument called the *Hemoscope,* which worked on a sort of nephelometric principle of light dispersion, was produced. This, too, failed to solve the problem.

Now, in addition to devices for counting of red and white blood cells, advanced instrumentation makes it possible to determine red cell volume and hemoglobin and to estimate, from these parameters, the various indices that describe the red cell. A device to give information similar to the red cell sedimentation is available. At least three companies have introduced highly automated systems to differentiate between types of normal white cells and enumerate them. It is probably only a matter of time before a complete blood count will be performed by one instrument and this information, along with the patient's identification, be entered directly into a computer for immediate reporting and storage. Some of the principles and ideas that make these things possible will now be examined.

PARTICLE COUNTING

The instruments now in common clinical laboratory use depend on one of two principles. The Technicon and some other, less advertised systems count by means of a light signal, using a magnifying lens with or without the dark-field principle. The Coulter principle uses cells to interrupt a flow of current between two electrodes and counts the signals thus produced. Several variations of these two general ideas have been made, and a great deal of research into the physics and mechanics of cell counting, sizing, and identifying has been conducted. Much will probably be done in this field in the next few years to further relieve the tedium of individual observation of cell and particle number, size, and type.

COULTER CELL-COUNTING DEVICES

Technologists are greatly indebted to Joseph and Wallace Coulter for the introduction and refinement of sophisticated methods of cell counting. The illustration and description of this system, which Wallace Coulter prepared for presentation to the National Electronics Conference in 1958, is of some historical interest and is a very lucid explanation. The principle, with many refinements, is still basically the same as it was at that time. With his permission the following excerpt is reprinted in detail and his original accompanying illustrations are used.

Figure 1 [our Fig. 9-1] shows a simple arrangement for holding the sample, establishing sample flow and "metering" the flow so that an electronic counter can be activated as a selected sample volume is drawn thru and scanned by the orifice. A dilute suspension of cells *(E)* is contained in a sample beaker. The tube *B* carries the aperture *A* thru which the sample is drawn. *C* and *D* are the electrodes. When stopcock *F* is opened, an external vacuum source (and waste discharge) *(P)* initiates flow thru the orifice and causes the mercury *J*

in the manometer to assume the position shown with the mercury in the open leg of the manometer drawn slightly below the horizontal branch. When stopcock *F* is closed, the unbalanced manometer functions as a syphon to continue the sample flow thru the orifice. As the mercury in the open leg rises into the horizontal branch, it makes contact with a wire electrode *(L)* sealed in the manometer wall and energizes a high speed decade counter which begins counting all pulses which reach or exceed the threshold level. A few seconds later the mercury column makes contact with a second wire electrode *(M)* which stops the counter. The syphoning action continues until the mercury column comes to rest at a level near that of the mercury in the reservoir. Contact *K* provides a ground return path for the start and stop electrodes. The contacts *L* and *M* are very carefully located so that the volume contained in the tube between the contacts is ½ milliliter. As a consequence of the arrangement the counter is actuated as ½ milliliter is drawn into the system. In practice the horizontal section is a ∪ tube in the horizontal plane so that contacts are near together. By this means the vacuum in the system at the start and stop contacts is kept substantially equal so that any elasticity in the system due to bubbles etc. will introduce less than 1/10th percent error in the syphoned volume under the worst conditions.

The function of inlet *O* and stopcock *G* which is normally left in the closed position is to allow rapid filling of the system when setting it up instead of depending upon the relatively slow flow thru the orifice.

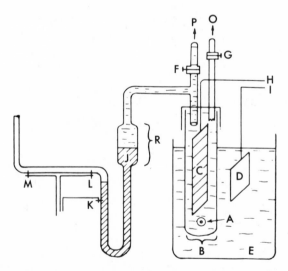

Fig. 9-1. Principle of the Coulter Counter as reproduced from *High Speed Automatic Blood Cell Counter and Cell Size Analyzer,* by Wallace Coulter, 1956. (Courtesy Coulter Electronics, Inc.)

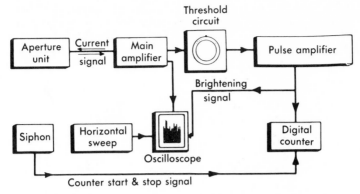

Fig. 9-2. Electronic circuitry of the Coulter Counter (as in Fig. 9-1). (Courtesy Coulter Electronics, Inc.)

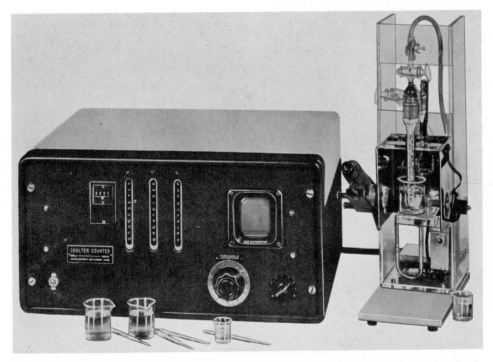

Fig. 9-3. Model A Coulter Counter (as in Fig. 9-1). (Courtesy Coulter Electronics, Inc.)

Figure 2 [our Fig. 9-2] is a block diagram of the electrical functions and Figure 3 [our Fig. 9-3] is a photograph of a model now in use in a number of laboratories. The pulses produced at the orifice are amplified and displayed on the oscilloscope screen and appear as vertical lines or spikes as shown in Figure 4 [our Fig. 9-4]. The height of an individual pulse spike from the baseline is a measure of relative size of the cell producing the pulse (except for coincident passage to be discussed) and

since the rate at which they are produced is several thousand per second, the viewer obtains an immediate impression of the average cell size and cell size distribution. The threshold control dial located below the oscilloscope screen enables the operator to select the height or level above the baseline which if reached or exceeded by a pulse will result in the pulse being counted. The height or level corresponds to a particular cell size. When the syphon activates the counter, all cells of this partic-

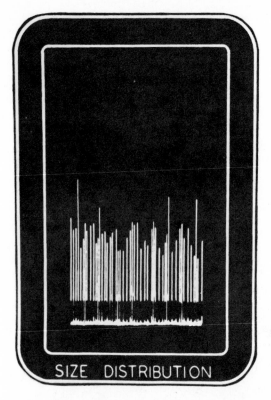

SIZE DISTRIBUTION

Fig. 9-4. Pulse pattern on oscilloscope screen (as in Fig. 9-1). (Courtesy Coulter Electronics, Inc.)

ular size or larger present in half milliliter drawn thru the orifice will be counted. Cells below this minimum size will not be counted. In addition to a display of relative cell size the oscilloscope also indicates the effective level or setting of the threshold control by brightening that portion above the threshold level, of any pulse which reaches or exceeds it and which of course would be counted. In Figure 4 [our Fig. 9-4] the threshold level is shown intermediate between the height of the smallest of the desired pulses and well above the small irregularities on the baseline which represent the passage of very small bits of debris and any extraneous electrical disturbances which may be present. The screen indicates, at a glance, a wide discrimination against undesired debris and electrical background noise and correct functioning of the threshold circuit in relation to the particles to be counted. For the particular sample represented the threshold control setting could be varied considerably without affecting the count. For routine cell counting the threshold control is left at a sufficiently low setting to count the smallest cells likely to be encountered and need not be reset for different

samples. The minimum function of the oscilloscope display is to provide a check of overall instrument performance in a manner which requires only an instants observation and is readily understood by the average medical laboratory technician.

The Coulter Counter pictured in Fig. 9-3 has become known as the *Model A*. It is hand wired and uses a total of 30 vacuum tubes. Many of these units are still in use and, aside from tube failure, do not have a great many repair problems. The units in more common use at the present time are the Model F_N (Fig. 9-5) and the Model ZBI. As can be seen, the manometer glassware and suction pump have been included in the case. The digital and mechanical registers of the Model A have been replaced, first by glow tubes in the Model F and then by numerical readout tubes in the models F_N and ZBI. The sensitivity controls have been mounted on the front panel. The viewing lens for observing the orifice (mounted on the manometer stand of the Model A) has been replaced by a viewing screen. The most important changes, however, have been in the electronics. All tubes have been replaced by transistors, and printed-circuit boards are used throughout. The Model F Counter has been one of the most trouble-free, sophisticated instruments in the clinical laboratory.

Two minor problems have occasionally come up with this counter. The first has to do with the adjustment of the vacuum supply to the mercury column in some of the older units. After some months of continuous use the pump may wear, the vacuum control valve may fail by clogging, or tubing may begin to leak. Once this occurs, the readjustment of the vacuum system, after repair is completed, may be an annoyance to the busy technologist. Changes have been made in the pump to virtually eliminate this problem. The new pumps are installed within the Model F_N and can be purchased for replacement in the Model F.

The second problem is concerned with the tendency of the Model F to pick up AC

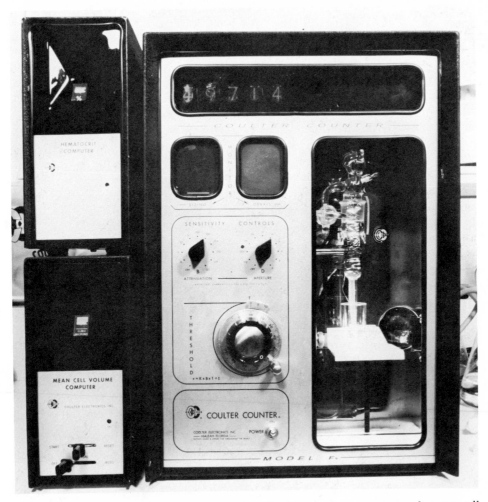

Fig. 9-5. Model F_N Coulter Counter shown with hematocrit computer and mean cell volume computer. (Courtesy Coulter Electronics, Inc.)

broadcast signals from brush motors, fluorescent lights, etc., causing a high background count. Although instruction manuals warn the user to avoid these devices, it is hard to imagine a busy laboratory without several dozen motorized instruments, fluorescent lights, and other static-producing equipment. A surprising number of these cause no problem, whereas the unexpected source may cause difficulty. Grounding the chassis of the instrument sometimes completely eliminates the trouble. Both of the problems described have

virtually disappeared in the more recently produced instruments.

All electrically powered laboratory equipment should be grounded, and laws in most states require a three-pronged plug on all units, the third prong being the ground. It happens at times that the third slot of the wall receptacle is not actually grounded. This can happen in old buildings especially and in parts of buildings where wiring has been haphazardly added. The grounding can be checked with a voltmeter by measuring between the hot side of the circuit and the ground line. If no current registers, the "ground" is not actually grounded.

In spite of the small problems that may occur with the Coulter models F and F_N these are highly reliable instruments, and problems are almost always attributable to diluent, glassware, or dilution error. Use of Coulter's Isoton Diluent, Isoterge Detergent for cleaning the instrument, and disposable plastic beakers, while slightly more expensive, almost guarantees immunity from these problems.

Coulter Counter Model B (Coulter Electronics, Inc., Industrial Division). This company manufactures a number of different devices for particle counting and sizing. One, the Model B, is used in conjunction with a particle size distribution plotter to chart Price-Jones red cell size–distribution curves automatically. For the di-

agnosis and study of certain types of anemias, the Model B and the distribution plotter constitute a very valuable tool. However, an appreciably large volume of work would be needed for these units to be economically practical, although they would save much time and provide extremely valuable information.

Coulter Counter Model S (Fig. 9-6). When the second edition of *Elementary Principles of Laboratory Instruments* was going to press, the Model S was just coming into production. At that time I predicted that it would have "a major impact on the clinical laboratory." That prediction seems to have been borne out. A large percentage of all clinical laboratories of any appreciable size are now using this equipment and it is considered a standard device in most hematology departments. Indeed, in most

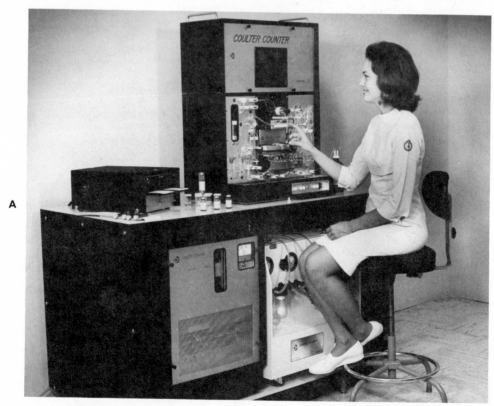

Fig. 9-6. Model S Coulter Counter. (Courtesy Coulter Electronics, Inc.)

laboratories, it is a black day when the Model S is out of service—which, fortunately, occurs seldom if proper maintenance and service are provided.

On first examination this seems to be a complicated system. Like most systems, when we examine it part by part, it is much simpler than we would first suppose. The electronics may be beyond comprehension for many, but the general idea behind each subsystem is easy to grasp.

In discussion of the Coulter principle of particle counting it has been explained

that a particle passing through a small orifice interrupts an electric current, giving a blip or signal that can be counted. Both red and white cells are counted in this way. Cells of each type are drawn, at a constant rate, through three apertures at once. The three internal electrodes, one in each aperture tube, are associated with one common external electrode immersed in the fluid that is being drawn through the apertures. Thus there are three *white cell counts* and three *red cell counts* performed during each cycle of the instrument. These

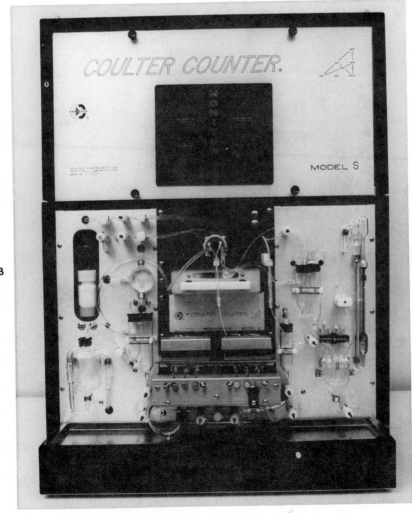

Fig. 9-6, cont'd. For legend see opposite page.

are compared and if results are within reasonable limits the three are averaged. If one count is out of limits, the other two are used; but if the three are widely separated, no result is reported. If a result is rejected, a red "voting light" over the oscilloscope screen, associated with that orifice tube, comes on so that the operator knows to check for foreign material in that orifice. Unless there is a problem with blood clots or a similar hazard, these lights seldom come on during the count cycle. The manner of preparing the blood dilution for red and white cell counts will be explained presently.

While the blood is being diluted for the white cell count, a hemolyzing agent is added. The bath from which the white count is drawn is optically clear and presents an optical path of about 1 cm from front to back. A small light at the front of the bath acts as an exciter lamp and, at the time the white cell count is being taken, a photocell behind the bath is measuring the optical density of the hemolyzed blood solution. From this information a *hemoglobin* value can obviously be obtained.

As pointed out, while cells are being counted, each cell produces an electric signal (which is actually the instantaneous decrease of the orifice current). The size of this signal is an accurate measure of the electrical resistance offered by the cell, and this is a function of the cell's volume. Measuring the total of all of these electric signals and then dividing their total by the number of impulses (or cells) provides a very accurate average signal that corresponds to the average cell volume. Applied to the red cell–counting sequence, this technique reveals the mean red cell volume (MCV).

Methods for obtaining four parameters—RBC, WBC, Hb, and MCV—have now been discussed. Three other parameters are calculated from these four measured values. To find the mean corpuscular hemoglobin (MCH), the hemoglobin value is divided

by the number of red cells per unit volume. This can be done electrically, using the electric signals just measured.

The hematocrit is defined as the packed cell volume, or the percentage of a blood sample that is red cells. This value is usually obtained by centrifuging a blood sample until cells are packed and measuring the volume of the red cell pack, as a percentage of the total. If the average volume of the red cells in the sample (MCV) and the number of cells (RBC) are known, multiplying these will indicate the total red cell volume in a given volume of blood. This is a highly accurate *hematocrit*. There is a problem, since we have not been able to measure this way in the past and the cell packing that we normally do leaves interstices between the spherical cells even if we have absolutely ideal centrifugation. Since we have only an electrical value from the Model S that is analogous to a value that is not too well defined, we simply assign the normally determined value to the electric signal; in other words, we standardize the instrument with a known hematocrit value. Much research has been done to better define this situation, but it is more an academic problem than a practical one.

The *mean corpuscular hemoglobin concentration* (MCHC) tells us how much hemoglobin there is, on the average, in a given volume of cell space. Obviously this can be determined from the electrical information corresponding to the mean corpuscular volume and the hemoglobin.

After this survey of the origin or all of these seven parameters, the system by which the sample travels to each measuring point will be examined. The fluid-handling system of the Model S is extremely accurate. The degree of automation and the number of operations involved present a very complex fluid-moving problem. All movement of fluid is either by pressure or by vacuum. There are a great many valves that, on signal, open or close to move diluted

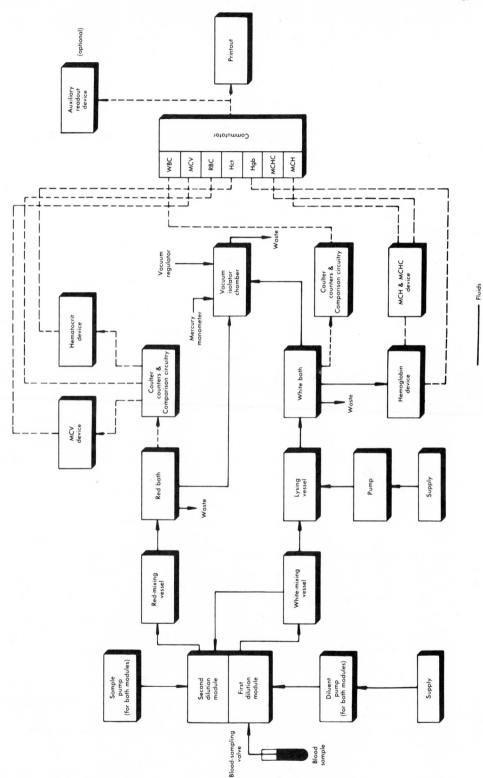

Fig. 9-7. Block diagram of the Coulter Model S blood-counting system. (Courtesy Coulter Electronics, Inc.)

sample in the right direction. The command center for all of these is a bank of small induction motors accessible from the back at about the center of the counting module. Vacuum is provided by the pump in a separate module under the counter.

Measurement of samples is by *segmented stream*. If the sample were in a tube having a very consistent and accurate internal diameter, a highly accurate sample could be measured by cutting off a precise, highly reproducible length of this tube. This is, in principle, what is accomplished by the measuring valve. The valve core is a metal cylinder, through which an accurate channel has been bored lengthwise. This cylinder is tightly fitted, at its ends, against plastic block faces. Holes in the block faces correspond to the holes in the cylinder, thus providing a pathway for fluid through one end block, through the channel in the cylinder, and through the other end block. If the cylinder is rotated on its center axis, however, a stream of fluid through this pathway would be cut off and an accurately measured sample would be retained in the channel of the cylinder.

Blood is drawn into this device by vacuum and the valve is turned, cutting off the accurately measured blood sample. As the valve turns, however, the sample channel is aligned with other holes in the plastic end blocks and a measured stream of diluent washes the blood along to its next position and performs the necessary dilution at the same time. In this way the blood sample is first diluted and moved to a chamber on the right side of the counting module. From this chamber an aliquot is withdrawn and similarly measured and rediluted for the red count. This sample is placed in a bath on the left side of the machine. Both the original sample (white cell dilution) and the rediluted red count sample are now swirled into an additional chamber to facilitate mixing. Before moving to the counting bath, the white cell dilution goes to a hemolyzing bath where a few drops of a hemolyzing agent are added. Both the red cell and white cell dilutions now proceed to the respective counting baths where the orifice tubes will draw off samples at a controlled rate for the counts previously described. Between counting cycles the counting baths and orifice tubes are well rinsed with diluent. The block diagram in Fig. 9-7 may make it easier to understand the counting cycle.

It is hoped that this condensed and simplified explanation of the Model S hematology system will make possible a fairly clear idea of the rationale involved. This system has proved to be very accurate and highly reproducible. The amount of laboratory work time saved is impressive and the improvement in accuracy in hematology, in general, is a substantial contribution to better patient care.

OPTICAL CELL COUNTERS

Fisher Autocytometer (Fisher Scientific Co.) (Figs. 9-8 and 9-9). In this instrument the sample is drawn through the capillary field by a glass and Teflon syringe operated by a relay. Dark-field lighting illuminates the field, and the cells show up as bright points against a black background. These light signals are converted into electrical impulses by a photomultiplier tube. A threshold circuit rejects signals lower than that of a blood cell, and an anticoincidence circuit corrects for the exact coincidence of cells passing through the field. The resultant signals are totaled and presented on the dial as a total signal for a given volume of blood that has been proved experimentally to represent a specific cell count. Both red and white cells can be counted and the same threshold used for both. Only a selector switch is changed between readings of RBC and WBC. This switch changes the counting ratio and illuminates the dial with a red light for the RBC and a white light for the WBC. Figs. 9-8 and 9-9 show the flow diagram and schematic detail of this system.

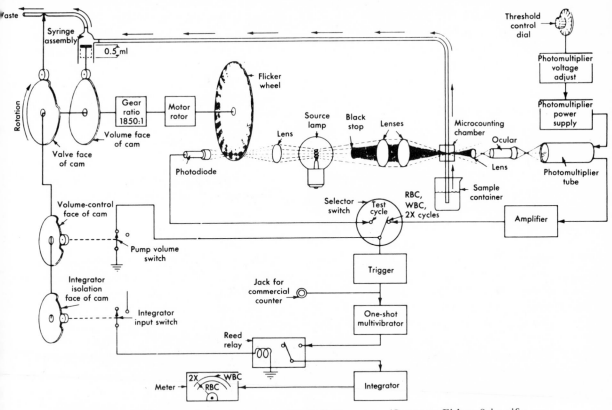

Fig. 9-8. Flow diagram of the Autocytometer Cell Counter. (Courtesy Fisher Scientific Co.)

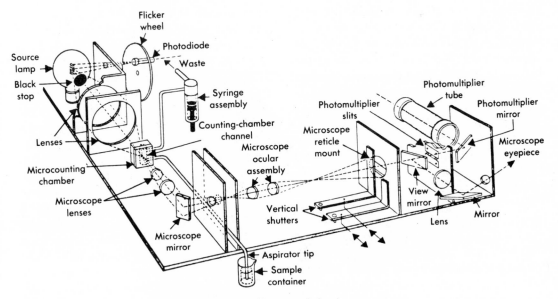

Fig. 9-9. Schematic diagram of the Autocytometer.

The instrument is transistorized except for the photomultiplier tube and two other small tubes. The electronics seem to be quite stable.

There is some difficulty at times when the capillary becomes plugged with clot or extraneous material. It is not particularly difficult to remove and clean the parts, however.

A built-in testing cycle for the electronics of the machine is incorporated in the Autocytometer. A signal of known frequency is presented to the circuitry to test its validity.

Fisher Scientific Co. has recently introduced the Autocytometer II, which has been modernized in design and improved in several ways. Readout is now a lighted digital display. The attractive built-in self-testing feature is still included and somewhat improved. This company also produces the Hem-alyzer, which performs red and white counts by the same general method as their other instruments but also does a cyanmethemoglobin. Whole blood samples are placed on a turntable from which they are automatically sampled. Samples are diluted, tests are done, and results are printed on a tape at the rate of about 35 an hour.

Hema-Count (General Science Corp.). This instrument would appear to have a similarity in principle to the Coulter systems. I have had little success in getting solid information from the company about operating details. Three models are advertised. The Hema-Count MK-2 can count red or white cells but performs on one channel only. The Hema-Count MK-3 can perform tests for four parameters—RBC, WBC, hematocrit, and hemoglobin. Two serial dilutions are prepared and from these the four values can be determined in about 2 min./sample. Very little information is given in advertising literature about the rationale of the equipment and, aside from a leaflet distributed by the company showing a comparison of a hundred counts done on this system and on the Coulter

Model S, I have seen no comparative studies of its accuracy, reproducibility, etc.

Hemalog and Hemalog-D (Technicon Corp.). Technicon has produced several hematology devices over the past several years. In the previous edition of this book the SMA-4A and SMA-7A systems were described. These systems have now been replaced by two new devices with greatly expanded capabilities. These are the Hemalog, which automates twelve parameters, and the companion Hemalog-D. Since these are still quite new and rather complicated, we shall review separately the rationale that Technicon has published for each of these systems. Some liberty must be taken in simplifying complex and detailed matters.

The Hemalog is designed to automatically render twelve different hematological values from two Vacutainers of blood. These parameters are RBC, WBC, platelet count, hemoglobin, packed cell volume (PCV), conductivity cell volume (CCV), PCV/CCV ratio, MCV, MCH, MCHC, prothrombin time (PT), and partial thromboplastin time (PTT). Some of these values are new to us, and their determination and their significance will be explained.

A digital clock, which is in reality a small computer, controls all of the various timed functions that occur as a cycle is in progress. A three-way mode switch allows one to select the ten parameters involved in a CBC and platelet count, the PT and PTT only, or all twelve values.

The Hemalog sampler has two round sample trays—one of which fits into the center of the other. They interlock in one position only; therefore sample numbers must always match. The inner tray contains the citrated Vacutainer tubes for PT and PTT determinations. This tray is removed and placed in a centrifuge before the run to separate the plasma, after which it is replaced. The outer tray holds the EDTA Vacutainers for the CBC and platelet count. The sample arm has a stirrer, which precedes the sample probe to mix the sample. There is a probe for each of the two tubes and each has a strainer at its tip to catch fibrin and debris. These strainers are back-flushed after each cycle.

There are two interesting changes from the standard AutoAnalyzer hardware. In place of coils, there are glass tubes with constrictions periodically placed. These provide better mixing in shorter time and distance. Also, most of the fluids are moved under carefully controlled air pressure instead of by the conventional peristaltic pump. This is a surprising innovation that sounds very promising, since tube fatigue with variations of flow, etc. are now practically eliminated.

The counting of cells and platelets is done in a manner similar to that used on other optoelectrical counters except that the flow cell has been redesigned and the forward-scattered light around a light target is collimated and counted. This improved design allows cells to be counted almost individually so that there is little coincidence.

An ingenious hematocrit centrifuge is built into the system to provide the packed cell volume or PCV. A J-shaped tube is built into the hematocrit head. Blood is forced into a central chamber by air and finds its way into the J-shaped tube where it is spun down at 20,000 rpm. The level of packed cells is read while the tube is in motion. Another sample then pushes the first out through the waste outlet and rinses it out by overfilling by about five times the required volume.

A current is passed through a column of whole blood to determine its conductivity. From this measurement the value called conductivity cell volume or CCV is derived. Normally this value should be quite close to the hematocrit or packed cell volume. However, when the two are compared (CCV/PCV), there is occasionally a difference apparent that may indicate some pathological change in electrolytes or protein.

The hemoglobin is read in a classic manner, using the cyanmethemoglobin method with Drabkin's solution as a diluent. The indices MCH, MCV, and MCHC are all computed from the derived values already discussed.

The method for determination of PT and PTT seems quite innovative and practical. A roll of Mylar tape, with small wells formed in it, is provided for each of the two parameters. Tiny particles of dry magnetic iron oxide are in each well. As the well approaches a probe, 0.03 ml of plasma is dropped into it. The iron oxide is suspended in the plasma, making the plasma opaque. Now 0.03 ml of thromboplastin and 0.01 ml of calcium chloride are added and the suspension is stirred by magnetic effect in a rotating magnetic field. Addition of the calcium chloride starts the timing cycle. As a fibrin clot is formed, it enmeshes the iron oxide in a tight clot, allowing light to pass and trigger the end of the timing cycle. Technicon claims excellent results with this system. Time will tell how it will work out in practice. It might be assumed that very long PTs would fail to produce enough fibrin to clear the field sufficiently. These tests could be repeated by hand, of course.

The entire system shows many new and promising ideas. As with any new system containing as many innovations as this has, there will certainly be problems and some redesigning. On the whole, however, the system offers much more promise than the SMA-4 and SMA-7, and its development will be extremely interesting.

The Hemalog-D is a totally automated leukocyte differential counting system. The general idea of the system is that cells, if they are differentially stained in solution, can be counted according to their staining properties as they pass detection points. To this end the Hemalog-D has been built largely around conventional AutoAnalyzer devices and effective differential stain techniques.

In general, a sample is drawn up, formalin is added for cell fixation, a hemolyzing solution is added to remove red cells, and the solutions are sent through four staining subsystems, from which they are counted. One of these staining subsystems uses neutral red to differentiate basophils. A second subsystem uses alpha-naphthol butyrate and basic fuchsin in a stain to distinguish monocytes. In a third system eosinophils and granulocytes are stained, using 4-chloro-1-naphthol at pH 2.5 for eosinophils. When the same solution is alkaline, neutrophils are stained. Lymphocytes are the balance of the total count.

A special flow cell has been developed that places the stream of stained cells in the center of another outer stream so that cells are not traumatized. The sample flow

through the counting beam has a laminar nature so that cells are easily isolated in the tiny point of focused light. Each stain used gives the specific type of cell a constant stain intensity, which can be differentiated by the detectors. Each cell is detected by both a scattered-light sensor and an absorbed-light sensor. This prevents either system from counting red cell stroma or other debris.

Differentially counting white cells in this manner is a technically interesting but difficult task to perform of which many details are omitted here for brevity. The system is ingenious and early work with it shows promise but there have been many problems. The Hemalog-D might be expected to be able to function soon, at least as a screening device, but it is a rather

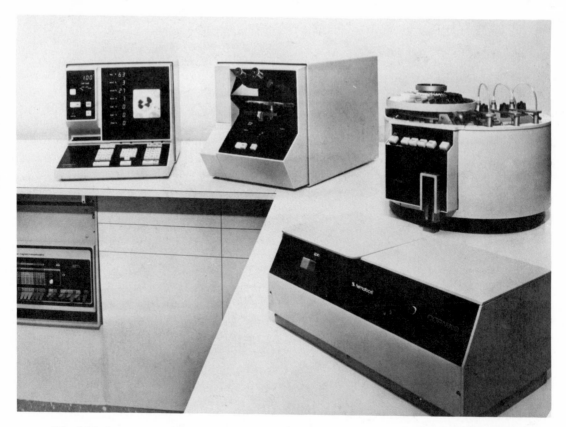

Fig. 9-10. Larc system for automatic differential cell counting. (Courtesy Corning Glass Works.)

intricate system with many potential sources of problems.

Some companies have been working on the automation of white cell differentials, using a system called pattern recognition. A stained blood smear is photographed by television camera. The image on the CRT is then scanned electronically; such characteristics as (1) shape and size of nucleus, (2) color and size of granules, and (3) shape, size, and intensity of chromatin pattern are measured. About 30,000 bits of information about one cell are collected in a hundredth of a second. The electronics of this acquisition of information is quite complicated; however, if the instrument's capability to amass this amount of infor-

mation can be accepted, it is not hard to conceive of a system with a remarkable capability in cell recognition. There are, of course, many technical problems to be solved but two systems have been widely demonstrated and show rather striking capabilities at this early date.

The two most prominent companies involved in this approach to the automation of differential counts are **Corning Glass Works** and **Geometric Design Corp.** (which is a subsidiary of Smith, Kline & French Laboratories). The Corning system has been named the Larc. No name has apparently been assigned by Geometric Design Corp. at this time. Fig. 9-10 shows the components of the **Larc system,** and

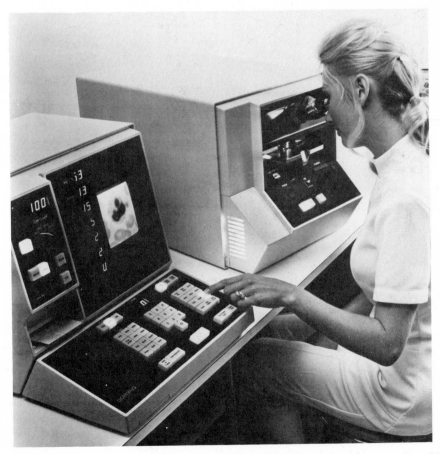

Fig. 9-11. Close-up of Larc scanning and reporting modules. (Courtesy Corning Glass Works.)

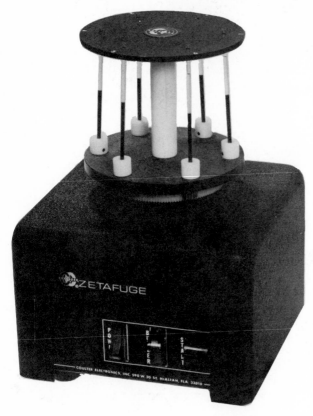

Fig. 9-12. Zetafuge. (Courtesy Coulter Electronics, Inc.)

Fig. 9-11 shows a closer view of the scanning and reporting terminals.

As this goes to press, **Coulter Electronics** has also announced a pattern recognition system that will automatically scan several slides in succession and recall abnormal cells for visual observation.

This approach seems to be an extremely valid one that will probably bring another small revolution to the world of hematology. Poor blood smears constitute some problem for the method, but Corning has devised a system of centrifuging blood across a slide and leaving a monocellular layer on the glass (upper right in Fig. 9-10). It will be most interesting to see the development of different types of automation for doing differential counts during the several months ahead.

AUTOMATED SEDIMENTATION RATE

Technologists and doctors often fret about the time that is required to complete a sedimentation rate. In an article on the zeta sedimentation ratio, published in the August, 1972, issue of *Laboratory Medicine,* Drs. Brian Bull and J. Douglas Brailsford have presented an interesting idea. The sedimentation of cells can be speeded up by centrifugation and, if all variables are properly controlled, a value can be determined that correlates well with traditional sedimentation values. Apparently the effects of temperature, vibration, etc. on the sedimentation rate are eliminated in this 3-minute method.

Zetafuge (Coulter Electronics, Inc.) (Fig. 9-12). Coulter's Zetafuge is intended to provide a means of properly performing this new test. The instrument is shown here, although no appreciable clinical trial of this device has been reported yet. The idea seems quite worthy of investigation.

REVIEW QUESTIONS

1. Name at least four sources of error in manual (microscopic) cell counts.
2. What two principles are used in automated cell counters?
3. If the mercury failed to rise in the manometer of the Coulter Counter, what would be the probable cause?
4. What causes the pattern on the oscilloscope screen of the Coulter Counter?
5. If the Coulter Counter failed to start counting when cycled, could you think of a mechanical reason why?
6. From earlier sections of the book, can you explain how the threshold of the Coulter Counter works?
7. What is the principle of the red cell count used by the Technicon SMA-7A?

10
Automated chemistry

During the 1950s many medical laboratory workers were putting forth efforts to simplify procedures and save work time. Some of these efforts led to automatic pipetters, sequential samplers, shakers, rotators, etc., which were the first tentative steps toward automation of methods. A small company called Technicon Corporation introduced a tissue processor that moved surgical specimens through the steps of fixation, dehydration, and embedding in a timed sequence. This was done rather simply by mounting a metal disc on a clock movement so that it completed one rotation in 12 hours. Notches along the circumference of the disc actuated microswitches, at specific times, turning small induction motors on and off. The motors, by a chain of gears and levers, caused the raising, lowering, turning, and agitating motions required.

These devices worked well and were quickly followed by others that performed mechanical functions in some sort of timed sequence in an automatic fashion without human involvement. There is really nothing particularly difficult or mysterious about these machines that do work by using gears, levers, cams, wedges, etc. in familiar ways. Almost all of the automation that will be discussed in this chapter involves this sort of mechanical function in conjunction with various electrical devices such as were discussed in earlier chapters. It is true that some of the modern marvels of automation seem mysterious but when each step is examined, in its function, there is very little that does not seem reasonably simple. Many of the instruments are incredibly sophisticated because of the number of individual simple tasks that are performed. Saying that each of these tasks is in itself simple does not in any way detract from the impressive engineering involved in combining them into an integrated and practical working tool.

As automation has progressed, it has become possible to perform large numbers of analyses and accumulate quantities of data. In many cases, the sophistication of analytical devices has brought out many details requiring complicated decisions. Both the orderly storing of data secured through automation and the making of complex decisions can be done well by computers. Automated systems present details—changes of time and temperature, variations in chemical concentrations, etc.—to computer circuits, for storage and retrieval at a later date or for use in further operation or computation. Modern automation makes use of mechanical ingenuity, electronic technology, and data handling.

Some of the specific devices and systems that are currently in use or are currently being introduced will now be discussed. For convenience they will be considered in groups of devices that attempt to solve the same sort of problem or operate on the same general principle. Also, the fairly simple devices that automatically pipette, dilute, record, sample, etc. will be omitted, since many of these are considered in a later chapter.

TECHNICON'S MOVING-STREAM PRINCIPLE

Historically the first real automation of clinical chemistry was done by the Technicon Corp. using a combination of clever, innovative ideas. The first idea involved in the Technicon approach is that samples can be picked up in a stream of fluid and moved along a tube by peristaltic pump, through various changes, and finally be analyzed colorimetrically. For this concept to work, steps must be taken to segregate the samples in the moving stream and assure that cross-contamination between samples does not occur. If a nonwettable plastic tube is used, there is a very small holdback effect if bubbles of air large enough to completely fill the lumen of the tube are introduced regularly. Mixed with diluents and reactants, the sample passes along the tube in small segments separated by air bubbles. This technique works well, and holdback with cross-contamination is effectively eliminated. There are a few places, such as in the colorimeter, where air bubbles cannot be tolerated. At these points the air is bled out of the tube through the vertical arm of a T-shaped fitting called a debubbler. Where the stream must run any distance without bubbles interspersed, a holdback is experienced. Keeping such distances very short minimizes this problem.

A second idea utilized by most of the Technicon systems is dialysis of the sample. Blood serum is, of course, rich in proteins. Proteins precipitate with heat or with strong chemicals such as acids. Precipitated protein would render a solution cloudy and would produce a substantial error in colorimetric readings. Since most of blood chemistry methods in use in the 1950s depended on heat or on acids, some way had to be found to eliminate protein. The Technicon solution was to pass the stream of sample across a membrane, parallel to a moving stream of fluid with a lower tonicity. As the two streams pass on either side of the membrane, certain substances dialyze across the membrane and pass from the sample stream into the new stream called the dialysate. It should be obvious that not all of a substance will pass across the membrane, but the amount that does pass is a

function of its concentration in the sample stream.

Since the concentration of material in the dialysate is not a linear function of the material in the original sample, some means must be found to correct for this error. If a series of standards are run through the entire system and a curve is constructed by plotting their concentrations against their absorbance values, unknown samples can then be read on this curve. If an infinite number of points could be plotted, the method should provide excellent accuracy. Since this is not practical, values must be interpolated between established points on the curve. The resultant values are not absolute by any means but are clinically acceptable by almost any standard.

These early AutoAnalyzer systems produced by Technicon Corp. consisted of several components connected into a train. A typical system might include the following:

1. A sampler that could insert a plastic sampling tip into a different sample each minute and hold it there for a given time while sample was aspirated at a constant rate.

2. A peristaltic pump that advanced a stream of sample, reagents, air, and diluent along separate plastic tubes by rolling steel rollers forward and pressing the tubes shut.

3. A dialyzer that allowed dialysis to occur between two moving streams in a temperature-controlled unit.

4. A unit where solutions passed through long coils to prolong their stay in a temperature-controlled bath.

5. A colorimeter where the absorbance of the test solution was measured in a flow cell.

6. A recorder that drew a curve, using the output of the colorimeter.

Later systems have utilized these basic components, modifying them as need dictated.

As the interest in automation increased, Technicon adapted its systems to perform multiple analyses on a single sampling, and numerous modifications and improvements have been made. It has been possible to reduce the sample size significantly with a parallel reduction in reagent consumption. The large and awkward dialyzers have been replaced by quite small modules using a small, easily replaced membrane. The once cumbersome and problem-plagued peristaltic pumps have been replaced by better-designed, smaller units. Many other modifications have been introduced that have improved flow characteristics. Many of these changes have been incorporated into the current AA II Series. In the mid-1960s various multichannel systems were introduced.

The most dramatic early multiple system was the SMA 12/30 (Sequential Multiple Analyzer), which could perform twelve simultaneous routine colorimetric tests on one sample and could introduce samples at the rate of thirty per hour. In due time this unit was replaced by the SMA 12/60 which doubled the number of samples per hour and again reduced the sample and reagent requirement substantially. The principal innovation that made it possible to do sequential tests was the Technilogger, which allowed the recorder to accept the output from the photocells of three colorimeters in rapid sequence as the appropriate analysis came to completion in that instrument. This process is then repeated as the next three tests are completed, etc. The obvious problem comes in phasing tests so that they come to completion and into the proper colorimeter flow cell at the correct moment. Since one sample is being tested for twelve constituents each minute, there is a period of only 5 seconds in which each result can be recorded. If the flow through the system, for one constituent, is slightly longer than for another, the test with the shorter line will come to completion, each test cycle, a little earlier; after a number of tests it may get considerably out of phase. Fig. 10-1 shows how the recorder charts sequential tests on a single sample.

Another Technicon system, introduced about the same time as the SMA 12/60, was the SMA 6/60. This system tests for glucose, urea nitrogen, chlorides, carbon dioxide, sodium, and potassium. The first four of these tests use classic colorimetric methods that present no particular problem of instrumentation. Sodium and potassium, however, are done by flame photometry. The sample is diluted in a lithium (internal standard) solution by the proportioning pump and fed directly into the flame. Although flame photometry is a pretty well developed science, there are many problems inherent in the continuous operation of a flame photometer in automated equipment. Maintaining a constant, even flow of fluid into the atomizer, maintaining flame characteristics, and eliminating carry-over between samples have all been problems. The present SMA 6/60 does these things relatively well but not without a considerable amount of maintenance and occasional problems.

Reading the colorimetric values in the moving stream of Technicon's systems has not been any particular problem, once the *flow cell* was perfected. The debubbled stream passes through a narrow, horizontal glass tube, the ends of which are optically clear. Light, focused exactly on the front of this tube, passes through the solution for a prescribed distance (usually about 10 mm) and exits at the back where it strikes a photocell. The fluid enters via a connecting arm at the bottom at one end and exits in the same manner at the top and at the opposite end. Except for the flow cell, the colorimetry is not remarkable. The exciter lamp is monitored by a reference photocell and the error signal between the photocells is amplified and activates a recorder pen.

Various other devices have been incorporated in Technicon chemical analyzers but the above, in essence, is the rationale of the system. Space does not allow for consideration of all the details of construc-

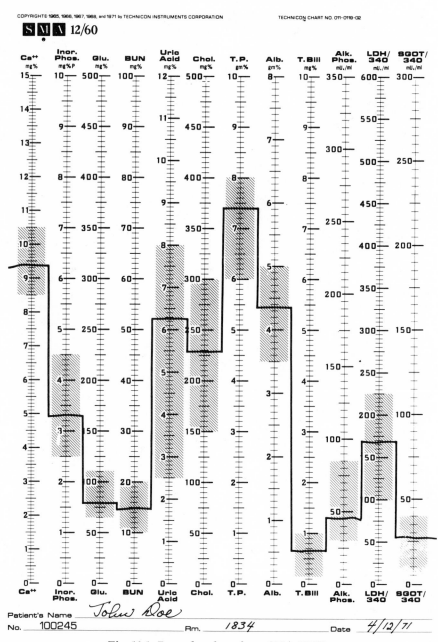

Fig. 10-1. Recorder chart from SMA 12/60.

tion, methodologies, and modifications of each of the systems to be discussed; each automation system could be the subject of a large volume.

Certain advantages and disadvantages should be considered in this survey. The AutoAnalyzer was the first really workable automated chemistry system and for many years it was virtually without competition. This fact alone has given this system considerable authority, and the company had years of experience in this field before most competitors entered it.

The idea of dialyzing the sample to get away from the problems of deproteinization is a solid advantage that other systems have had difficulty overcoming. Newer methods that can be performed successfully in the presence of protein are being developed; therefore this is a less important point than it was at one time but the advantage is still significant.

A principal disadvantage of the system is that plastic tubes become fatigued and distort, and they fail to carry the same volume, especially when pump characteristics change. The system requires a great deal of maintenance and a thoroughly competent analyst still requires a rather lengthy training on the system before he becomes proficient. There is no selectivity, and all tests must be done on each sample. Consequently there is no saving of reagents if tests are not needed. Also the system is not easy to activate for a small number of tests or for a single sample.

DISCRETE CHEMICAL SYSTEMS

Other than the moving-stream systems of Technicon Corp., the principal automated chemistry devices involve discrete chemistry tests. In all of these methods, each sample is kept discrete or separate from all others, and the reactions take place in individual tubes. **Hycel Corporation's Mark X** system will be discussed as more or less typical of these, since this was among the first significant challengers to the AutoAnalyzer approach.

The rationale of the chemistry tests done by the Mark X is identical to that of the manual methods in most cases. Deproteinization is not possible. The various mechanical systems are all concerned primarily with performing functions that are normally done by hand. The Mark X is pictured in Fig. 10-2.

The first system to be examined here is the reaction tube transport system. Ten test tubes are solidly mounted in line in a slat. Each of these tubes will be the site of a specific methodology. There are sixty identical slats of this sort in the transport. They are arranged around a belt, very much like the cleats on a caterpillar tractor are. While they are on the top of the belt, the tubes are upright and contain test materials. As they move to the end, they tilt forward, pouring out their contents, and then pass along the bottom of the belt in an inverted position during the washing cycle. Each 90 seconds the tubes advance one position. As clean tubes come into the upright position, sample and reagent are added. Incubation and color development proceed for about 30 minutes and colorimetric readings are taken just before the tubes reach the end of the top section where they tilt over to empty. This tube transport system is mechanically reliable, and failure of this feature is almost unheard of. Details can be seen in Fig. 10-3.

The sampling system consists of a carousel or sample wheel that will hold sixty samples. Each 90 seconds it advances a new cup into the sample position. At that time an arm swings over the cup and a sample probe slides forward and lowers into the cup. The sample that is picked up will depend on how many tests have been ordered. The arm now moves over the slat of ten test tubes and the pickup probe proceeds to deliver serum into the tubes corresponding to the tests that were ordered. At the end of the delivery cycle, the probe lowers into a wash cup where it is washed, inside and out. Vacuum and air pressure control sy-

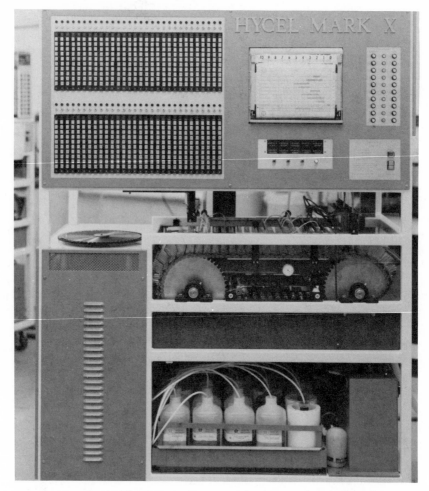

Fig. 10-2. Mark X automated chemistry system. (Courtesy Hycel, Inc.)

ringes or pistons that move the arm and the probe and also cause pickup and delivery of samples. A complicated system of relays is used to control the command system, telling the probe how much sample to pick up and where to deliver it.

The reagent delivery system transfers a predetermined quantity of reagent from the reservoir in the bottom of the machine to the reaction tube by way of a preset syringe at the back of the Mark X. These syringes are operated by vacuum and air pressure at the command of a relay in the control system and function only when that test is ordered. Delivery tubes for the

reagents are directly over the reaction tubes. If reagent is added directly after serum is introduced, it will be in contact with the sample for about 30 minutes. If it is introduced in the position prior to the colorimeter, it will react for only 90 seconds. On older systems reagent syringes gave problems after wear set in. The newer syringes seem to be excellent.

When the tubes arrive at the readout position, a colorimeter bar lowers ten probes into the respective reaction tubes and draws the colored test solutions into glass cells located between small exciter lamps and photocells. A switching arrangement

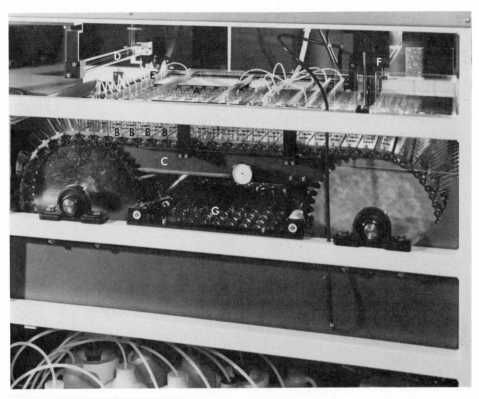

Fig. 10-3. Closer view of the Mark X: *A*, reaction tubes; *B*, slats with 10 tubes each; *C*, water bath; *D*, sample arm; *E*, reagent lines; *F*, colorimeter bar with pick-up tubes; *G*, reaction tubes in wash position. (Courtesy Hycel, Inc.)

sequentially directs the output of each cell to the recorder, where a pen draws a line corresponding to the absorbance of that solution. The recorder paper is especially printed to assign an area on the paper to correspond to each test in the sequence that the colorimeter reads. The pen draws across a scale of values for the test that it is recording. A shaded area on each scale indicates normal values. The chart looks similar to the Technicon chart shown in Fig. 10-1. After the test is read, the colorimeter bar discards the solution and purges itself in preparation for the next sample. Movement of the bar and displacement of fluids are by vacuum and air pressure.

On the front of the Mark X there are two panels of buttons. There are eleven of these buttons for each sample entered.

One button orders all tests to be done on this sample. The other ten provide for ordering individual tests selectively. Depressing the buttons sets a complicated series of relays in the command system. These tell the sample system where serum is to be delivered and commands the reagent system to deliver as indicated.

Baths are provided for the tubes during the reaction cycle. These are lowered away from the tubes each time the tubes are moved forward and raised again when movement stops. While the tubes are in the inverted position, they are drained, washed, rinsed, and dried.

This summarizes at least the salient features of the Mark X. The system functions extremely well, mechanically, with almost no down time or problems. The chemistry tests have to be selected from those not requiring deproteinization and this is a handicap. Also, only forty samples per hour can be processed. This would not be a disadvantage in any but the larger laboratories, and the economy of performing only those tests that are ordered is an attractive feature. This also allows tests to be done even if inadequate serum sample would preclude an entire profile. Hycel has established an enviable reputation for service, and these systems are rarely down for any significant time.

The discrete nature of each test provides a definite advantage over the flowing-stream idea, in my opinion. The lack of mechanical means of reliably measure and move samples and reagents has kept discrete systems from developing, but these deficiencies seem now to have been largely overcome by the introduction of new types of metering pumps, valves, etc. New discrete systems are in advanced stages of development and some of these will surely become very popular. Some of these will be discussed presently.

Hycel Corp. has more recently introduced an advanced model called the **Mark XVII**. This instrument has added a flame photometer and has increased the channels to sixteen (one test is calculated). The flame photometer's very compact burner assembly is located at the right end of the chassis after the readout block. It is mounted in such a way as to allow it to swing out to one side, for better access to the readout block. A small propane tank is mounted at the back and the compressed air supply built into the instrument for operation of the reagent system is used as an oxidant for the flame. The electronics of the flame system is built into the main central electronic system over the tube transport system.

Rather than have one small exciter lamp for each channel, there is one larger lamp with fiberoptic "light pipes" that carry the light to the sample. Also, the reagent

storage area is refrigerated and thus prevents the time-consuming chore of refrigerating leftover reagents at the end of each run.

The sample volume has been reduced. On the Mark X, 1.4 ml of serum was required for ten tests. On the Mark XVII, 1.19 ml is sufficient for the seventeen tests. There is a saving in reagents because of the decrease in reactant volume, of course.

There are eighteen sets of zero and standard calibration knobs to be used for setting these values for each test and a blank. On the Mark X there are ten sets. This advanced instrument is designed to accept a sample identification label that is machine readable. Sample ID systems are discussed in the next chapter.

At this time there has not been enough evaluation of the Mark XVII to provide basis for a reasonable judgment of its ultimate position in the field of automated chemical systems. Many laboratory directors have felt a little overwhelmed by the constant parade of newer, more sophisticated, and more expensive systems and have delayed changing expensive first-generation automation for more expensive second-generation equipment for fear of obsolescence when the ever more sophisticated and expensive third generation arrives. This dilemma has probably affected the market for automated chemistry equipment to a considerable extent.

Another recent innovation is the **Programachem 1040** produced by **American Monitor Corp.** This is a system designed to run one method at a time but to convert to other methods very quickly with a few simple steps. A punched program card is used to select the proper reagents, volume of serum, mode of operation, reagent volume, sequencing of reagent dispensing, mixing, incubation time, temperature, etc. After insertion of the program card, the wavelength and standard value are selected and the selector switches are depressed opposite sample cups. Reports are printed out on a tape showing sample number, type of test, results, and reporting units. Printout is at the rate of fifteen tests per minute.

For some situations the Programachem 1040 would be an ideal solution to high-volume work problems. Some tests can be performed at the rate of 1040 tests per hour and changeover is quite rapid. Perhaps the task of profiling a large number of analyses of several types might be done more easily on a profiling system such as Technicon's SMA 12 or Hycel's Mark X. This instrument does appear to be very well conceived and well engineered.

Beckman Instruments' DSA 564 is a model that supersedes the Model 560 which has been operated successfully for the past few years in an appreciable number of laboratories. The two instruments are quite similar but the 564, of course, is modified to improve operation and give added flexibility. This is a modular instrument in that a number of functions can be added rather easily by adding pipetting towers, deproteinizing module, etc. The system is built around a reaction cup transport system. Samples are transferred from a carousel into cups at the first station, and a diluent is flushed through to rinse the delivery tip. After this, reagents may be added at any point. Cups come into contact with a temperature-control block and travel on top of it for a predetermined period of time. At the end of the run, probes remove the test and blank and draw them into the flow cells of a double-beam ratio-recording interference colorimeter.

This is a micro system, capable of doing many of the tests on 20 microliters. This is an economy as far as reagents are concerned but the volume is almost never small enough to utilize a fingerstick to obtain the necessary sample. Thus it has the disadvantages of a micro system without the ultimate advantage.

The entire system is computer controlled, after the initial setup, by a PDP 8 computer which also has some data-handling capability and some quality control function.

The DSA 564 has not had an excessive amount of down time or repair and seems to function well mechanically. More than one channel can be set up at one time and the system can be changed over to additional methods. The changeover is not difficult but requires several manual manipulations. The system is apparently liked by users but it shows little evidence of becoming one of the most widely used systems.

E. I. DuPont de Nemours & Co., Inc., has had the **Automatic Clinical Analyzer (ACA)** on the market for some time (Fig. 10-4). This system takes an approach to chemistry automation that is different than any other system on the market. The reagents are prepackaged in a small plastic package or kit, which acts as a reaction vessel as well as a cuvette for reading the colorimetric test at the end of the run. These units are remarkably complex packages as may be seen in Fig. 10-5. Serum samples are placed in rectangular sample cups and a card on the side of the cup is filled out with the test identification. Anything written on the card is photographically reproduced on the final report form. The analytical packs, for the tests requested, are entered in the rack directly behind the serum sample. Each pack header carries a binary code that identifies the test for the analyzer and instructs it as to the steps it is to take with this method. As soon as the system is activated, a sample is picked up by a needle and injected into the test pack or packs as they advance into proper position. Detailed steps of the analytical operation will vary with the test pack in question. In a typical situation using a chromatographic column, the diluent is injected into the column immediately after the sample. From the filling position the pack is carried by a transport system through the various steps involved—

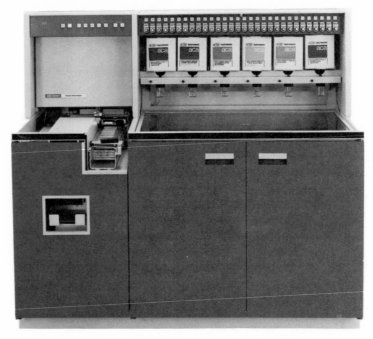

Fig. 10-4. Automatic Clinical Analyzer. (Courtesy E. I. DuPont de Nemours & Co., Inc.)

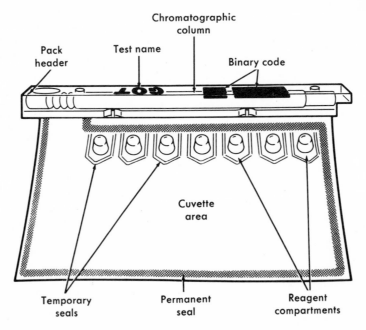

Fig. 10-5. The "pack" used on the Automatic Clinical Analyzer. (Courtesy E. I. DuPont de Nemours & Co., Inc.)

which may be preheating, breaking of various seals between reagent packs, mixing, incubation, and finally reading of absorbance value. An area of the pack is designed in such a way that the thickness remains constant at 1 cm during reading. The material is transparent and optically consistent. Absorbance is read through this area in an interference filter colorimeter. Results are printed out on a report slip that carries a photographic image of the identification information written on the sample label.

This is, of course, a very simplified explanation of an intricate process performed by a highly engineered instrument. The precise planning and construction of all details, from the pack design to the photograph processing of labels, is fascinating to the student of automation. The system had a slow start in the laboratory market as the system evolved and problems were solved. Reliability at this point seems to be high and comparisons of test results with other methods indicates good accuracy and reproducibility. A self-check system detects many potential errors in instrument operation. The computer monitors processing sequence and acts as a command center for initiating steps in each test cycle. It also processes the photosignal and converts it to a digital test result.

This is a highly automated method in which the operator has very little to do with the actual processing of the test. One would suppose that a person could be trained to operate the ACA in a short time with relative safety if the system was already in reliable operation. There is no extensive start-up procedure, operational check-off, or standardization run prior to the start of actual sample testing. Cost of supplies would make the ACA expensive to use to profile several tests on each patient. For certain situations, such as performance of stat cholinesterase tests at night, the cost of supplies would be completely offset by the saving of the work

time of a skilled technician. Approximately sixty tests are done per hour on the average, and elapsed time averages 7 minutes. About thirty methods are available. As a stat instrument for a large hospital, this would seem to be an excellent choice.

Instrumentation Laboratory, Inc., and **Harleco** have collaborated in a small, economical semiautomated system called the **Clinicard Analyzer.** This system uses a plastic, three-part cuvette with reagents in a kit form to do several chemistry tests in a partially automated fashion. Most methods have some manual manipulations to prepare the cuvette and reagents for insertion in the instrument. A punch card, when inserted, controls the amount of standard and specimen pipetted, wavelength, type of reaction (sequence of cuvette reading), and selection of computer program for calculations and sets an "error limit" at which an alarm sounds. Coding on the cuvette determines the temperature and time of incubation. The cuvette is manually placed in the incubator and removed to the colorimeter. The colorimeter has a quartz iodide lamp and five interference filters and the detector is a photodiode. Three readout modes are available. In the *standard mode* the test is read against a blank and standard. In the *reference mode* the test and blank are read against an arbitrary reference signal. In the *rate mode* the reaction cuvette is monitored for 1 minute and the electric signals for the last 48 seconds are averaged and used to determine enzyme rate reactions. All photosignals are processed through the computer program and results presented on a Nixie tube readout as digital concentration units or International Enzyme Units.

The system is new and has not had extensive routine use. It would seem that the system lacks the degree of automation of the larger, more expensive instruments and the cost, per test, of cuvettes and reagents is rather high. No doubt this sort of low-cost system would speed work and provide more reproducible results, especially where trained personnel are in short supply. At this moment about ten tests are available for the system. It is too early to make a judgment of its operation.

MORE HIGHLY AUTOMATED NEW SYSTEMS

Several advanced instrument systems for the automation of clinical chemistry are in late stages of planning and will, no doubt, be in routine use in the next 2 or 3 years. Technological developments are such that they come to market about as fast as books. The best I can do, in this case, is to present these systems with appropriate comments and hope that they indeed come to market, that they are not unduly altered, that he has had sufficient, good information and that his crystal ball is not cloudy.

Technicon Corp. has apparently nearly finalized plans for its **SMAC** system. The letters stand for Sequential Multiple Analyzer with Computer. This is a continuous-flow system in roughly the fashion of the SMA 12 and SMA 6, but the physical arrangement is much different and a great many innovations will provide faster and more accurate tests, more tests, less reagent consumption, and considerable computer control. The system is large in size and scope, and this brief summary must touch on only the more striking changes. Fig. 10-6 shows a prototype of this system.

The chemistry portion is enclosed in a cabinet about the size and shape of a large, two-door refrigerator with a small counter projecting at the front for the sampler. Individual cartridges are arranged like drawers above the sampler level in two tiers. There are twenty of these cartridges in the basic instrument with plans for two additional blocks with ten cartridges each.

The sampler takes up to nineteen carriers that hold eight samples each. Technicon's ID system is used to automatically recognize samples from a binary code on the labels. The sampler can search for the next sample if the rack is not filled. Serum samples are immediately diluted and bubbles are introduced. The diluted stream

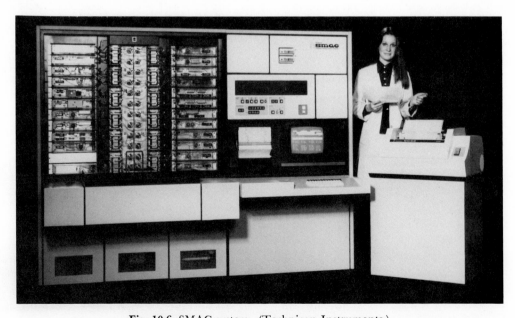

Fig. 10-6. SMAC system. (Technicon Instruments.)

now mounts to the various cartridge manifolds through a *riser* at the center of the system. At each level, part of the sample is drawn off by pumps on each cartridge. These pumps are quite small and are run by a common drive from a motor at the bottom. All lines are very small—about 1 mm in diameter. Dialyzers have a smaller bore to increase velocity, and a thinner membrane is used.

When the reaction is completed, the colored solutions pass through very small flow cells, which have a capacity of about 2 microliters. A common light source is used and light pipes (optical fibers) lead the light to the cuvettes. After the beam passes the cuvette, light pipes carry it to a common photomultiplier that continuously and sequentially monitors all channels. The bubbles are not removed from the stream of fluid, since the computer is able to recognize and disregard them. The computer takes the continuous scan of all cells and, from the composite information, selects significant information and calculates concentration or activities for each channel.

All of these results are printed out on a single report form. The computer is not designed for test data storage but controls all of the operation of the system, handles patient and test identification, and monitors for many sorts of errors and malfunctions. It also performs necessary calculations and reporting functions.

Sodium and potassium are to be analyzed by ion-selective electrodes rather than by flame photometry. A separate system has been designed and is being field-tested to measure pH, P_{CO_2}, sodium, and potassium by electrode. (See Fig. 10-7.) A dilution of the serum is made, presented to the electrodes, read, flushed out, and rinsed away. When all details are worked out, this system is to be incorporated in the SMAC. This would seem to be an attractive idea, since automated flame systems, in general, have had many maintenance problems. Unfortunately, the electrode technologies are not without problems. If this system can be made to work reliably, it will be a most worthwhile contribution to instrumentation.

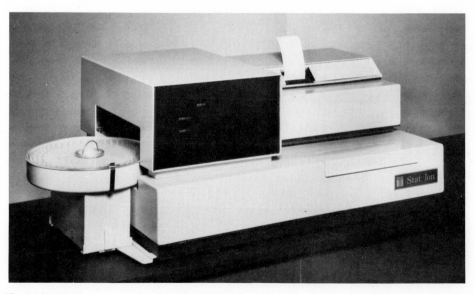

Fig. 10-7. Stat Ion system for flameless determination of sodium, potassium, chloride, and CO_2. This automated system will use ion-selective electrodes for all four parameters. (Courtesy Technicon Instruments.)

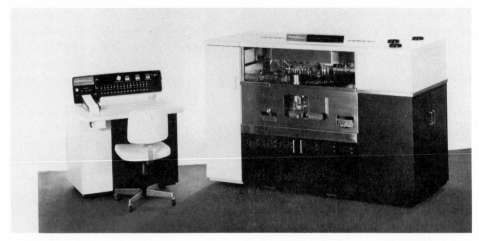

Fig. 10-8. AcuChem Advanced Automated Chemistry System. (Courtesy Ortho Diagnostic Instruments.)

The SMAC system is highly automated, and contains many innovations and many engineering successes. The system is not ready for mass distribution as this is being written, and it may be some time before it is. It should be a valuable tool to the highly automated laboratory when it is ready. Technicon's fine engineering and maintenance capabilities guarantee that it will be a functional, practical instrument. It will not be without competition, however.

Ortho Diagnostic Instruments is well along with plans for the **Acu-Chem Microanalyzer** (Fig. 10-8). The features of this system that seem different and possibly advantageous are listed here.

1. The idea of using a very small sample for many tests. They propose to do this by diluting 200 microliters of serum to 4 ml with water and then passing it through a stream splitter to various channels. The splitter exerts equal pull on tubes of different size to arrive at proper fractionation of the diluted sample.

2. Reagent dispensing and measuring is rather complicated. Air pressure pushes a stream of fluid through a tube to a point at which a photo-

sensor detects it and activates the reversal of a double-diaphragm valve that closes to interrupt the stream. The segregated sample is then blown into the sample by air pressure. This system is unique. In principle it should work well but it is untried.

3. The photometer arrangements are interesting. There is a sort of photometer tree. One quartz-iodide light source provides the beam, via quartz fiber optics, to five cuvettes. Fluid is passed into a cuvette and allowed to stabilize before the reading is made. Cuvettes from 10 to 50 mm in path length may be used. All channels on this tree are chopped at different frequencies and fed to the same detector, along with a reference beam. After mixing and amplification the signals are decoded and converted to give concentration values.

4. Standard values are dialed in at the console before standards are introduced. The system equates the light signal from the standard with the value introduced and compares samples to these standards.

5. It is not possible to select a different test pattern for each sample with any

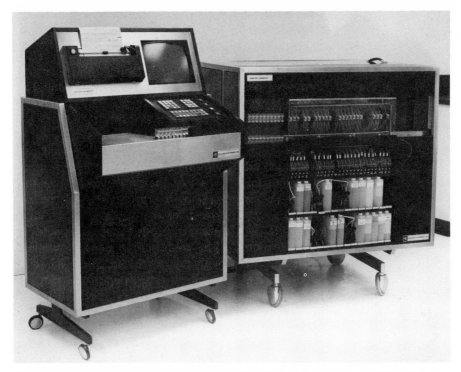

Fig. 10-9. New ACS (Automated Chemistry System). (Courtesy Coulter Electronics.)

practicality, but controls can be set for a pattern of tests to be done on a series of samples. Then the pattern can be changed for another series. This is somewhat less desirable than test-by-test selectivity, obviously.

6. Specimen ID number is printed out with concentration values. This is the work list number introduced at the console panel.

7. Two-point automatic calibration is offered.

8. Automonitoring is continuous and visual and audible signals show malfunctions. I believe that work with the system will be needed, to see how effective it is.

9. Chemistry tests offered are all standard, and sixteen methods are available.

This system is quite innovative and several of the ideas seem interesting. Some

features would seem to present developmental problems that may require considerable work before the AcuChem is ready for mass distribution.

The **ACS (Automated Chemistry System) of Coulter Corp.** (Fig. 10-9) is possibly somewhat further advanced than the SMAC or the Acu-Chem system. At this writing, the first production models are being shipped. This system is to be operated almost entirely by computer after the association of the sample with the patient information. There are twenty-two chemistry channels, one of which is a blank. All tests done on one sample will require 1.6 ml of serum and will require 29 minutes from introduction of sample to printout. A new sample may be introduced each minute. Tests may be individually selected from the entire profile, and the time for a single test will depend on its location in the testing train. Thus a blood sugar or a sodium-potassium test could be done as a stat in 5 or 6 minutes. The reason for this will become apparent as the system is described.

The system consists of two movable consoles. The first is the electronic console with the computer functions and the second is the processing console with all of the chemistry equipment. The electronic console is about 30 by 42 inches and stands at counter height. There are a keyboard and a CRT screen in the top and a gate for sample identification. Each sample rack has binary code at each cup position, which can be read by the processor electronically. The rack is placed in the identification bridge. As patient identification is entered on the keyboard, it appears on the screen for checking against the request slip. The test requests are entered and checked for correctness. When this brief procedure is finished, the sample rack is placed in the processing module. Racks can be stacked so that new samples can be continuously added. The rack is picked up by a transport, which carries it along a track below the sampling heads. There is a 1-minute delay between sampling positions. Tests that require the longest time are sampled first. Those that can be completed quickly are near the end of the transport's track. If there is no rack in the transport that would interfere, a new rack can be inserted at any point along the transport and it will be sampled as it comes to the appropriate sample head. These heads are computer controlled and sample is picked up only if it is programmed in. Sample measurement is by segmented-stream in a manner similar to that described for the Coulter Model S. The segmented sample is drawn into the reagent stream by Venturi action and deposited with reagents in the reaction tube. These tubes are carried along in a transport mechanism similar to the one described for the Mark X. The volume of reagent is between 3 and 5 ml per test. Reagent addition, mixing, incubation, and sampling at the colorimeter are all performed by mechanical methods controlled by computer. Most mechanical functions are pneumatic.

The colorimeters use a small exciter lamp like that used in the Model S for each cuvette. There is an interference filter for each and a silicon photocell as a detector. The cuvettes use a combination of a sort of windshield wiper effect and air blast to eliminate carry-over.

All of the fluid handling in the ACS is similar to the very excellent pneumatic system of the Model S, using air and vacuum controlled by valves and solenoids. The combination of this excellent system with the proved accuracy and reliability of Coulter's segmented-stream sample measuring should prove very effective.

The computer in the electronic console takes care of calibration and blanking. Standard values are entered on the keyboard at the time the standard solution is in the identification gate, and the computer is advised that these are standards. All samples are then automatically read against these values. Blanking is similarly performed. The computer has various other operational functions such as warning of impending depletion of reagents and unacceptable deionization of water by the built-in deionizer.

Reports are printed out at the electronic console and may be passed directly to the Status I computer, which will be discussed in a separate chapter. The report contains the identification information previously entered, the result of each test ordered in units of concentration or activity as indicated, and the time the analysis was completed. The normal report is about 7 by $4\frac{1}{2}$ inches and is suitable for charting.

This discrete sample, computer-controlled system is extremely impressive. It is too early to make a valid judgment about it but the excellent planning, engineering, and maintenance of this company would recommend this as a system to watch.

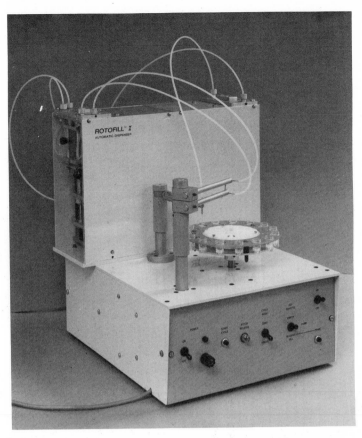

Fig. 10-10. Rotofill I, the dispensing unit for the Rotochem. (Courtesy American Instrument Co.)

Three companies have approached the automation of chemistry tests from a different direction. These three have introduced centrifugal systems that spin sample and reagents to provide a fast mixing and reaction rate. Reactants are thrown by centrifugal action into transparent cuvette areas toward the periphery of the rotor. A light directed through this area is absorbed by each sample solution as its cuvette passes between exciter lamp and detector. Each photosignal produces a peak, which is displayed on an oscilloscope screen. These peak heights are evaluated by a computer and translated into digital concentration or activity units.

All three centrifugal units operate on essentially the same principle and most

details of the systems are the same. Each has a pipettor that loads serum samples and reagents into the rotor (Fig. 10-10). Each has a small computer system and printout that produces a report giving sample number and digital results. All of the systems use samples between 1 and 50 microliters and a total reagent volume of 250 to 500 microliters. Since there are so many similarities, it is easier to consider a few differences.

The **GEMSAEC** is produced by **Electro-Nucleonics, Inc.,** and was invented at the Oak Ridge National Laboratories by Dr. Norman Anderson. This unit has a 15-place head. A 4K, PDP-8 computer is used for computation. The spectrophotometer uses a high-quality diffraction grating with

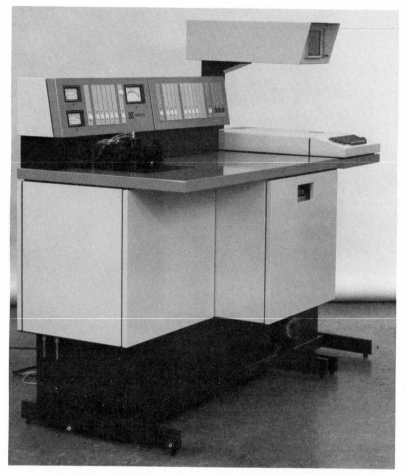

Fig. 10-11. Rotochem system. (Courtesy American Instrument Co.)

a band pass of 5 nm. The spectral range is from 320 to 785 nm. Printout is by teletypewriter.

The **Union Carbide Centrifuchem system** can handle thirty samples at one time. The spectral range is 340 to 720, using interference filters. A special-purpose computer is used and printout is by a digital printer.

The **Rotochem,** produced by the **American Instrument Co.** (Fig. 10-11), has a rotor with fifteen positions. Programming is by magnetic tape cassette and the computer is an 8K, PDP-8 unit. Reporting is by teletypewriter. The spectrophotometer uses grating ruled at 600 lines/mm and spectral

range from 200 to 800 nm. A nice feature of this system is its ability to rinse and dry the rotor automatically in place on the centrifuge.

A closer scrutiny of these systems would reveal other differences, of course. The Rotochem is the most expensive of the three and the Centrifuchem the lowest in price. These prices probably reflect the differences in the type of components offered, more than quality. A number of these systems are in use and users, in general, are pleased with their performance.

Analysis by these systems is very rapid once the sera are separated from the clots, in the cups, and identified. Two of the systems do only fifteen samples at a time while the other does thirty. Only one type of test can be done at a time. Conversion to another method is fairly fast, requiring from 1 to 5 minutes. In spite of the claims of speed for these systems, I doubt that these systems will save an appreciable amount of time in actual laboratory use. Actual analysis is not the most time-consuming part of most automated procedures. Sample handling, setting up, transposing data, etc. take more time and it does not appear that these systems are substantially superior in this regard.

There are numerous other automated systems that have received attention in the past few years. A complete listing of these would be time-consuming, and an adequate description of each would require a separate book. Mention is made here of a few other systems. The **AGA Corp.** distributes a very elaborate system called the **Auto Chemist.** This instrument is produced in Sweden. It performs about 135 samples per hour and has a large repertoire of procedures. It is a highly computerized system. Total cost is nearly $500,000. Operating costs are reputed to be low. There are only a few of these in use in the United States. The **Medi-Computer Corp.** is the American distributor for the **Vickers Multi-Channel 300 Automated Analysis system,** which is produced in England. It is capable of processing up to 300 samples per hour and is capable of simultaneously performing sixteen determinations. This is a modular arrangement and in the **300-M** configuration there are ten modules interconnected. A small computer controls the operation of all modules and handles all computations, reporting results on two teletypewriters. The system seems quite complex. The system is just now being presented in many areas of United States. **Joyce-Loebl & Co., Ltd.,** of England also has a system which is much less automated, called the **Mecolab Clinical Laboratory Analysis system.** In the United States it

is distributed by **Tech/OPs Instruments.** This is a single-channel modular system. Switching from one method to another is rapid and easy. **Cecil Instruments,** another English company, produces a less automated system called the **CE 404 Colorimeter system. Bausch & Lomb Analytical Systems Division** produces an **Automatic Sample Processor** that can be used in conjunction with their **Spectronic 400** spectrophotometers. Perkin-Elmer Corp., Honeywell, and various other companies distribute systems that contribute something to the automation of clinical chemistry.

An interesting semiautomated chemistry system, just introduced as this goes to press, is the **Kiess DMA-16/P,** which does sixteen chemistry tests and a prothrombin time. Prepackaged reagents are sealed into a cuvette. The sample and other reagents, in some cases, are added. After mixing, incubation, etc. as required, the tube is inserted in the cuvette well and the button for that test is pressed. Automatically the correct filter is chosen, photosignal electrically compared to a stored standard signal, and the test result reported on an electronic digital display in appropriate units.

The prothrombin timer is automatically activated when plasm is added to the reaction tube, and results are shown on digital display when the clot occurs.

This unit is remarkably small to have the automatic features it contains. Fig. 10-12 shows the unit, which is only about 14 by 18 inches and 4 inches high. No reports of any kind are available on the performance of this unit, at this time. Since this is entirely new, one would anticipate some problems. The concept looks good for the very small laboratory where well-trained personnel are not available.

ENZYME SYSTEMS

There is some question about the logic of discussing enzyme systems in the chapter on chemistry automation. Most of these systems are not very highly automated. For

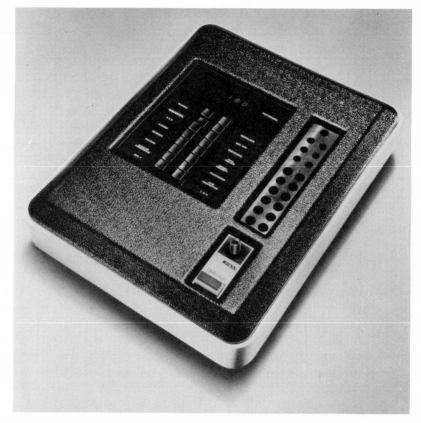

Fig. 10-12. DMA 16/P Blood Analyzer. (Courtesy Kiess Instruments, Inc.)

lack of a better place to present this material as a single subject, let it be considered here.

An enzyme is a protein material that is able to catalyze a chemical reaction. In an appreciable number of cases the rate of reaction and thus the concentration or activity of the enzyme, are measured by the change of nicotinamide adenine dinucleotide (NAD) to its reduced form (NADH) or the reverse reaction (NADH to NAD). At 340 nm NADH absorbs light strongly, but NAD absorbs much less. Hence the change of absorbance at 340 nm is a good measure of NAD/NADH conversion. Most of the enzyme systems discussed here are instruments set up to measure absorptivity change at 340 nm during a timed interval. In some cases, different wavelengths may be

chosen to facilitate measurement of other reactions. Some of these instruments were designed for routine photometry and adapted for some degree of automation of enzymes; and others were primarily enzyme analyzers, to which end-point colorimetric functions were added.

The Gilford Instrument Laboratories were probably the first to introduce some measure of automation to enzyme analysis. The first steps in this direction involved using a Beckman DU monochromator for the isolation of the 340 nm light beam. This light was directed through cuvettes in a sample changer capable of alternately moving four cuvettes, in sequence, into the light path. A photomultiplier detected the absorbance value and a recorder drew a short line each time a cell was positioned

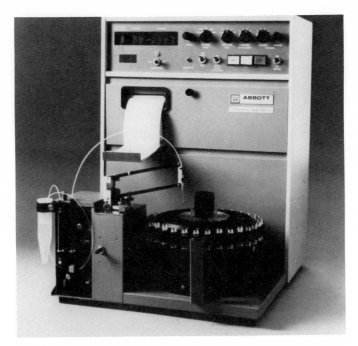

Fig. 10-13. Bichromatic Analyzer (ABA-100). (Courtesy Abbott Scientific Products Division.)

for a short interval. Between cells, the recorder pen returned to base line. The recording, after a number of cycles of the sample changer, showed a progressive change of absorbance readings for each of the samples. A straight line, drawn through the pen traces corresponding to each sample, produced slope lines that could be used to figure ΔA per minute and hence enzyme activity for each of the samples. Thus more than one reaction rate could be measured with a single photometer and recorder at the same time. A number of other refinements were included in this system but the basic concept was one of looking at more than one reaction at the same time, using one set of basic equipment. This is the concept of **Gilford Instrument Laboratories, Inc., Model 2000 Multiple Sample Absorbance Recorder.**

Since the time of their first system, Gilford Instrument Laboratories has produced many instruments and modifications. Their current enzyme system is modular

and is built around the Model 300 spectrophotometer described earlier. In its most complete and most automated form the system is called the **3400 Automatic Enzyme Analyzer.** Prepipetted samples are placed in a test tube rack in a temperature-controlled bath. An automatic dispenser adds a predetermined amount of substrate, after which the test is mixed by an air blast and permitted to pass through a predetermined lag phase. A probe then picks up the sample and draws it into the spectrophotometer, where readings are taken every 10 seconds, for 2 minutes. The six data points of the first minute are subtracted from those of the second minute. This absorbance change is multiplied by a factor that has previously been determined and entered in the calculating circuitry. The enzyme activity is then printed out in whatever units have been chosen. Up to a hundred tests can be run in this manner, virtually without operator attention after the initiation of the test run. Temperatures can be changed, lag phase can be selected, sampling times can be programmed and various multipliers can be used to produce the reporting unit desired. The spectrophotometer, as noted earlier, has a wavelength range of 340 to 700 nm to accommodate various kinetic reactions.

Abbott Scientific Products Division has introduced a system that is primarily aimed at kinetic enzyme reactions but is also able to do end point reactions. This instrument is called the **ABA-100** (Abbott Bichromatic Analyzer) (Fig. 10-13). It is called a bichromatic analyzer because absorbance measurements at two wavelengths are used for each reading. The difference in absorbance at the two wavelengths is designated as A_d. The change in A_d between the initiation of the reaction and each timed repetitive reading determines the rate of reaction and hence the enzyme activity. This bichromatic approach is used to minimize the effects of turbidity, hemoglobin, protein, etc.

Since an absorbance sensitivity of 0.0001 A is acheived and temperature control is about 0.1° C, very slight changes in absorbance are significant, and a shorter reaction time can be achieved. Reactions take place in a round 32-section plastic disposable cuvette. The lamp is in the center and, as the cuvette rotates, light passes successively through each section. The cuvette normally makes one complete revolution in 5 minutes, dwelling at each cuvette for 9.6 seconds. In the normal mode a sample of 5 microliters of serum is picked up from a sample cup and washed into a cuvette section with 250 microliters of substrate. A 5-minute period is required for this operation initiating thirty-one test reactions and one blank. When the cycle is completed, absorbance readings are taken each cycle (every 5 minutes) for as long as the operator needs to satisfy himself of linearity. Absorbance changes (A_d changes) are printed out and can be compared for each sample to assure linearity of reaction (zero

order of kinetics). In another mode, a single sample can be held in one position and readings taken at 15- or 30-second intervals.

An end point mode is also included. In this mode, a single absorbance reading can be made after 5 minutes, or at 10 or 20 minutes. In all cases, the computer circuits built into the system can calculate concentration or enzyme activity units in whatever terms required. A blank correction is routinely done automatically. A tungsten-halide lamp is used as a source and interference filters are provided. About 100 kinetic reactions can be read in an hour. This system has been in use for some time. It has proved itself to be accurate, reproducible, trouble-free, and rapid. Most users have been pleased with its operation. In addition to the enzyme determinations, it has been primarily used for stat glucose and BUN tests.

The **Zymat 340,** produced by **Bausch & Lomb Analytical Systems Division,** has a sample carousel that fits into the center of a larger cuvette wheel. A sampling probe picks up a sample, which may be as small as 0.2 ml and transfers it to the corresponding cuvette. Two reagents may be added through separate syringes. The serum mixture is allowed to come to equilibration for 12 minutes while the carousels make a complete cycle before the substrate is added. After an appropriate interval, measurement begins and is printed out at 50 and 100 seconds as activity in International Units. The sample wheel holds forty-seven samples and the total elapsed time to run one load is 108 minutes. The double-beam filter photometer uses a photomultiplier as a detector. Reference and sample beams pass through separate 340 nm filters. No reagent or substrate blank is used in the reference beam.

Photovolt Corp. produces an **Enzyme Rate Analyzer** called the **ERA II** (Fig. 10-14), which automates only the reading and calculations of enzyme testing. Serum and substrate are mixed and placed in the ERA

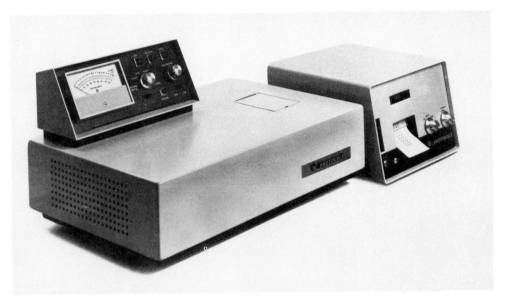

Fig. 10-14. Enzyme Rate Analyzer (ERA II). (Courtesy Photovolt Corp.)

II along with an appropriate blank. A 15-second delay for equilibration is allowed, after which timing begins. After 15 or 60 seconds a second reading is taken and the $\Delta A/T$ is converted to units of choice and printed out. The instrument is calibrated against controls of known activity. The very short time span is possible because of the 0.0001 A sensitivity of the photometer, according to the company. Temperature equilibration is available, using an external circulating water bath, and the company suggests that this method of operation is favored. I would certainly agree with that. The ERA II would be a practical choice in a laboratory where large numbers of tests for the same enzyme are not anticipated.

FUTURE TRENDS IN CHEMICAL AUTOMATION

The automation of clinical chemistry procedures has occurred almost entirely within the past 15 years. The process seems to accelerate each year as more breakthrough occurs in electronics and other fields. Many of the techniques of space exploration have been translated into faster, smaller, more accurate instruments in other fields, and it is no accident that the fallout of the space program has been realized during the years of fastest development in laboratory automation. As mentioned earlier, some hesitancy is being noted on the part of administrators and laboratory directors to invest heavily in today's automation—in anticipation of next year's developments. Many thoughtful laboratory people are wondering what is the prudent course in the present situation.

Several points seem obvious. With almost 80% of laboratory expense relating to personnel costs, automation that saves any appreciable work time is a good investment. At the same time, one wonders at the logic of writing off the largest percentage of a $50,000 to $100,000 investment in 3 to 5 years because of obsolescence. This practice has been ingrained into our thinking. At the same time, the public is asking for increasing amounts of free or low-cost medical service. Public funding, however, seems almost inadequate to finance the service promised or desired. There is continuous criticism of the cost of medical services. Pressure on hospitals to cut costs is increasing at the same time that the demand for improved services is being voiced.

As we increase our capability to perform large numbers of atuomated tests, the demand for other tests is stimulated and there is often a lag period before these new tests are ordered in quantities sufficient to stimulate the production of automated equipment. Many people have tended to project the increase in total numbers of tests, types of analyses, etc.—to prophesy infinity in these areas. While progress will no doubt continue to be made, there is reason to doubt that straight-line projections of laboratory activity are valid. Most explosions of knowledge ultimately tend to simplify problems rather than render them more complex.

The roles of computers and data handling in the laboratory have not yet been discussed but it is difficult to think about the future of laboratory automation without taking their influence into account.

As more data is accumulated, more time is consumed also in identifying patients, collecting blood, and processing and reporting information. It would seem, then, that the most fruitful field for development would be in these areas. The next chapter will point out that automated devices for fast processing of requests, more certain and rapid patient and sample identification, and faster data handling are being built into complex systems that integrate with chemistry, and other, processors. This would seem to be the immediate direction of development. Many of these devices are modular in concept but flexible enough to tie in to different configurations.

It would seem that the best system will be the one that can handle the largest volume of tests the most rapidly and that is the most flexible, the most economical, and the most capable of automating the entire laboratory performance. Competition will probably largely eliminate systems that are not satisfactorily accurate or reliable. As time goes on, it seems imperative that preoccupation with numbers, volume, data flow, and techniques be overcome and that there be a thoughtful evaluation of the cost effectiveness of all this, as it relates to patient well-being and care. Maybe then we will start to differentiate many of the meaningful observations from the trivia.

REVIEW QUESTIONS

1. What is the function of the dialyzer in the Technicon AutoAnalyzer?
2. What is meant by discrete analysis?
3. What is the advantage of using a dialyzer in blood chemistry determinations?
4. Name three automated enzyme systems.
5. At what wavelength are most enzyme tests now done, and why?
6. What is continuous-flow analysis?
7. How does a peristaltic pump work?
8. Name four automated chemistry systems. Which are discrete sample analyzers?
9. How is carry-over avoided in the Auto-Analyzer?

11

Data handling and other automation

Everyone who has worked in clinical laboratories during the past decade has seen the phenomenal increase in laboratory work. The number of hospital beds has increased. The number of different tests that each laboratory can do has increased. The utilization of tests in diagnosis has exceeded all projections. With the automation discussed in the past two chapters, profiling of patient data has become an accepted procedure. It is not uncommon for each patient's laboratory record to contain forty to fifty bits of information, and this amount is often required as an admission profile. This mass of information presents problems of many kinds. It is much easier for mistakes to be made. Much time and space are required for filing and storage. The retrieval of information becomes a burdensome problem. Indeed, in a large hospital laboratory the ability to render fast accurate results is impaired by the very volume and diversity of tests. Obviously some means must be found to organize information and streamline communications if we are not to flounder in the rising sea of information.

PATIENT INFORMATION

Various devices for solving the problems of data handling have appeared. One of the most urgent problems is the correct identification of patient samples and reports throughout their processing, from collection through reporting to the doctor or on the patient's chart. Typically several people are involved in this process and many steps are taken. When blood is drawn, the wrong patient may be stuck or the tubes may be mislabeled in any of several ways. In the laboratory, blood or serum may go through one or more transfers to new tubes where identity must be maintained. Transferring to sample cups or

reaction vessels, pouring into cuvettes, and recording results may all be steps fraught with the possibility of error. Transposition in recording data is especially a source of error. Many studies of errors of this type have been made, and each study reports frightening figures. Most technical errors contribute some percentage of change in test results but a transcription error can raise the magnitude from bad to catastrophic. For example, a 50% error on a 40.0 mg% blood sugar would make it 60 mg%. A transcription error could make 40.0 mg% become 400. mg%, and heroic treatment would probably kill the patient.

Several systems of sample identification have been attempted. One of these is **Technicon Corporation's Sampler T 40** used with precoded cards bearing human- and machine-readable sequential identifying numbers. These cards are attached to the patient's serum sample and inserted into a card holder adjacent to the sample cup. A card reader in the sampler reads the coded six-digit number and stores it in an electronic buffer until it is printed out along with the test result. When a computer system is used, **Technicon's Computer Data Acquisition system** provides the means of printing out a complete report with the patient's name and other pertinent information.

The **PosIdent system** of **Hycel, Inc.,** has gone a step further by starting the

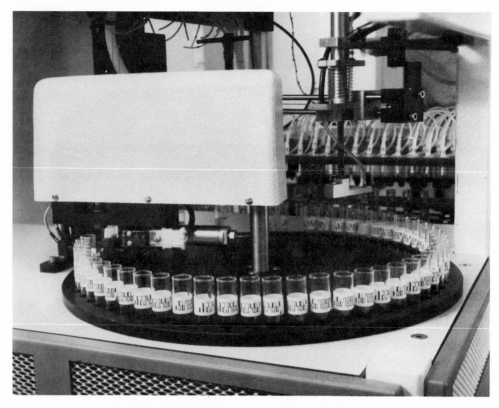

Fig. 11-1. PosIdent label reader. (Courtesy Hycel, Inc.)

identification procedure at the patient's bedside. This is a most promising development, since many errors are made at the time the sample is drawn or at least before the sample gets to the analyzer. The PosIdent provides for a patient wristband containing a packet of twenty labels bearing a preprinted, machine- and human-readable identifying number. When blood is drawn, one of these labels is attached to the blood tube, using a tube holder called a *go/no go* device, which positions the label so that a label reader can properly index it. When blood is centrifuged, the serum is left in the sample tube, which is transferred to the specially designed sampler carousel. As an alternate method the samples can be placed in a sample cup that can sit in the top of the original sample tube. In either case, the identifying number is read electronically and the num-

ber printed onto the recorder chart. Thus the identity is maintained from patient to report through all steps. The PosIdent label reader is pictured in Fig. 11-1.

American Science & Engineering Co. has recently introduced a device that looks promising. A plastic tag attached to the patient's wrist carries binary code of the patient's identifying information. At the time the blood is drawn the plastic tag is slipped into a hand-held encoder that is attached to a printer by a small cable. The encoder reads and transmits the identifying information to the printer, where a label is prepared.

None of these systems seems to give the ultimate in patient/sample identification but they are all very worthwhile, tentative steps toward the elimination of errors in identification and transposition. As this sort of device is perfected and adapted to the computer and multichannel analyzer, errors will, no doubt, decrease considerably.

SIMPLE DATA-HANDLING SYSTEMS

Several companies have produced a variety of devices that interface with automated equipment to convert analog information to a digital form and present it in some more usable form. Analog-to-digital converters with a printer or an electronic display are produced by several companies. **T & T Technology, Inc.,** produces systems designed to interface with an analyzer, convert analog signals to digital, and print out results, in any of several sequences, properly identified with the original sample. The **SMART** system is designed for the Technicon SMA analyzers. The **DART** system is used with the Hycel Mark X. **COURT** interfaces with the Coulter Model S hematology system. In each case a work list is prepared, using a teletype that will also punch a paper tape. Up to sixty characters may be used for patient identification. The paper tape is loaded into a tape reader associated with the analyzer and is indexed with the lead sample cup. As the testing cycle progresses, the ID information is printed out, in any desired format, along with test results. The commonest format used is a label that attaches to the recorder chart to show the ID information and values for each test under the corresponding tracing on the chart paper.

Another system is **Intec., Inc.'s, Tec-12 Analyzer Data Terminal.** A log of the work to be done is prepared, using a teletype. The teletype, in addition to typing the printed work list, also produces a machine-readable paper tape. This tape is loaded into a tape reader at the analyzer and indexed with the first test cups. Intec's Re-Tran Potentiometer receives the signal from the analyzer recorder and a typed label showing the patient's name, identifying information, and test result is prepared for attachment to the recorder tracing.

Hycel, Inc., has developed an accessory called **HYCOMP,** which allows their chemistry analyzers to be placed directly on line with a centralized hospital computer. The computer can then be accessible to more than one teletype and provide reporting service to remote locations. In addition to interfacing the analyzer and computer, the HYCOMP provides automatic calibration for the analyzers, automatic correction for drift, and automatic detection and correction for various interfering substances.

Infotronics, Inc., has developed a series of interfaces for automated systems, which print out results on tape labels. These are actually small computer systems dedicated to the instrument in question but able to perform many functions. The model **CRS-1000** is a very economical computer with a 16 K core in the CPU. It is designed to handle all kinds of analyzers and serve as a general-purpose calculator.

Nothing has been said about minicomputers such as the **Sony ICC 2500 W (Sony Corp. of America).** These devices are primarily high-level calculators capable of performing certain functions on data entered via the keyboard, using very limited stored information. They are convenient for situations in which a calculator would be heavily used. Presumably the average, routine clinical laboratory would have rather limited application for such a system if a good calculator were available.

COMPUTERS

Computers have become a way of life for most Americans. Many of our bills are prepared by computers; college class schedules are prepared and grades reported automatically. Airline reservations, business accounts, train schedules, and manufacturing routines are controlled by large data-handling computers. Although we take them for granted, it may be useful to review briefly why a computer might be of value in the laboratory and what functions it might serve there.

It has been widely reported that, in laboratory reports prepared by hand, there are errors in 10% of cases examined. No one wants to believe this of his own laboratories, but close examination always shows an appreciable number of mistakes of the sort that a computer would not make. Another widely reported statistic is that from 10% to 15% of laboratory revenue is lost as a result of billing documents being erroneous, illegible, or lost. In a properly operated computer installation, this sort of error would be almost nonexistent. We have already noted the volume of laboratory reports and the retarding effect that such volume tends to have on urgent reports. For all of these reasons and more, the computer would appear to be desirable, at least in situations where it can be economically justified.

Functions that the laboratory computer is generally supposed to serve are the following:

1. Processing of requisitions
2. Identification and label preparation
3. Preparation of work lists and organization of blood collection sequences
4. Automatic operation, correction, and control of analyzers
5. Collection of data
6. Collation of information and reporting in any of various forms
7. Record keeping
8. Quality control
9. Billing
10. Elimination of obviously erroneous reports
11. Storage of data

Not all systems perform all of these functions, and some may perform others. All of these, however, are within the capabilities of most systems. As discussion proceeds, it should become apparent that present methods of doing many of the above tasks

are poor and that automation can often improve the situation. This is not to say that all laboratories can justify the considerable expense or properly utilize these systems, however.

To consider the various systems and properly evaluate their possible utility, it is essential to understand a few rather simple terms. In these few pages it is quite impossible to present in detail the working of these complex, technical devices, but a quick review of some salient features and concepts seems necessary.

A computer is a mechanical and electronic system that is able to automatically control apparatus or processes of a complicated nature without human intervention. Most computers collect, process, store, and report data or information according to prescribed programs of instruction and may mechanically initiate or control mechanical devices in response to such data and instructions.

The heart of the computer is called the *central processing unit* (**CPU**). In this console are the circuits that control the translation and execution of coded instructions. There is also a section that performs the arithmetic and logic sequences, as well as a main storage unit for holding the instructions and data immediately being processed. If time were available to examine each step in each system, it would be found reasonably understandable. Obviously many things are happening simultaneously or in fast sequence and the total operation is quite complex. To simplify study of the functions of the CPU it might be said that the *control unit* consists primarily of various switching functions that choose between pathways within the system. The *storage unit* is composed of *registers,* each of which is made up of a large number of tiny magnetizable particles that can be given a positive or a negative charge to indicate 0 or 1. Each of these magnetic positions holds one *bit* of information. Since we are working with binary numbers, or numbers on a base 2 system, any number can be expressed in these terms. Letters can also be expressed by combinations of numbers. Every computer has a capacity to handle information in "words," which are groups of *bits* of a given size. These groups are called *bytes.*

In the *arithmetic and logic* unit various types of gates and circuits are supplied to perform specific functions. These devices consist primarily of semiconductor diodes and transistors in configurations that allow current to pass under specific conditions. An arrangement that allows a current to pass when two similar signals are presented is called an *AND gate;* one that will allow either of two signals to pass is called an *OR gate.* Similarly there are other types, such as not-and or *NAND gates* and not-or or *NOR gates.* This section also includes circuits that add, subtract, multiply, and divide.

Usually separate from the CPU there are various types of *terminals.* These are the devices that can send instructions to the CPU to initiate some process and/or to receive back information from the computer. These terminals may be *on-line,* which means they are connected in such a way that signals are directly conveyed, or they may be *off-line,* suggesting that someone must initiate the process of communication each time information is to be entered. Smaller computers have the capability of handling only a fairly small number of on-line terminals at any one time.

Terminals may be *input, output* or both input and output (I/O). They may also be *unit record devices* that may punch, read, sort, or list cards, etc. Also it is necessary to have storage on *magnetic discs* or *magnetic tapes* that are located in *external storage terminals.* While the CPU is performing some operation, it is usually necessary for it to store certain information externally for brief periods of time. This is done in *buffer storage.*

All of the devices so far considered above would be considered as *hardware* of the computer system. But the problem of putting data into storage and asking for information, solution of problems, retrieval of information, etc. must be accomplished in some manner. Words and numbers must be converted into some sort of code that the circuits and gates of the computer can act on. Also the instructions to the computer, as to what function or process is to be initiated, must be put into a code that the control unit can understand. All of this arrangement of codes, which is required to make the computer hardware functional, is called *software.* Each set of instructions that initiates a sequence of functions is called a *program,* and the person who prepares the program by converting human-readable problems into computer language is called a *programmer.* To simplify this preparation of machine-readable code several types of *"languages"* have been worked out. *Machine language* is the code the computer understands. *Low-level languages* are close to machine language and use *mnemonics,* or shortened forms of words. These abbreviations are usually specific for the system on which they are used. This sort of communication is called *assembly language. High-level* languages like *Cobol, Fortran,* and *ASCII* are closer to standard English and are adaptable to almost any computer. These languages are all *alphanumeric,* meaning that they include both numbers and letters of the alphabet.

A common error made by laboratory directors who are not well informed about computers is to assume that the best system for their laboratory is the one that has the finest hardware. In fact, the very best hardware is quite useless without software; and much hard work by programmers who understand the clinical laboratory thoroughly, is needed to make the system functional. For this reason, the best-known computers in the business world may be very poor choices for laboratories. In the following listing of a few computer systems for the clinical laboratory, an attempt has been made to include only those that have reasonable software for such use.

Turn-key operations or installations are those in which almost all responsibility for software and equipment maintenance resides with the vendor. It is my personal opinion that this sort of system is preferable in the hospital laboratory. Whereas it is true that we should always be prepared to learn as much as possible of other disciplines, to make our own more meaningful, it seems that the skills necessary for properly preparing and maintaining software are somewhat foreign to patient care and analytical procedures. Outside of research facilities, the time spent in computer operation could probably be better spent in activities more closely related to patient care. The weakness in this position, of course, is the fact that there are not many turn-key systems for clinical laboratories that are really tried and proved effective.

Several companies have advertised their capabilities in the hospital and medical laboratory field but a close examination of their advertising, in many cases, reveals very little in the way of software and specialized terminals for the routine clinical laboratory. In terms of total competence in the field of clinical laboratory computerization, DNA (Diversified Numeric Applications, Division of Avnet, Inc.) seems to have a slight edge. This company has designed a very complete laboratory system with highly specialized terminals for the input of manual and automated test results in hematology, chemistry, urinalysis, and bacteriology as well as a special SMA interface. Programs have been made for admission and discharge of patients, unfinished work, reporting, cumulative summaries, outpatient files, etc. to cover a great many of the laboratory functions that are amenable to computerization. It is quite obvious

that laboratory people have been intimately involved in planning of the software. *DNA's* systems are called *Uni-Lab Computer systems.* There are several configurations, varying from about $50,000 to $350,000 depending on the equipment involved.

Digital Equipment Corp. (DEC) has a computer called the **Clinical Lab-12.** This, like the DNA is a *dedicated system,* meaning a system that is totally dedicated to the laboratory and is not used by others. It uses a PDP-12 (12,000-word core memory) for the central processing unit. Storage is on a disc that can provide 524,288 bytes of memory. Each byte is twelve bits on this system. Two discs can be used with one CPU. Up to six teletype terminals or similar units can be accommodated. High-speed printer, tape unit, card reader, and interfaces to the Technicon Auto-Analyzer, Coulter Counter, Hycel Mark X, etc. are available. Programs include administrative update, patient inquiry, requisition entry, work sheet generation, accession number entry, summary reporting, test updating, and delete data as well as those necessary for analyzer interfacing. To protect the system from losing information during a power failure, magnetic tapes of all data are run twice a day and may be taken more often if a shutdown is expected.

The **Coulter Electronics, Inc.,** has recently entered the laboratory computer field with the **Status I system.** This system is a dedicated, time-sharing system using a PDP 8 for a CPU. The basic equipment is manufactured by the Digital Equipment Co. It will interface directly with the Coulter Model S Hematology system and the 22-channel Coulter Chemistry Analyzer. It would seem to be an advantage to interface analyzers and computers manufactured by the same company. Teletype terminals have CRT screens where information being entered is immediately checked for accuracy before being released into the computer.

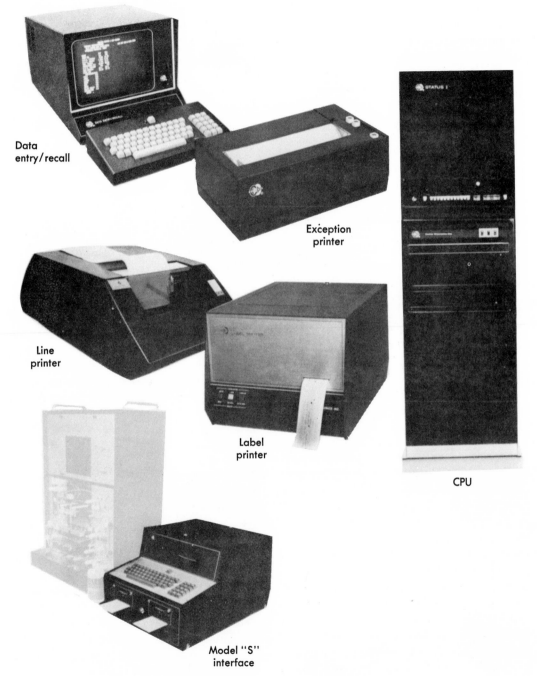

Data
entry/recall

Exception
printer

Line
printer

Label
printer

CPU

Model "S"
interface

Fig. 11-2. Status I computer system. (Courtesy Coulter Electronics, Inc.)

The system also has a high-speed line printer, a label printer, and an exception printer where reports that exceed prescribed limits may be printed out. Every patient entering the hospital is admitted to the Status I system immediately. Requisitions are entered as received. Labels are printed immediately on "Stats" or any tests to be made immediately. All others are stored and labels are printed on command—for example, at 6 A.M. for morning pickup. Labels are printed as a pickup list, with each nursing station printed separately with beds in sequence. A summary of Vacutainers required for each nursing station is also printed. Programs include census, available bed list, pickup list, requisition entry, and data entry for each department—including batteries, various summary reports, unfinished test reports, tests out of control, patient discharge, statistical counting, etc. The system is advertised as having capacity for a 1000-bed hospital with comfortable safety factors. A fail-safe system makes it impossible to lose complete data or program during a power failure. The concept of the system is to allow inquiry as to the status of any patient at any time via the teletype with CRT screen. This would seem to be a highly desirable feature. Fig. 11-2 shows the various components of the Status I system.

Spear Medical Systems, a Division of Becton, Dickinson & Co., has produced a system called **CLAS-300 B.** This is a large, sophisticated system with a very large capacity. The CPU is a 4 K memory of twelve-bit bytes, which can be expanded to 32 K. Storage can be on four magnetic tapes with 500,000-byte capacity in this optional unit. The random access disc has a storage capacity of 2,560,000 bytes and an extremely rapid access speed. Up to sixty-four devices can be selected and addressed by the CPU. A wide variety of interfaces and other terminals are available. Programs include all of those previously mentioned for other systems. This would seem to be

a system capable of almost any laboratory operation but rather expensive.

Many other companies have hospital systems with some attention paid to the laboratory. Most of these have limited software for laboratory or are otherwise limited. Technicon Corp. acquired Lockheed Aircraft Corp.'s Hospital Information Systems Division in 1971 and is working on improving the MIS-I system. This is a total hospital system but there will, no doubt, be much emphasis placed on the laboratory applications of the system as Technicon develops it. Xerox Corp. and Honeywell Corp. both have sophisticated hospital systems but have not gone heavily into laboratory-dedicated computers or laboratory software.

Several companies, including Addressograph Division of Addressograph Multigraph Corp., as well as Hewlett-Packard, have developed terminals that are able to read imprinted identification information and checked boxes on prepared forms. These are still subject to some problems but much progress is being made. When these devices become completely reliable, a great saving in work will be accomplished and almost any transaction can be made with the computer with very little effort expended.

AUTOMATION OF URINALYSIS

Several companies are known to be working on systems for automating the routine analysis of urine. It is amazing that this fairly simple, venerated set of tests should take so many years to automate. The problems, however, are somewhat larger than might be first imagined, since urine is anything but a simple solution. Seemingly simple reactions show interferences when automation is attempted. Thus urates, phosphates, drug metabolites, vitamins, and other substances cause problems that are either not recognized or are overcome by various manual procedures.

The only automated urinalysis system

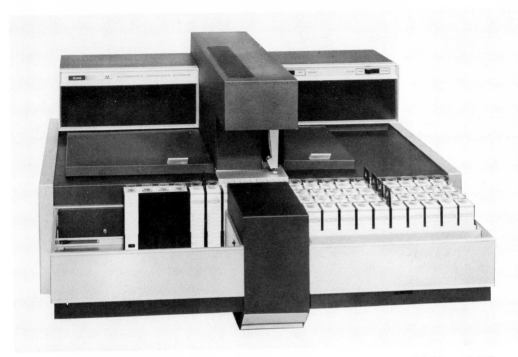

Fig. 11-3. Automated urinalysis system, Clinilab. (Courtesy Ames Co., Division of Miles Laboratories, Inc.)

that has had any appreciable success, at this writing, is **Ames Co.'s Clinilab.** This instrument tests seven parameters: pH, protein, glucose, ketones, bilirubin, occult blood, and specific gravity. All of these except the specific gravity are colorimetric reactions performed in a cellulose strip attached to a plastic background. Color is read by reflectance and translated into classic urine report format, which is printed out on an identification tag attached to each urine sample. Specific gravity is done by the falling-drop method familiar to most technologists but is read automatically. The chemistry tests are quite similar to the well known dipstick tests successfully used by Ames for many years. The output of this system can be fed directly to any computer and an interface is available to translate ID information into ASCII computer code. The Clinilab is still fairly new and there are a few interferences and lim-

itations that require occasional rechecking. Basically, however, the idea is sound and nearly all tests are more accurately performed than they would be by manual methods. Many human mistakes are certainly obviated. The system costs around $30,000, which would seem to make its use feasible in only the very large laboratories at this time. Almost certainly this system or one like it will come into routine use in due time, however, as the economics are worked out. The Clinilab system is pictured in Fig. 11-3.

AUTOMATION OF BACTERIOLOGY

Bacteriology has been an area that modern instrumentation and automation have bypassed until now. At the present time, however, a number of devices are being researched that would change bacteriology considerably and speed diagnosis. These vary from the very simple to the extremely sophisticated. A few of these are already reasonable and there are almost certainly a few that will never become practical. A quick review of these may suggest what the future may bring.

At the very simple end of the spectrum is a plating device that inoculates plates very rapidly and with absolute uniformity. A drop of inoculum is placed in a loop and the plate rotates as the loop moves from the center to the outer edge. Material is distributed in an Archimedes spiral in ever decreasing concentration.

Another chore of bacteriology that has been considerably simplified is the counting of colonies on a petri plate. This is a process that can be done electronically fairly easily. Although other companies have units performing the same task, it should be sufficient to review the **Artek Automatic Bacterial Colony-Counter system** produced by **Artek Systems Corp.** Colonies as small as 0.25 mm can be counted and the colonies may be as close as 0.5 mm to each other. The total plate count can be up to 999, and the time for the counting process is less than $\frac{1}{2}$ second. The report is an electronic digital display, but teletype is available and paper tape in ASCII code can be produced for off-line computer use. If large numbers of plate counts are made, this system could probably pay for itself at a price under $5,000. The American Instrument Co. has a similar unit called the Petri-Scan.

A related device is a scanner, working on the same principle, which is able to measure the size of the zone of inhibition around an antibiotic sensitivity disc. One system that is available, **The Millipore Zone Analyzer,** produced by **Millipore Corp.,** measures the zone around each antibiotic disc and prints out the name of the antibiotic and the designation that is appropriate—resistant, moderately sensitive, etc. The technician need only index the plate to the proper disc and start the sequence. One system allows the operator to indicate the periphery of the zone with a light pen. This might be necessary where a zone is equivocal.

Another system for measuring antibiotic sensitivity is **Technicon Corp.'s TAAS** system (Technicon's Automated Antibiotic Susceptibility). In this system the bacteria are actually counted through a particle counter. Sterile broth is pipetted into fifteen chambers and inoculated with the organism to be tested. After a short lag phase, thirteen of the wells are presented with discs impregnated with different antibiotics. The fourteenth chamber grows uninhibited to serve as a positive control; in the fifteenth, growth is arrested by the addition of formalin. Particle counts, taken after about 3 hours, are a very sensitive measure of inhibition of growth. The rationale of the system seems logical enough. Critics point out that solubility of antibiotics from the discs is not the same in all cases and, also that, once the organism is isolated, inhibition can often be detected on an agar plate in a little more time than that of the TAAS. (They fail to mention that the plate sensitivity has the same problem of antibiotic solubility and diffusion.) As for the time required, it seems obvious that a great deal of technician time could be saved by this system that reads thirteen susceptibilities of an organism at the rate of forty specimens per hour. The system is still relatively untried and no judgment can yet be made concerning its practical operation. It is, of course, expensive and rather complex.

Other approaches to the automation of sensitivity testing are being examined and some prototypes are out. It will probably be some time before any one system is established and proved but almost certainly an efficient and feasible system will be developed in due time.

A spin-off from space exploration is responsible for a method that is getting attention. When luciferin and luciferase come into contact in the presence of adenosine triphosphate (ATP), a flash of light is produced. ATP is present in bacteria, as in all other living things. In urine, the ATP of human cells can be chemically blocked so that only the ATP of the bacteria can cause the light-emitting reaction, which can be detected and quantitated rather easily. The idea is intriguing and has shown experimental success.

Johnson Laboratories, Inc., have produced a system called **Bactec,** which works in a different way to detect bacterial growth. Glucose and certain other substances are tagged with the carbon isotope C^{14}. Almost all organisms metabolize glucose with the formation of at least some trace of carbon dioxide. When the tagged glucose is used, $CO_2{}^{14}$ is produced and it can be drawn out of a sealed culture bottle and detected. If there is no growth, no gas will be produced. The company claims to have a perfect score in detecting all the positives found in a parallel study with 2500 blood cultures. In fact, fourteen more positives were found by the Bactec system and these were later proved to be true positives. The point was further made that most positives are found between 1 and 6 hours after inoculation. This system certainly seems promising for the large laboratory where much time is spent in examining negative blood cultures. The price of the equipment and labeled blood culture media would make the system practical only for the large laboratory. Perhaps this situation will change if the technique becomes popular enough to lower production costs. Much experimental work remains to be done, however.

A method that has excited a great deal of interest has involved the examination of the metabolic products of various bacteria by gas chromatography. Some of the first work was done on the gases released by anaerobes grown on certain media. More recently careful work has demonstrated that many, if not most, bacteria produce gases or volatile acids that are characteristic enough to identify them when studied by gas chromatography. Body fluids of animals infected by some bacteria can be shown to contain characteristic substances that are diagnostic. Virus infections in some cases can even be occasionally demonstrated in this way. Certain characteristic volatile acids and alcohols are the chief chemical components that can be identified by gas chromatography in this technique. This approach, while still experimental, would seem to offer considerable promise. The project seems huge now, but it indicates possibilities of growing, extracting, and chromatographing in an automated device and of identifying organisms, by computer, using gas chromatograms along with other detectable characteristics. Fig. 11-4 shows the AnaBac Gas Chromatograph designed specifically for bacteriology.

Along this line, Patrick Burns has prepared a master's thesis (Mississippi State U., 1972) titled *Identification of Microorganisms Using Computer Programs,* in which he has evolved a rudimentary computer program for identifying most of the human pathogens and many other infectious organisms by means of certain common diagnostic criteria. Certainly this approach promises to simplify the identification of many organisms when good programs can be worked out in a format compatible with most computers. Other computer programs of this sort have also been developed by other workers.

Other studies have been involved with automated techniques for separating the bacteria in a mixed culture using size and electric charges. If this technique proves practical, the same characteristics that allowed separation may prove useful as criteria for identification.

Many other studies are progressing in such areas as the measurement of heat produced bacterial growth, the plotting of growth curves, using absorbed and scattered light, and the release of radioactive

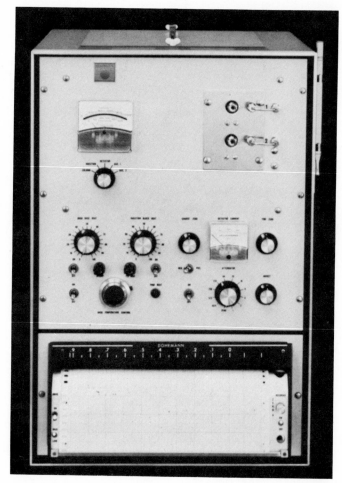

Fig. 11-4. AnaBac Gas Chromatograph designed specifically for bacteriology.

materials form media variously tagged to demonstrate metabolic characteristics of diagnostic significances.

From all of these projects and studies, it seems certain that the means to automate much of the tedium of microbiology will certainly be found and that feasible systems will be produced in the next few years.

Laboratories, being places for study and examination, will never be completely automated There will always be new horizons for exploration and new information to examine and collate into the body of knowledge with which work is done. But it seems inevitable that a great deal of the study of human exudates, transudates, and tissues occupying us today will certainly be automated and computerized in the near future.

REVIEW QUESTIONS

1. What laboratory tasks are computers designed to perform?
2. What is a byte?
3. Name some ways that people are using to automate bacteriology.
4. What functions do mini-computers perform?
5. Define or explain the following: on-line I/O, bit, N OR gate, mnemonic, alphanumeric, turn-key, machine language, CPU, and buffer storage.

ISOTOPES AND RADIANT ENERGY

Isotopes are forms of an element having the same atomic number and similar chemical properties but differing in atomic weight and, often, in radioactive behavior. *Stable* isotopes vary in atomic weight but possess no imbalance of electric charge and, hence, exhibit no radioactivity or instability. An atom that possessed an additional or deficient neutron, for example, would change in weight but would still possess very similar properties.

Radioactive isotopes have an electrical imbalance that causes the atom to emit characteristic particles or energy forms that may be detected easily, even in rather small quantities.

Naturally occurring isotopes have been known for many years. It was not until the explosion of the atomic bomb, in 1945, that quantities of these radioactive materials became available for study. Construction of the cyclotron and the chain-reacting pile made possible the preparation of various radioactive isotopes of nearly all the elements. Recent advances in chemistry have made it possible to substitute radioactive elements into a large variety of molecular structures. These "tagged" molecules can be used to follow the course of various physiological phenomena by the simple device of detecting the characteristic radiation in the tissues, exudates, etc. after ingestion. Thus it is possible to follow many physicochemical processes occurring in an organism without interrupting or disturbing its physiological functions. The advantages of this sort of technique are obvious.

Depending on the molecular physics involved, several different particles and forms of energy may be emitted by a radioactive isotope. The energy of these is generally rated in terms of two capabilities. The first of these is the *ability to penetrate.*

Relatively heavy alpha particles may be capable of penetrating only a few centimeters of air, whereas more energetic gamma rays can penetrate many materials for some distance and can even pass through an inch of solid lead.

The second capability considered is the *ability to ionize* other atoms that are encountered. This capability of the particle is related to its energy, which is measured in *electron volts.* An electron volt is the measurement of power equivalent to the energy of one electron accelerated through a potential difference of one volt. This value is 1.6×10^{-16} erg. It is a very tiny measurement, and the measurement *million electron volts* (MEV) is more commonly used. The smaller term *thousand electron volts* (KEV) is also commonly used.

Alpha particles are doubly ionized helium atoms with very high energy levels but very low penetrating power. Preparations emitting alpha particles are not commonly used as tracers for obvious reasons.

Beta particles are high-energy electrons or positrons. They have slightly more penetrating power than alpha particles but are stopped by a few meters of air or very light shielding. Their ionizing potential is relatively low but varies, depending on the decay reaction that produced them.

Gamma rays and *X rays* are both energies of the electromagnetic spectrum. X rays are much less commonly produced by isotopes and are of little value in isotope measurement.

Gamma radiation is the form of energy that is most commonly used in tracer studies in biological tissues. Radiation of this type is characterized by wavelengths of less than 1 Å. Compared to ultraviolet or visible light, these waves have very high energy; but compared to the ionizing potential of alpha particles (around 10 MEV), they are fairly weak However, they have high penetrating power, as mentioned earlier. The combination of these characteristics makes gamma radiation convenient for biological work. A gamma-emitting isotope injected into, or ingested by, a living organism will not cause a great deal of ionization, with resultant tissue damage. At the same time, the gamma ray energy will penetrate the tissues and utensils sufficiently well for their position and concentration to be easily detected.

The exact energy (wavelength) emitted by a particular isotope depends on the quantum mechanics of the atom in question, and only discrete energy levels are possible. It is thus possible to identify an isotope by its energy level or spectral emission. This identification process might be compared to spectral scanning in the visual region. By noting the amplitude of the energy at the characteristic wavelength (energy level), it is possible to quantitate the isotope by comparing the energy reading with suitable standards. This process is quite similar to that of spectrophotometry in the visible range.

Unfortunately, the energy peak for the isotope of an element is less clear-cut than the emission or absorption maxima of visible light. The gamma ray, with a very specific energy, may communicate all of its energy to an electron that is ultimately the source for our photoelectric measurement. In this process, called the *photoelectric effect,* the energy of the photoelectron is equal to the energy of the gamma ray. In a considerable number of cases, however, the gamma ray may *collide* with an electron. The energy available for measurement in such a case is the net energy that will be dispersed. This process, called the *Compton effect,* yields a scattering of energies somewhat lower than that of the original gamma ray. Compton scatter and various other sources of radiation cause the definition of the specific energy of the gamma ray to be more difficult. In spite of this problem, the istopic element can be quite definitely identified and quantitated with adequate instrumentation.

Radioactive isotopes are atoms in their excited states and, as such, are unstable. Over a period of time the atom returns to ground state, at which time emission theoretically ceases. Since this radioactive decay is a geometrical progression (first-order rate), the end point is infinity and there is no such thing as a time at which the atom has returned to ground state. To describe the decay rate for various radioactive isotopes, the term *radioactive half-life,* or *physical half-life,* is used. This is the time required for the given isotope to lose one half of its radiant energy. Table 4 lists the half-life span of a number of common isotopes. Note that one element may have more than one isotopic form and each form may have its own radioactive characteristics.

Table 4. Half-life of various radioisotopes commonly used as tracers

Name of element	Symbol	Half-life
Iodine	I^{131}	8 days
Iodine	I^{125}	60 days
Gold	Au^{198}	2.7 days
Mercury	Hg^{197}	2.7 days
Mercury	Hg^{203}	48 days
Chromium	Cr^{51}	28 days
Cobalt	Co^{57}	270 days
Selenium	Se^{75}	127 days
Strontium	Sr^{85}	65 days
Technicium	Tc^{99m}	6 hours
Indium	In^{113m}	1.7 hours
Xenon	Xe^{133}	5 days
Iron	Fe^{59}	45 days

The *biological half-life* of a compound is a measure of the disappearance of the compound itself from the organism and has no relation to its radioactive properties.

UNITS OF ACTIVITY AND STANDARDS

The activity of a radioactive isotope preparation is measured as the number of nuclear disintegrations occurring per second. The *curie* is the unit of activity commonly used. One curie is 3.7×10^{10} disintegrations per second. This is a great deal of activity, and smaller units such as a *millicurie* and a *microcurie* are much more commonly used.

Exposure to radiation is measured in *roentgens*. One roentgen is the amount of radiation that, when passed through 0.001293 gram of air under standard conditions, will produce one electrostatic unit of electricity per centimeter, or 1.61×10^{12} ion pairs per gram of air.

In the calibration of devices for the detection of radioactivity, standards are necessary. Since all active isotopes are constantly in the process of decay, it is necessary to establish the activity of the standard in question at the time of use. Commercially available isotopes of all sorts, including standards, carry a label giving activity at a specific date and hour. If the half-life is known, the decay rate can be applied and the current activity determined. Manufacturers often supply convenient decay charts that give the approximate activity at a particular time interval after assay.

Most of the commercially available preparations are given an assay value and decay rate that are quite adequate for clinical use. Absolutely standardized solutions are more carefully assayed and are hence more desirable for calibration purposes. They are, naturally, considerably more expensive. A *reference solution* is a solution that has been carefully measured in comparison to an "absolutely standardized solution."

Certain *solid standards* are available. These may be thin wafers of a long-lived isotope that allows the setting of the spectrometer at a given point with good accuracy. They may also be *mock standards* whose radiation simulates the radiation of a commonly used element. For example, barium 133 and cesium 137 in a 12:1 ratio have an emission closely resembling that of iodine 131 if a filter is used to screen out extraneous levels.

MEASURING DEVICES

There are several ways of measuring radioactivity but relatively few of these have been used in practical working instruments in the biological sciences. Many specialized devices have been developed, using a few basic principles.

The simplest means of detecting radiation is undoubtedly by the use of photographic plates or film. The familiar *radiation-monitoring badges* worn by all personnel in x-ray and radiosotope work are the commonest application. Copper and cadmium filters are placed over the film. If gamma radiation is present, the film will be darkened over its entirety. If only the cadmium filter protects the film, the radiation is X ray. If both cadmium and copper protect the film, beta radiation is present.

The localization of an isotope in tissue can be demonstrated by a film process called *autoradiography*. If the tissue is placed on a film for a few minutes, the radiation from the isotope will cause the film to blacken in the area adjacent to it.

The *ionization chamber* is another radiation-sensing device. If an electric field is applied across a chamber filled with gas, radiation (charged particles) entering the field will form ion pairs, adding to the saturation current. This small additional electron flow can be measured by an electrometer in any of several ways. Small pocket chambers (*dosimeters*) that store the charge until the device is inserted into a meter socket are available. As the chamber discharges, the meter is deflected to indicate the absorbed charge. Many types of survey meters for detecting stray radiation, spilled radioactive material, etc. are made, using the idea of the ionization chamber. These chambers measure various types of radiation, depending on what gas is used in the chamber.

Recently *metal oxide semiconductors* (MOS) have been found to provide an accurate and reliable means of measuring radiation. Meters using MOS detectors are economical and sensitive and are finding wide application.

The *Geiger counter,* so well known to the public, is constructed in a manner similar to that of an ionization chamber. The cathode is in the form of a metallic cylinder around the anode. A high potential (1000 to 2500 v) is applied. Ion pairs result from this very high potential, and other ionization is produced as high-velocity charges strike gas molecules. An avalanche effect is produced. As the cumulative charge is released at the anode, a pulse is produced and the process may be repeated at a rate dependent on the intensity of the radiation. There is a brief dead time between discharges, and practical counting rates are not in excess of 15,000 per minute. This type of counter is best for beta radiation.

For detection of gamma radiation, *scintillation crystals* are the method of choice. The most widely used crystal of this sort is the *sodium iodide* crystal, activated with 1% thallium. *Anthracene, stilbene,* and several other organic crystals are also used. These crystals are optically clear and are usually 2 or 3 inches across. As the gamma rays strike the crystal, a very tiny scintillation, or flash of light of short duration, is produced. The time is usually a fraction of a microsecond and the total energy released may escape detection by the eye.

The scintillation crystal is enveloped in a foil that protects it from extraneous light and helps reflect the scintillation. The end of the crystal is sealed to the face of a high-quality photomultiplier tube that detects and amplifies the impulses.

The crystal and photomultiplier are usually enclosed in a lead-shielded *probe* along with a preamplifier circuit that further amplifies the output of the photomultiplier. At the front of the probe, a thick sleeve of lead is usually placed in such a way that the crystal is protected from all radiation except that approaching it from an area determined by the opening in the sleeve. This protective lead shield is called a *collimator,* since its function is to collimate radiation onto the crystal. If the collimator is shaped like a funnel, all the radiation in the angle of the funnel will strike the crystal. If a series of very narrow holes is bored through a thick lead plate at the front of the crystal, only radiation that comes from directly in front of the crystal will reach it. *Counting wells* are, essentially, probes in which a crystal is hollowed out to permit a test tube to be inserted. This more intimate contact between the radiating substance and the crystal allows better counting sensitivity. A lead collar over the top of the crystal allows only an opening for insertion of the test tube. A high-voltage DC source of excellent quality is necessary to operate the photomultiplier tube. One of the leads to the probe or the well will be of high voltage—probably around 1000 v.

Signals from the probe or well are relayed to the main amplifier, where they are further amplified and may be processed to a discriminator and scaler.

The *pulse-height analyzer* or spectrometer is the part of the system that allows identification of the isotope from its energy level. The lower discriminator is designed to reject all pulses below a given level. The upper discriminator rejects impulses higher than the lower discrimination level plus those in the *window* or *channel* width. By the use of the two discriminators, only the voltage analogous to the MEV of the isotope in question is passed through the discriminator or spectrometer. The number of emissions at this MEV range provides quantitation of the isotope, and stray radiation and radiation from other elements are eliminated. This device, although operating on a different principle, functions as a monochromator similar to that used in the visual range.

The *scaler* is a device that combines several individual signals, by means of capacitors, to make them count as a single impulse. Two common types of scalers are in use. One is the *binary scaler*, in which the impulses are divided in each phase by two, giving multipliers of 2, 4, 8, 16, 32, 64, etc. The other is the decimal or *decade scaler*, which passes each tenth pulse. The latter is obviously much simpler to use, but the former is more adaptable.

Various readout mechanisms are used. Glow tubes or Nixie tubes are now very common. They allow fast accurate counting. Decade tube arrangements are sometimes used in conjunction with mechanical counters. The problem often becomes one of devising an economically feasible system that is capable of the considerable counting speed required with acceptable accuracy.

An *anticoincidence circuit,* with the function of compensating for the coincidence of two scintillations at the exact same time interval, is included. The probability that two scintillations will coincide can be determined mathematically, and an appropriate signal correction is made. The various elements of a typical pulse-height analyzer are schematically shown in Fig. 12-1. This may help to clarify the components and relationship just discussed.

Many detectors are equipped with timers, which are simply electrical devices that open and close the counting circuits, permitting the counting of emissions per minute or other time interval.

Radioactive isotopes are used in medical situations, principally as *tracers;* that is to say, some radioactive element is "tagged" onto a molecule or other entity that is given to the patient. Since the element continues to radiate, it can be located in the body by means of collimated probes or be found in the blood, urine, stool, etc. and identified by its characteristic radiation. Gamma emitters are best suited to medical work, since they have low ionizing poten-

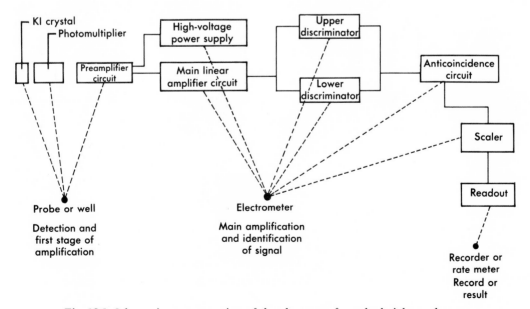

Fig. 12-1. Schematic representation of the elements of a pulse-height analyzer.

tial and hence cause less tissue damage. They also have considerable penetrating power and can be measured through greater thicknesses of body tissue. Fortunately it is possible to measure very small amounts of gamma radiation with excellent accuracy, and spectrometers that can accurately identify the radiation as characteristic of a given element are available.

Many special devices for measuring gamma radiation under certain circumstances have been developed.

It is possible to use the total number of emissions (or the cumulative "signal") passing through the window as one ordinate for a recorder, with time as the other function. This is the sort of arrangement often used for *renograms,* which record the emissions over the two kidneys, against time, to obtain a graph of kidney function.

Rectilinear isotope scanners are being used frequently in medicine and biology to map areas of the body where an isotope may be concentrated (or excluded). An arm carries the probe containing the detector crystal back and forth over the area to be scanned in a regular mapping pattern called a raster pattern. At the other end of the arm is a tapper, recording the signals from the crystals as dots on a paper. The result is a map of the area, showing the loci of heavy or light isotope concentrations. The signal from the crystal may also be fed to a tiny light bulb that flashes to produce exposure of an x-ray film after the same general pattern. Various companies manufacture a scanner with two crystals. These detectors scan both sides of the patient simultaneously to speed up the total scanning process and to define areas more sharply.

The rectilinear scanner provides a means of producing an image or map of the area under observation but it has limitations. The time required to perform a scan makes it impossible to observe fast changes in isotope concentration. Also, the study of different areas or levels in an organ is very time-consuming and tiring. Some method

has been needed for visualizing isotope distribution very rapidly. Also, a means of visualizing distribution in three dimensions was needed. The *gamma camera* and various refinements and additions have gone a long way to answering these needs.

The construction of a single detector has already been reviewed. In this detector a crystal was cemented to the face of a photomultiplier tube. The gamma camera has one very large crystal with nineteen photomultiplier tubes cemented in a symmetrical pattern to its upper side. Each scintillation will be sensed by more than one photomultiplier. The strength of the photosignals originating on the various photomultipliers will depend on the proximity of the tube to the scintillation. With simultaneous signals of different strength from different locations, it is possible for the computer circuitry to locate the position of the flash on X and Y coordinates and position a light dot on a CRT. With hundreds of scintillations being plotted in this fashion, the CRT becomes a map of the radioactivity of the area under examination. If a *persistence scope* (a CRT with a phosphor coating that continues to glow for some measurable time) is used, this map can be examined while it is showing a large number of scintillations. It is possible to place a photographic film in front of the CRT and produce a picture for later, detailed examination. Polaroid pictures can be made rapidly and easily in this way.

Since this sort of information can be gathered easily and quickly, it is possible to do sequential pictures (with a time-lapse camera, for example) at very short intervals and thus get a time-lapse pattern showing the progress of an event. By the same token, it is also feasible to focus at different levels of an organ and thus obtain some depth perception.

Tomography is the technique involved in getting views of radioisotope distribution and concentration at various planar sections within an organ. Various devices and techniques have been proposed recently to accomplish this. Most of these involve some device for rotating a collimator with parallel holes drilled at the same angle. By triangulation the concentration of isotope at a given depth can be located. This idea may require a moment's thought. If a rod were pushed through one of the holes of the collimator and the collimator then made to spin, the rod would appear to be a cone. The point of such a cone will be farther from the collimator if the hole used is close to the edge of the collimator. As the holes approach the center of the collimator, the point of the cone (or focus of radioactivity) is seen closer to the collimator. By using the information received from all of the photomultiplier tubes of the gamma camera, equipped with such a rotating collimator, the computer circuitry can establish the level of concentration of isotope. This technique is not perfected for routine use, but it shows promise.

Another recent advance in isotope imaging has been development of the *data storage* and *playback systems* that can be used with gamma cameras. The circuitry of the camera locates a scintillation as an X-Y plot, and this information is then fed to the CRT to locate a point of light at an analogous position on the screen. It is also possible to store this electrical information on magnetic tape and play it back in the same order it was received. Thus it is possible to

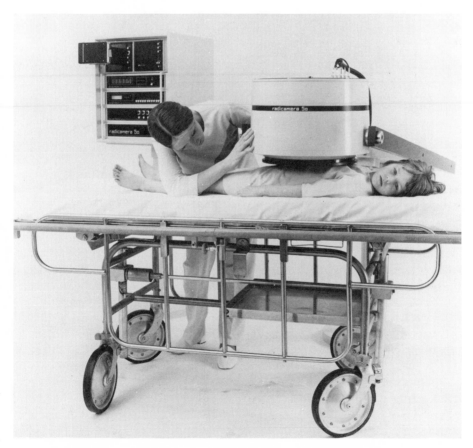

Fig. 12-2. Radicamera gamma camera. Technician is positioning detector head over patient. Electronics console is in background. (Courtesy Nuclear Data, Inc.)

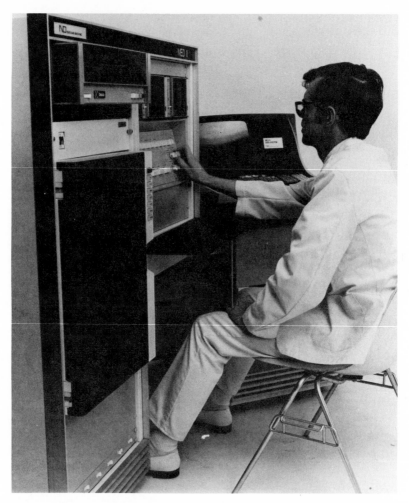

Fig. 12-3. Med II system for data storage and retrieval, designed to function with the Radicamera. (Courtesy Nuclear Data, Inc.)

watch the kinetic accumulation of information on the screen and to reproduce it at will. Also, it is possible to isolate a specific *area of interest* on the matrix when the stored information is being played back. These characteristics make the gamma camera a valuable diagnostic tool with great flexibility.

Fig. 12-2 shows the **Radicamera Scintillation Camera system** made by **Nuclear Data, Inc.** In Fig. 12-3 the data storage and retrieval system designed to operate with it is presented.

The field of nuclear medicine is growing rapidly and several manufacturers are producing devices for utilizing isotopes for diagnosis. The single probe, the rectilinear scanner, and the gamma camera have been mentioned. All of these are primarily used *in vivo*. There is also a great deal of work being done with isotopes *in vitro*. Most of this work is done in well counters of some sort.

Some techniques call for chromatographic separation on paper and scanning, with a probe, to locate radioactivity. Since there are now many techniques in which a liquid sample is used, it has become practical to use automatic sample changers and printers. These are able to monitor tubes during a preset period of time, for a specified isotope, and print out the scintillation count on each specimen. Some of these systems have become very sophisticated, allowing great flexibility in monitor time, channels of radioactivity, etc.

Some of the tests done in vitro are blood volume, T-3, T-4, and T-7 tests for thyroid function, the Shilling test for vitamin B_{12} deficiency, and numerous radioimmune procedures. The possibilities of radiochemistry are just beginning to be realized.

Specialized instruments have been manufactured to perform single functions. Many companies, for example, have introduced *blood volume apparatus* that measures radioactivity of a tagged substance before injection into the body and, later, the radioactivity of a blood sample from the patient. By calculating the dilution that has occurred between the two readings, the blood volume can be estimated. Since only one element is involved and the activities will be within about the same range, the equipment can be rather simple. The circuitry for the simple calculations is also quite elementary.

Since this is a rather specialized area, individual instruments will not be discussed here. Nuclear Data, Inc., Ohio Nuclear, Inc., Packard Instrument Sales Corp., and Searle Analytic, Inc., Subsidiary of G. D. Searle & Co., are principal suppliers of hardware for nuclear medicine.

REVIEW QUESTIONS

1. What is an isotope?
2. Are all isotopes radioactive? If not, what would make some isotopes radioactive while others were not?
3. What form of energy is most commonly measured in medically utilized isotopes? Why?
4. What sorts of detector are most commonly used for detecting isotopes in the clinical laboratory?
5. Why is the rate of radioactive decay expressed as "half-life"?
6. What does the "window" setting of a pulse-height analyzer represent?
7. What characteristic of a radioactive element is used to identify it? What units of measurement identify the element?
8. What is the function of a scaler?

13

Miscellaneous instruments and devices

A walk through any medical laboratory reveals a large number of devices that have still not been discussed here. A complete cataloging and description of these would require a considerably larger book, and new gadgets each year vie for a place in the medical market. This chapter will provide a quick look at a few of the more significant of these. Devices for heating and cooling, centrifuges, recorders, coagulation-measuring devices and dilutors are all important. These and a few other selected devices will be discussed.

HEATING AND COOLING

Water baths, incubators, ovens, refrigerators, chilling baths, etc. are vital to the laboratory. Heat is generally produced by passing an electric current through a high-resistance wire or heating block. Heat production requires considerable electricity. A 2- or 3-gallon bath may draw 10 or 15 amps when it is heating up rapidly. Exposed wire coils are rarely used for resistance now, since they become oxidized or corrode and break easily after heavy usage. Where a block or panel of metal is used, the element rarely becomes bad.

Heat, once produced, must be transmitted to the area to be heated and evenly distributed there. In blood pH and blood gas analyzers, as well as in equilibrated sample compartments, the heat is often distributed by pumping water through tubes,

around the samples. Circulating pumps are required to move the water. An impeller may be used to push the water forward or a positive pressure pump may be used. Valves are necessary to allow the fluid to continuously flow forward as it is pushed along by pistons, peristaltic rollers, or vibrators.

In conventional water baths the water may circulate simply by convection current. An agitator, mixer, or pump may be used to provide better mixing and more even temperature distribution, however. (See Fig. 13-1.)

In ovens, incubators, and air baths, the heat may be radiated through large metal surfaces, the air may move by convection, or a fan may be provided to maintain circulation. The accuracy of temperature control required will dictate the method used.

Several means are available for controlling the heating process. The oldest and simplest of these is the *bimetallic strip thermostat*. Two metal strips with different expansion coefficients are fastened together at either end. When they are heated, one metal expands more than the other and causes the sandwiched strips to bend (Fig. 13-2). This distortion is used to close or open a contact to a heater. In older ovens, heaters, etc. and in some cheaper models the current was passed through the bimetallic element to the heater. This resulted in considerable arcing at the contact points, with dire results: either the contact points fused, causing the heater to stay on until a fuse blew or the unit burned up, or the surfaces of the contacts got so rough, blackened, and corroded that they would not conduct and the circuit would not close. In an attempt to correct this deficiency, manufacturers used silver or platinum contact points, but this did not completely solve the problem.

Where these devices are used in newer controls, current is passed through a micro-

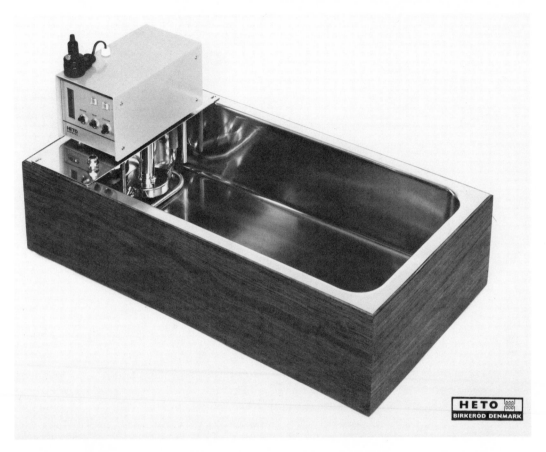

Fig. 13-1. Heto water bath. This bath uses a ram-jet type of pump to provide excellent mixing and temperature equilibration. A high-quality mercury thermoregulator controls heating. It is finished in a durable and attractive wood cabinet. (Courtesy The London Co.)

switch that is closed or opened by pressure of the distorted bimetallic element.

Wafer elements or expansion elements are composed of two circles of metal, fastened together to form a wafer. The outside of the wafer is constricted by a heavier ring. As the material expands, the metal discs buckle outward so that the thickness of the wafer increases. This expansion is used to depress a microswitch that opens or closes a circuit.

Fluid-expansion elements are used in many water baths. A liquid-filled probe is immersed in the water. The probe is connected to an expansion element in the con-

trol panel by a very fine capillary. As the fluid is heated, it expands, causing the expansion element to inflate, which, in turn, depresses the plunger of a microswitch. Corrosion or mechanical damage may cause leakage of the fluid from these elements. In most baths the liquid-containing unit can be replaced or the entire thermostat assembly can be replaced.

With all these devices, the microswitch may become defective and have to be replaced. This is usually a fairly simple task and many microswitches are standard items that are available in electric supply outlets.

All the above devices for temperature

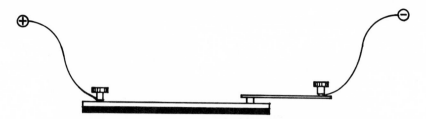

Bimetallic element at room temperature (contact to heater closed)

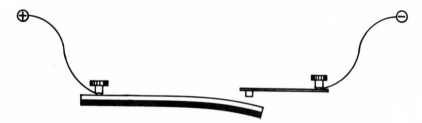

Same element at 37° C (contact to heater opens as element is distorted)

Fig. 13-2. Bimetallic thermostat.

sensing are purely mechanical in nature. The *thermocouple* is slightly different. When two metals are brought into close contact, there is a rearrangement of electrons on their surfaces that produces a difference in electric potential between them. If a circuit between them is completed, a flow of electrons can be demonstrated with a sensitive meter. This effect is very marked in the case of certain metals; the rate of electron flow through such a circuit will vary considerably with temperature. This characteristic is used as a sensitive indicator of temperature change in the thermocouple. A very weak current can be amplified and used to activate a switch or a relay to control a heating cycle.

As explained earlier, the *thermistor* is a semiconductor component that allows current to pass at a rate dependent on the temperature. The current passed can be used to actuate an ammeter to indicate the temperature or to control the heating process itself. Newer instruments are using thermistors more than mechanical thermostats.

Gas heat is, of course, used for some de-vices where high temperatures are required and exact control is not necessary.

Cooling is done, in almost all cases, by refrigerator compressor, which uses the cooling effect of expanding gases. Cold spot platforms, for pouring paraffin blocks around histology specimens, have expansion coils embedded in an aluminum block. As the gas expands and cools the coils, the block is chilled. A thermostat in the block controls the compressor to produce more cooling or to discontinue it.

CENTRIFUGES

Various types of centrifuges, for separating solid components from liquid suspensions by centrifugal action, are used in the laboratory. They are relatively simple. A few words on their construction and maintenance might prove helpful, however.

The centrifuge consists of an electric motor to which are attached a head and accessories for carrying samples. Usually the head turns on a spindle, which is an extension of the motor shaft. To this basic instrument various devices may be added. A *safety shield* around the rotating head is a necessity, since a broken head or similar disaster could throw fragments at a velocity of 500 mph according to International Centrifuge manuals. An *on-off switch*, to interrupt the current to the motor, is an obvious requirement. A *timer* is commonly incorporated. Either a simple spring-driven clock mechanism that opens a switch at the end of a preset time cycle or an electric timer that performs the same function may be used. There is usually a switch that gives the operator a choice between continuous operation and operation using the timer.

A *brake* is often supplied. Some models make use of a *mechanical* brake, consisting of a leather shoe pressing on the rotor at some point. It is activated by holding down a lever or knob. Other centrifuges have an *electric* brake, which reverses the polarity of the current to the motor. When such a brake is held down past the time needed to stop the motor, the motor reverses direction and spins backward.

Tachometers are provided on many instruments to indicate speed, in revolutions per minute. A cable or flexible shaft attached to the motor spindle turns inside a flexible housing. It is attached to the meter movement at the other end. As the cable turns, it causes the needle to move upscale. If the cable is twisted or if it becomes dry or corroded, it may cause a ticking noise and the needle may jump erratically. Eventually the cable may break. Some centrifuges use electric tachometers in which a magnet rotates around a coil, producing a current that may be measured.

The speed of the centrifuge is controlled by a potentiometer or a *Variac,* which raises and lowers the voltage supplied to the motor. The potentiometers may become defective and fail to provide a smooth transition between speeds, or they may open entirely and fail to function. The Variac has a graphite brush or *wiper* that moves across its windings. This brush may become worn and may occasionally cause damage to the

windings unless sufficient care is taken. Many small centrifuges have a multiposition switch that selects voltage steps by connecting taps on a transformer.

Most centrifuge motors are series-wound DC motors that turn faster as the voltage is increased. Diodes and capacitors are used to rectify the alternating current normally available. Some centrifuges use AC motors in which the speed is adjusted stepwise by reducing the number of poles in the magnetic field.

Electrical contact to the *commutator* (Chapter 1) in nearly all centrifuge motors is provided by *graphite brushes.* These gradually wear down as they press against the commutator turning at high speed. If the graphite is allowed to completely wear away, the retainer spring of the brush will make contact with the smooth soft brass surface of the commutator and cut grooves or scratches in its surface. A rough commutator surface will cause excessively fast wear of new brushes; and the graphite that is worn away may deposit about the contacts and cause arcing and burning; this decreases the efficiency of the motor and may damage it or, in extreme cases, may even start a fire in the motor.

If the commutator becomes scratched or worn so that there is excessive brush wear, it may be "turned down" on a lathe. A few thousandths of an inch of the soft brass is shaved off until the surface is smooth again. The metal is usually only sufficiently thick to allow this process to be repeated two or three times before the armature is destroyed. It is very important that brushes be checked frequently and replaced before damage occurs. Be sure that the proper size brush is used. A brush that is too small may become lodged between the brush housing and the commutator and cause considerable damage.

When an *armature coil* burns or short-circuits or wires become broken, it can be rewound by an electric motor shop. Also, new commutator plates can usually be installed. Depending on the type of motor, difficulty in finding the proper replacement, and general condition of the rest of the motor, it may be cheaper to replace the motor. In general, small, standard motors can better be replaced. Occasionally the *field coils* of a motor may become damaged. They can also be replaced by an electric motor shop fairly easily in most cases.

The *shaft* of the motor, to which the head is attached, turns within *sleeve bearings* at the top and bottom of the motor. These bearings are designed to very close tolerance and must be kept well lubricated to prevent wear. Loose bearings may cause vibration and loss of motor efficiency. A dry bearing increases the load on the motor considerably, slowing the speed of the centrifuge and producing heat. Some centrifuges have sealed bearings with lifetime lubrication. The instruction book for the instrument should be read carefully to determine which bearings need grease or oil and where the lubrication points are located. The lubrication schedule should be followed religiously. *Ball bearings* are used in some motors. This type of bearing is somewhat more expensive and reduces friction considerably.

Badly worn bearings can be replaced, but this is generally a job for a careful electric motor shop or knowledgeable repairman. High-speed motors, in particular, are troublesome in this regard. Tolerances are very close, and centering and alignment are critical. Hematocrit centrifuges are especially troublesome, and the instrument with replaced bearings is often quite noisy.

Centrifugal force depends essentially on three variables. These are *mass, speed,* and *radius.* Since aqueous solutions or other solutions with a specific gravity close to 1.000 are usually involved, only the speed and radius must be considered.

The *relative centrifugal force* or **RCF** is calculated according to the following formula:

$$RCF = 0.00001118 \times r \times N^2$$

where r = the radius in centimeters and N = the number of revolutions per minute. The radius is measured from the center of the shaft to the inside bottom of the tube.

The speed is dependent on the voltage in most centrifuges, but efficiency (speed) is lost as resistance is increased. Resistance may include such items as air resistance and turbulence, dry or worn bearings, brush friction, and electrical inefficiency inherent in the design of the motor. The same centrifuge will achieve different speeds with different accessories and in varing states of repair. The calibrations often furnished on the speed control are only relative voltage increments and can never be taken as accurate indicators of speed. A tachometer or strobe light should be used to accurately determine speed. (A *strobe light* is a light that very rapidly turns on and off. When it is held over the spinning centrifuge head, it is adjusted to the frequency at which the head appears to stand still. At this frequency the light is on at exactly the instant when the centrifuge head is in the same position, during each revolution. The speed of the centrifuge in revolutions per minute is then obviously the same as the frequency of the strobe light. Allowance must be made for harmonics, of course.)

When the revolutions per minute have been determined, the RCF can easily be determined, by use of a nomograph (Fig. 13-3). This is faster and easier than using the formula and is sufficiently accurate for clinical use.

It cannot be overemphasized that proper maintenance is vital to the efficiency and long life of the centrifuge. The following rules are very important and are listed here for emphasis:

1. Check brushes often and replace according to the manufacturer's instructions well before they are completely worn away.

2. Be sure the proper brush is used. A brush that is too small may wedge

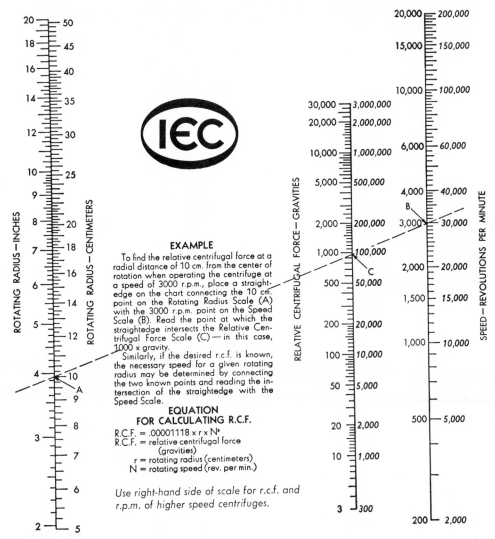

Fig. 13-3. Nomograph for computing centrifugal force. (Courtesy International Equipment Co., Division of Damon.)

between the brush holder and commutator and cause serious damage.

3. Keep the motor clean and free of carbon dust and debris.

4. Clean the inside of the bowl frequently and thoroughly. Always remove all traces of broken glass. Replace cushions in shields where glass has broken. Waxing the inside of the bowl helps keep down dust and dirt and reduces drag.

5. Lubricate bearings according to the manufacturer's directions. Never let a bearing become dry.

6. Use proper accessories and cushions for the instruments. Never run a centrifuge when it is out of balance or is vibrating.

7. Check the balance of accessories often. Numbering helps keep them in the proper position.

Several special-purpose centrifuge sys-

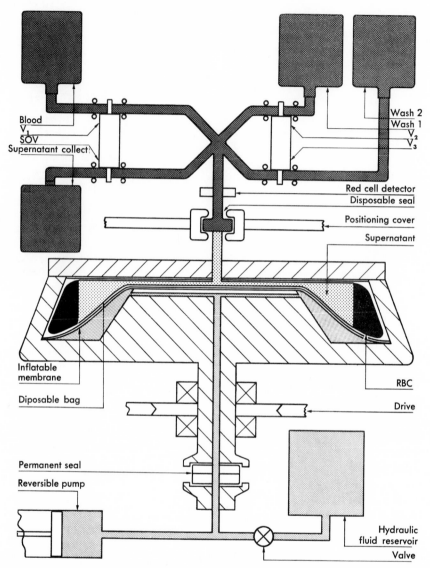

Fig. 13-4. Blood cell–washing scheme of IBM Model 2991 Blood Cell Processor. (Courtesy IBM.)

tems are available. *Refrigerated centrifuges* are required for some enzyme analyses as well as other temperature-sensitive procedures. A compressor unit is provided in the base of the centrifuge, and the bowl of the centrifuge is maintained at a temperature low enough to more than compensate for the heat of air friction. Although they are necessarily moderately expensive, there is nothing complicated about them.

Various *cell washers* and continuous-flow *plasma* and *blood cell separators* are on the market. These are centrifuges equipped with pumps, valves, sensors, etc. to allow them to cycle through the various steps of separating, discarding, washing, etc. The blood cell–washing scheme of the **IBM 2991 Blood Cell Processor** is presented in Fig. 13-4 as an example. The rationale of each of these instruments may seem com-

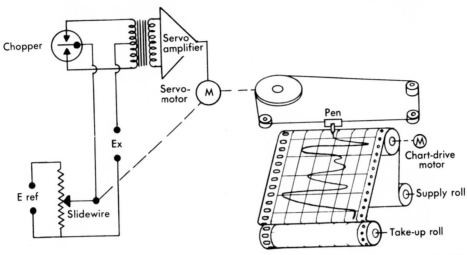

Fig. 13-5. Schematic diagram of recorder operation. (Courtesy Sargent-Welch Scientific Co.)

plicated but, once examined in detail, they are really fairly simple.

RECORDERS

Recorders have become almost as common as colorimeters in the clinical laboratory. They are essentially simple and relatively trouble-free, but there are a large number of types in use and the terminology to describe them can be confusing.

The recorders that will be discussed here are devices for marking on a chart certain phenomena as a function of time. There are two mechanisms involved. The first is the chart-drive motor that feeds the paper under the writing pen at a constant speed. The second is the pen drive that translates the incoming electric signal (from the photometer, thermometer, etc. that is being monitored) into a displacement of the pen corresponding to the signal size (Fig. 13-5).

The chart drive is a simple electric motor geared to move the paper forward. Fig. 13-6 is an exploded diagram of the paper drive of a **Sargent SRG Recorder.** Different chart speeds may be supplied by one of two mechanisms. Some recorders provide one motor and a clutch assembly for chang-

ing speeds by engaging gear trains with different gear ratios. Other instruments use a separate small motor for each speed desired, as can be seen in Fig. 13-6. Newer recorders provide simple mechanisms for changing chart speeds, whereas older models often require a time-consuming change of motors or gears.

The pen displacement may be done in any of several ways. Two general types will be considered here. One of the simplest types is used in the galvanometric recorder. The input signal is fed to a galvanometer that has sufficient force to move a pen or stylus. In effect, these recorders work very much like a d'Arsonval meter movement with a writing pen at the end of the meter needle. Most electrocardiographic machines use galvanometric recorders, and the record is burned into a plasticized paper by a hot wire or stylus. Some recorders that operate in this way describe an arc when the pen moves either up or downscale, since this is the way the tip of a pointer moves. Paper with curved time lines is used to correct the arc error. For some types of records this pattern is no particular disadvantage. Other galvanometric records employ vari-

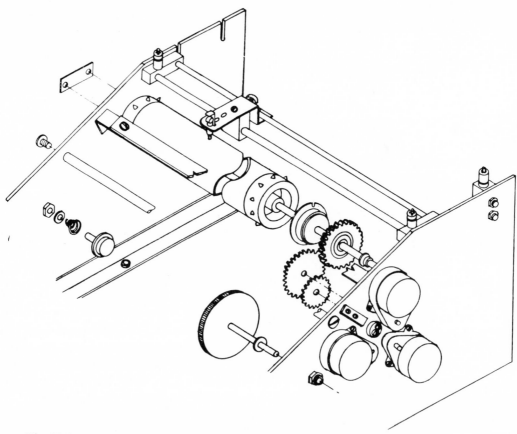

Fig. 13-6. Exploded diagram of the chart-drive assembly of a Sargent SRG Recorder. The clear, detailed sketch illustrates how carefully the manual is assembled to allow the untrained person to maintain and repair this sort of equipment. (Courtesy Sargent-Welch Scientific Co.)

ous mechanical tricks to translate the arc-shaped movement into a straight line.

The most common type of pen displacement in laboratory recorders is that of the servo potentiometer. This is an automatic null-balancing device. The recorder has a reference source, such as a mercury cell or a Zener diode, that supplies a reference voltage against which the signal is measured. The error signal between the two currents is fed to the servo amplifier. The amplified current, in turn, drives the potentiometer to its null point and, at the same time, moves the pen a distance relative to the correction made.

By adding resistance to either side of the measuring circuit, the zero setting can be moved to the right or the left; and by adjusting the bias to the servo amplifier, the span can be increased or decreased. The error signal is usually direct current and must be chopped for good amplification without drift. An electrical filter is placed in the input line to screen out extraneous signals of high frequency that would cause noise in the recording.

In evaluating a recorder, there are a number of terms used that apply only (or primarily) to recorders. A review of these terms may help to explain differences between instruments.

The *input signal* is the current that is to

be measured. The *input span* is the voltage range that the recorder is capable of recording. Most general-purpose recorders have an *input-selector switch,* which allows the use of any number of different input spans. The input selector is a resistor substitution bank that permits selection of the resistor needed to accommodate the desired signal. The *chart speed* is the speed with which paper is moved forward under the pen and is usually measured in inches per minute. Most general-purpose recorders allow several choices. *Pen response* is the speed with which the pen moves and usually measured in terms of the time it takes the pen to move from one edge of the paper to the other when an input signal greater than the input span is used. *Deadband* is the amount that the input signal can be varied without moving the pen. *Accuracy,* usually expressed in percent, is the limit that errors will not exceed when the instrument is used in accordance with the manufacturer's instructions. *Interference* is any unwanted current or voltage occurring in the instrument. *Common mode* is interference appearing between the measuring circuits and ground. *Null balance* is the situation in which the error signal between the input and the reference does not exceed the deadband. *Span* is the algebraic difference between the ends of the scale values. *Range* is the span expressed in terms of the values of the ends of the span.

Reproducibility is the measure of the instrument's ability to return to the same point on the scale when the same input signal is applied. *Normal mode* is the spurious volage that occurs between the measuring terminals. *Step-response time* is the time required for the pen to come to rest after an abrupt signal change. *Input divider* is a resistor or resistors installed in such a way that only a specific portion of the signal is measured. For additional information on terminology of recorders, refer to the literature of various recorder manufacturers. Texas Instruments' Bulletin no.

007, from which many of the above definitions were taken, is particularly helpful.

Many recorders have the capability of recording either a linear signal or a log signal and are called *linear-log recorders.* Normally a signal (from a photometer, for example) will displace the pen a given distance for each millivolt of signal. In many cases it would be very handy if absorbance units (which are log values) could be used on the recorder paper as a straight-line function so that concentrations would be immediately obvious. (If this is not entirely clear, the discussion of Beer's law in Chapter 2 may give some help.) The recorder may be able to make this translation. If a cam-drive gear is fashioned to describe a log curve, it will modify the pen movement so that the distance traveled is a log function of the input signal. See Fig. 13-7 for a comparison of the normal-drive gear and a log-drive gear. Other recorders make the linear-to-log translation electronically.

Integrators. A number of recorders are equipped with integrators. These are of little value in spectrophotometry but are extremely convenient in gas chromatog-

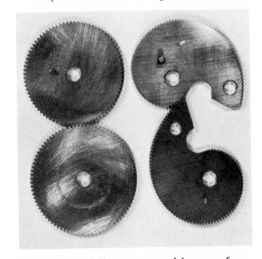

Fig. 13-7. Normal linear gear and log gear from a Sargent SRL Recorder. This log gear causes the pen's movement to be modified so as to effect the translation of charted values from linear to log.

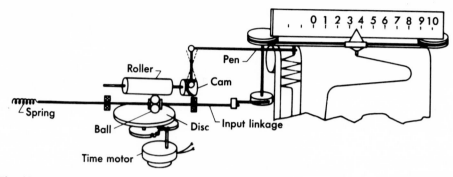

Fig. 13-8. Mechanical principle of the Disc Integrator. (Courtesy Disc Instruments, Inc.)

raphy and electrophoresis scanning, as indicated in discussion of these techniques. In such situations the quantity of some component is determined by multiplying the amplitude of the signal from a detector by the length of time the signal is produced. If both the flow rate of a gas in a tube and the time that this rate of flow continues are known, it is easy to calculate the volume, for example. Both the rate of flow and the time interval might vary in a random manner. If this information were charted on a recorder, the increase in flow would produce a peak on the chart paper. The height of the peak would represent the rate of flow and the width would represent its duration in minutes. Hence the area under the curve would represent the quantity of gas that had passed through the tube. An integrator is a mechanical or electrical device for translating the area under the curve to unit values.

Mechanical integrators. Most mechanical intergrators work on the principle of the **Disc Integrator,** pictured in Fig. 13-8. This type of integrator can be understood if we think of the disc, which is moving at a constant rate of speed, as the platform of a merry-go-round. If a midget were to pedal a tricycle at the outer edge of the platform fast enough to stay opposite the ticket booth, he would have to pedal very fast. If he were closer to the center, he could pedal much more slowly; and if he were

in the exact center of the platform, he could stay in the same position with no effort. The speed with which the tricycle wheels turned would be a function of the tricycle's position on the merry-go-round platform. The ball in the illustration may be compared to the tricycle wheel. Its position is determined by the position of the pen on the chart paper. The spiral-in and spiral-out cam is a device to push the integrator pen up and down on the edge of the paper each time the ball turns. This device is purely mechanical and has been relatively trouble-free.

On the older **Beckman Analytrol Densitometer** the integrator uses a small wheel with notches in place of the ball; by a different type of linkage, this wheel causes the pen to move up and down very slightly ten time for each revolution of the wheel. One large notch on the wheel causes the pen to make one large peak for each full revolution. This integrator is good in principle but has considerable mechanical trouble, which often makes peaks hard to interpret.

Electronic integrators. Many modern recorders use electronic integrators. These consist of very accurate capacitors that store a representative portion of the output signal and then discharge into circuits, that record this current fraction as an event, such as a pen stroke. This capacitor discharge may be recorded as blips on the edge of a recorder paper, as digits on a dial, or as some other form of record. High-quality electronic integrators are rather expensive but possess the advantages of having very few moving parts and being relatively trouble-free.

Types of recorders. The situations in the laboratory in which some parameter needs to be recorded are so numerous and varied that a large book would be necessary to detail them all. Many special-purpose recorders are designed to serve an immediate need. A few of these merit some mention.

Temperature-measuring recorders. These sometimes consist simply of a revolving drum, with a recording paper wrapped around it, and a pen attached to a sealed bellows. As the temperature of the bellows increases, the contents (gas or liquid) expand, moving the pen upward on the recording paper. The paper can be replaced each time the drum makes one complete revolution, providing a separate record for each time period.

Pressure recorders. These may work on a similar principle, with the pressure of a gas or liquid working against a spring or other resistance, activating the pen to move up or down on the paper. In pulmonary function–measuring devices the volume of an expiration is recorded as the bellows is filled with air and the attached pen moves up the paper, which is attached to a rotating drum.

Vibration recorders. These may rely on vibration of the pen assembly to move the pen, or the vibrations may be mechanically amplified. This sort of device is used in some seismographs for measuring earthquakes.

• • •

Certain types of recorders may have two or more pens and pen-drive motors, allowing more than one parameter to be measured at the same time. One pen may also be equipped to record the output of more than one detector by the simple device of a sequencing switch, which connects the pen-drive motor to each of the detectors in sequence either manually, as a function of time, or on stimulation by another circuit, such as a peak-height detector. As instruments become more automated, this last device is becoming much more common. Such devices, though precisely engineered, are relatively simple in principle, relying on the reversal of the error signal to activate the desired sequence of events.

X-Y plotters. X-Y plotters are recorders that record points on a graph as functions of two parameters. Time is usually not one of these parameters. Two pen-drive motors are required. One moves the pen along the abcissa while the other moves it along the ordinate of the graph. Such a system might plot the interrelationship of vibration frequency of a motor versus speed, or air temperature versus moisture content.

• • •

More than a cursory mention of some of the commoner recorders is impossible here.

Servo/Riter II (Texas Instruments, Inc.) (Fig. 13-9). One very reliable series of recorders is Texas Instruments' Servo/Riter II. This instrument uses a null-balancing servopotentiometer. The reference voltage is from a Zener reference circuit. Texas Instruments claims its recorders have no measurable deadband. The servo amplifier uses integrated-circuit components. (See Fig. 13-10.) Integrated circuits are made up of more than one transistor function designed into one chip or crystal. Thus an NPN and a PNP transistor or several stages of amplification may be incorporated into one semiconductor structure. This innovation provides greater reliability and ultimately may allow reduction in the size of the electronic portions of the instrument. The Servo/Riter II instruments are all completely solid state. This allows considerable simplification of design. In Fig. 13-11, notice how this reduction in space required for electronics has been used to provide

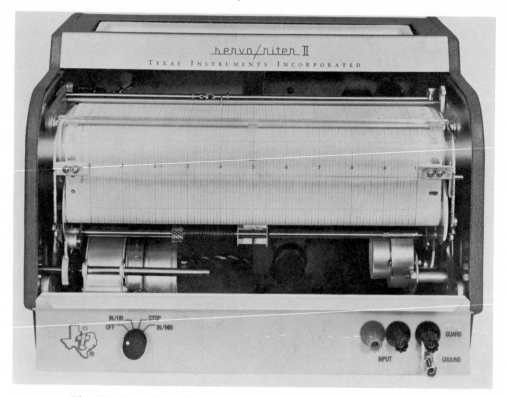

Fig. 13-9. Servo/Riter II Recorder. (Courtesy Texas Instruments, Inc.)

large chart space on a relatively small instrument. The same is true of the somewhat more compact portable instrument in Fig. 13-9. Here the chart is not displayed as liberally, but a wide chart is available in a very compact, lightweight recorder.

Controls on these recorders are extremely simple and clearly labeled. A large number of options in this series of recorders provides almost any input possibility that could be desired and any paper speed. Pen speeds as high as 0.4 second full scale are available. Recorders of this series have been widely used in clinical laboratories for several years and have proved themselves to be very reliable.

Sargent models SR, SRL, SRG, and TR (Sargent-Welch Scientific Co.). This company has produced several excellent recorders that are used considerably in medical laboratories. The SR, SRL, SRG, and TR models have all proved to be popular and

are quite reliable. The SRG is one of the newer instruments, and it might serve as a good example of this company's instruments. The physical configuration of these recorders is designed to provide a slanting desktop sort of chart surface to facilitate examining the record and making notations or measurements. All controls are on a panel on the same plane as the chart to allow any sort of adjustment to be made quickly and conveniently. Where space is not a large consideration and operators know their instruments well, this arrangement is excellent.

The SRG is fully transistorized. It is an automatic, self-balancing potentiometer. A Zener voltage supply is used as a reference. Deadband is less than 0.1% and reproducibility is better than 0.1%. Pen speed is less than 1 second full scale. Input signals may vary from 1 to 100 mv. Filtering is good. Three chart speeds are available by turn-

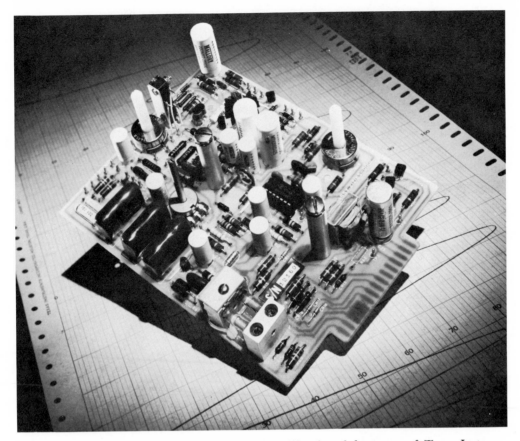

Fig. 13-10. Sophisticated solid-state recorder amplifier board from one of Texas Instruments' recorders. Integrated circuits have allowed additional miniaturization. Note size of the board compared to the chart. (Courtesy Texas Instruments, Inc.)

ing a switch on the front panel. Sargent recorders have proved themselves to be accurate, rugged, and reliable in use.

Electronik no. 16 Strip Chart Recorder (Honeywell, Inc., Industrial Division). This instrument is typical of all Honeywell's instruments. It is a continuously balancing servopotentiometer, using a Zener diode source as a reference against the signal to be measured. The circuitry is solid state and uses printed circuits for ease of repair. Honeywell has an excellent reputation in this field and has incorporated several excellent features in this instrument. Published specifications for the Electronik 16 claim the instrument will perform within a voltage variation of 100 to 130 v AC. An

accuracy of 0.25% of span is claimed, and the standard instrument is designed for operation with source resistances of 0 to 10 megohms. Deadband does not exceed 0.1% of full scale in normal operation. Nominal step-span response times of 15, 5, and 1 second are available on standard production models.

Accessibility of all working parts is one of the advertised features of this recorder. The entire mechanism slides forward out of the case, on runners, for easy service and repair. Another outstanding characteristic is the extreme versatility of input. By changing the range card and by combining resistors, almost any input voltage can be used.

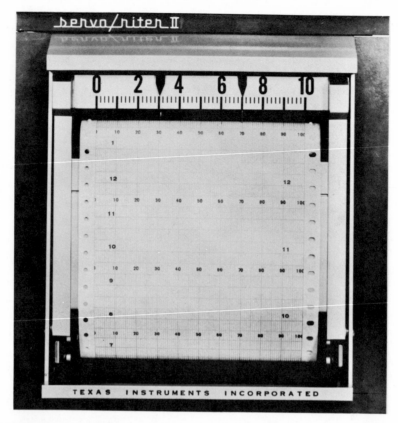

Fig. 13-11. Example of the large chart display available on a relatively small recorder, thanks to circuit miniaturization. (Courtesy Texas Instruments, Inc.)

These recorders are versatile, reliable, and well designed.

Beckman Strip Chart Recorder (Beckman Instruments, Inc.). This instrument is frequently used with several pieces of Beckman equipment and should be mentioned as one of the commoner ones found in the clinical laboratory. It is a small recorder (5 inches) that is lightweight and handy for tabletop use or wall mounting. It is economical and adequate for many laboratory functions. The input span is from 10 to 100 mv without step attenuation and is adjustable with a single control. Three chart speeds are available by use of a slide switch. A 5-inch chart paper is used.

COAGULATION DEVICES

The phenomenon of blood or plasma coagulation occupies a considerable amount of time and attention of the technologist. The principles involved are, of course, complex and not within the purview of this book. The measurement of the actual coagulation process is somewhat less complicated and, within some limits, is amenable to instrumentation. There are a number of problems, however. The nature of the clot formed and the sensitivity of occult activators and inhibitors that may affect coagulation render the process somewhat less concise than colorimetric analysis, for example. Certain fairly arbitrary tests of a general nature may usually be done safely by these devices. Specifically, prothrombin time measurement and partial thromboplastin time measurement are relatively reliable with automatic devices.

Any of several characteristics may be used to establish the fact that coagulation has occurred. The clot changes the viscosity, electrical conductivity, transparency, and fluidity of the sample. The clot has a cohesiveness and tensile strength and all or any of these characteristics can be measured. In practice, most of the devices produced in the United States work on one of three principles. The first of these depends on detection of the change in conductivity that occurs when a clot forms. The second detects a change in viscosity as the clot affects the motion of a mass or particles placed in the reaction tube. The third directly senses the change in optical density when clotting occurs.

For the past several years the **Fibrometer,** which is a product of **Bio-Quest (Division of Becton, Dickinson),** has been the leader in the field of automated coagulation procedures. The test is performed in a plastic cup that is held in a thermostatically controlled block. A gun-type measuring pipette is used to rapidly introduce the patient's serum into the reagent mixture. An electric switch activated by the pipette's plunger causes a timer to start and also causes a mixing head to lower over the cup. Two small sensing agitators mix the test solution at a regular rate until coagulation occurs. Normally the coagulum appears precipitously, causing a sudden change in conductivity of the test solution. The change in the very small maintenance current between the probes causes the timer to stop.

In general the device works well. Very little maintenance is required. A small amount of grease on the pipette plunger of the gun helps keep it functioning smoothly. The metal barrel of the gun comes off the plastic handle with a slight pull, exposing the plunger. If the plunger knob is turned in the 0.2 ml position and depressed, the tip, with a small O-ring seal, will protrude enough to allow light lubrication.

At times, the Fibrometer head fails to drop into place as it should. A very light application of grease and thorough cleaning of the drop shaft under the mixing head help to keep it functioning smoothly. Bio-Quest has been extremely good about keeping these instruments in repair, and the instruments have been almost trouble-free in service.

The **Clotek system** produced by **Hyland,** a division of **Travenol Laboratories,** works on a different principle. Reaction tubes with thromboplastin and a small steel ball are supplied. When the reaction is initiated and the test started, the tube moves up and down but the ball is held, suspended between magnets, where it aids in mixing as the reactant solution flows around it. When the clot is formed, the ball is trapped in the fibrin and moves up and down with the tube, intermittently interrupting a light beam. This photosignal causes the timer to stop.

A system that works on a similar principle is the **Hemochron** produced by **International Technodyne Corp.** This instrument is designed to measure blood coagulability as a substitute for the Lee-White clotting time. Whole blood is placed in a tube with a moving magnet, the position of which is sensed electronically. As the clot restrains the magnet, the electronic sensor stops the digital clock movement and sounds an audible signal. Temperature control of the unit is within 1.0° C. The manufacturers claim good correlation with the Lee-White technique, but much shorter and more reliable clotting times.

The coagulation system used by Technicon Corp. on the Hemalog system has previously been discussed, in Chapter 9.

Many of the newer systems rely on the photodetection of the clot itself, without magnets, steel ball, iron particles, etc. One interesting new model is the **Bio/Data Coagulation system,** produced by **Bio/Data Corp.** (Fig. 13-12). This unit has incubation space for forty samples and the reagents. As the automatic pipette is discharged into the reaction mixture, the timer is activated by a photosignal. The increase in optical density caused by clot formation stops the automatic timer, and

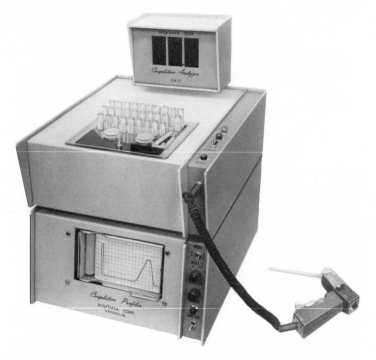

Fig. 13-12. Bio/Data Coagulation system. (Courtesy Bio/Data Corp.)

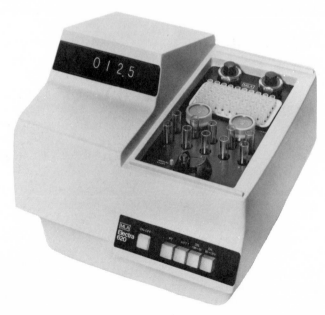

Fig. 13-13. Electra 620 Coagulation system. (Courtesy Medical Laboratory Automation, Inc.)

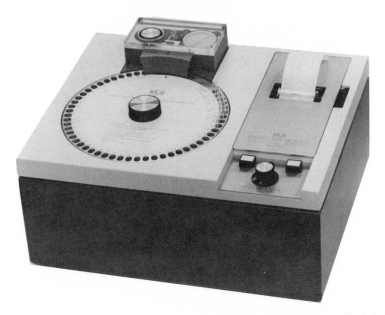

Fig. 13-14. Automatic Coagulation system, Electra 600. (Courtesy Medical Laboratory Automation, Inc.)

results can be read on a digital electronic display. One of the more interesting aspects of this system is the optional 3-inch recorder that shows the change in optical density. The company claims that a reasonably accurate fibrinogen level can be calculated from the slope and length of the curve plotted on the recorder as the clot forms. Work done on this technique, in my laboratory, has proved disappointing. The instrument has functioned well, but good correlation with fibrinogen values was not established to our satisfaction.

Medical Laboratory Automation, Inc., has introduced two optical-electronic coagulation systems that seem quite promising. The smaller and less automated system is the **Electra 620** (Fig. 13-13). Reagents, plasma samples in cuvettes, and sampling tips are all held in a temperature-controlled area. The pipettes are automatic but are not connected to the unit. Discharge of sample, through a light path, triggers the timing, mixing, and reading cycle. A double detection system is used to eliminate false end points. Readout is by electronic digital display. The unit is attractive and appears to be well planned and sturdily built. It has been introduced recently and little experience with it has been reported at this time.

The larger unit produced by MLA is called the **Electra 600.** This supersedes an earlier **Electra 500.** The Model 600 automates most of the coagulation functions. Up to fifty plasma samples can be pipetted into a sample carousel where they are held at 8° C until they approach the test station. As the sample arrives at the pretest area, the temperature is raised to 37° C. In the test position, reagents at 37° C are added automatically and the test cycle begins. As in the Electra 620, the change in OD of the reactants is measured and monitored by a second detector. The result is printed onto a paper tape with the sample identification number. A computer jack is also availabel for on-line testing. The unit is pictured in Fig. 13-14. A number of these units are in use and have proved satisfactory. Results are highly reproducible unless the reagents are inconsistent. The saving of time is probably somewhat less than one would suppose unless large numbers of prothrombin times and PTTs are being performed. This might be said about many automated systems that are underutilized, however.

Sherwood Medical Industries, Inc., has two instruments that compete with those named earlier. These are the **Coagulyzer, Jr.,** and the **Coagulyzer.** The smaller instrument is not remarkably different from the Electra 620. Pipette action electronically actuates the timer. Little detail is given concerning the photoelectric clot detection.

The Coagulyzer is designed to hold sixty samples in the unrefrigerated carousel. Reagents are pipetted automatically and the final pipetting triggers the timing cycle. In most details the instrument is similar to the Electra 600. Two separate, swinghead pipetters dispense the reagents, whereas the Electra dispenses through a stationary tip over the test station. I have no knowledge of comparison studies using these two automated systems. Since the operation is largely a fairly precisely defined mechanical sequence, there is little reason to suppose that large differences would be demonstrated.

Coagulation studies are highly technical in nature because of the complexity of the factors—activators, inhibitors etc.—and their labile natures. The consensus seems to be that direct photodetection of clot formation is the method of choice because no foreign materials are introduced into the test. Probes, magnets, and other particles can introduce physical or chemical factors that are difficult to assess. Unfortunately, the various means of detecting coagulation do not give prothrombin times of equal length; thus direct comparisons cannot be made between different types of instruments.

All of the devices described above can be used for prothrombin time, partial thromboplastin time, and factor assay tests. None are highly accurate when the clot is very poorly defined. It is likely that coagulation studies will be very difficult to automate further.

ADDITIONAL INSTRUMENTS

IL Hemoglobinometer, Model 231 (Instrumentation Laboratory, Inc.) (Fig. 13-15). There are many special-purpose colorimeters on the market and a number of these are designed specifically for reading hemoglobin. The Model 231 is particularly well designed and uses a slightly different rationale. The *isosbestic* wavelength of 548.5 nm is used. This is the point at which oxyhemoglobin, carboxyhemoglobin, and reduced hemoglobin all read at the same concentration. (See Fig. 13-16.) An artificial standard is used to calibrate the instrument. A blood sample is automatically aspirated, diluted, and read at 548.5 nm and the resultant concentration is exhibited on a digital dail. The process requires about 15 seconds. A narrow–band pass interference filter is used. The interference filter, isosbestic point, and automatic mechanical dilution provide accuracy that exceeds the accuracy of most hemoglobin methods. The instrument has the further advantage of flushing itself automatically a few minutes after the last sample is read. The IL Model 231 Hemoglobinometer is an outstanding example of special-purpose colorimeters designed for one specific function.

IL Co-Oximeter 182 (Instrumentation Laboratory, Inc.) (Fig. 13-17). A natural outgrowth of the Hemoglobinometer has been the Co-Oximeter 182. This instrument is able to record total hemoglobin at 548.5 nm. By ratioing the absorbances at 568 and 548.5 nm, the carboxyhemoglobin is measured. Oxyhemoglobin is measured in like manner, from the ratio of absorbances at 578 to 548 nm. This instrument is of particular value in cardiac catheteriza-

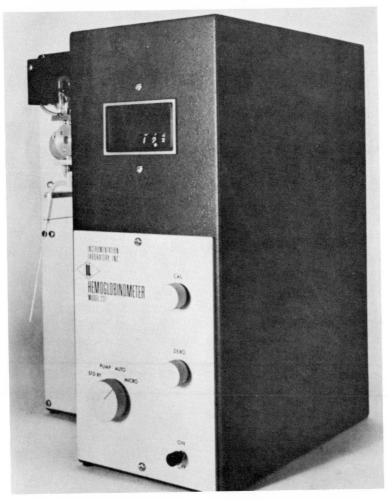

Fig. 13-15. Hemoglobinometer, Model 231. (Courtesy Instrumentation Laboratory, Inc.)

tion, distinguishing between the output of the right and left sides of the heart and differentiating conditions in which there is mixing. A review of Fig. 13-16 will facilitate understanding the instrument's operation.

An earlier instrument, the **American Optical Corp. Oximeter,** works on a similar principle. This device reads total hemoglobin at an isosbestic wavelength of 805 nm as reflected light passes through an interference filter of that wavelength. Since oxyhemoglobin is predominant at 660 nm,

reflected light from the sample also passes through an interference filter at 660 nm. The two photocurrents are nulled by means of an occluding disc calibrated as percent saturation (Fig. 13-18).

Fragilographs. These instruments have not become commonplace as yet, but they may receive more attention in the next few years. They are devices for measuring the fragility of red cells or other cells when exposed to solutions of differing tonicity. The principle is very simple. Whole blood is diluted in isotonic saline and introduced into

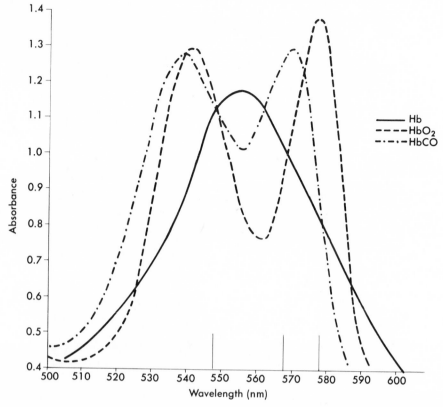

Fig. 13-16. Spectral scans of oxyhemoglobin, carboxyhemoglobin, and reduced hemoglobin. Note that any of the three would read the same absorbance at 548.5 nm if present in the same concentration. This is called the *isosbestic point* for all three. (Courtesy Instrumentation Laboratory, Inc.)

a cell whose walls on two sides are dialysis membranes. The cell is immersed in distilled water between a light source and a photocell. As dialysis occurs, the saline becomes gradually more hypotonic and the cells are lysed. This allows more light to reach the photocell. The photosignal is fed to a recorder as a function of time. The change in salt concentration, resulting from diaylsis, may also be described as a function of time so that the curve of cell destruction may be easily plotted against changes in salt concentration. Individual tests can be performed in 5 or 10 minutes. The fragilograph is manufactured by **Elron Electronics Industries of Haifa, Israel.**

Microtomes. There are many instruments in use in histology that might deserve men-

tion. Since microtomes are straightforward mechanical devices, we shall say nothing further about them except to emphasize the obvious but critical and often neglected point that lubrication is extremely important in their maintenance. The feed mechanism, in particular, is seriously damaged by wear when not kept properly lubricated. Aside from trivial mechanical annoyances this is about the only common problem with microtomes.

The cryostat microtome contains its own refrigeration unit to provide greater ease in handling frozen sections. It consists of a standard microtome mounted in a refrigerated cabinet and provided with an intensely cold block for quickly freezing the tissue block to be cut. The refrigeration sys-

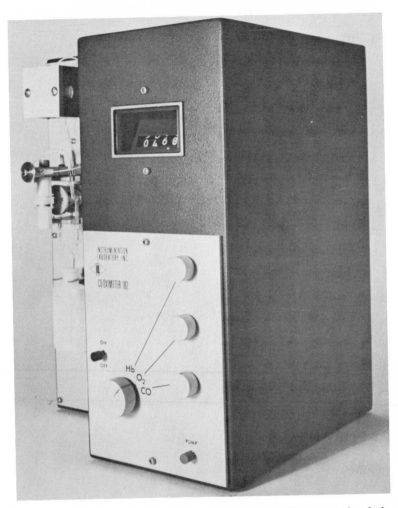

Fig. 13-17. Co-Oximeter, Model 182. This unit was a natural outgrowth of the Hemoglobinometer, which it resembles. Two additional filters (568 and 578 nm) provide the necessary information for calculation of the three forms of hemoglobin. (Courtesy Instrumentation Laboratory, Inc.)

tem is not remarkable, and any refrigeration repairman can attend to its problems. The quick-freezing block is seldom entirely satisfactory and is almost always supplemented by *Freon* gas in spray cans or some similar device. Because of the cold state of the microtome, either lubrication is often neglected or the oil does not get where it should go. When the instrument is defrosted, it should be wiped clean and dry and carefully lubricated. Circumstances may vary considerably, but this should

never be neglected longer than 3 months in any circumstance.

Tissue-processing equipment. Tissue-processing equipment is in use in practically every hospital laboratory. Technicon Corporation has been the leader in this field since its inception over 40 years ago. Lipshaw Manufacturing Co., Fisher Scientific Co., and others also produce devices of this sort. The instruments are all purely mechanical arrangements to move tissue samples or fluids from place to place ac-

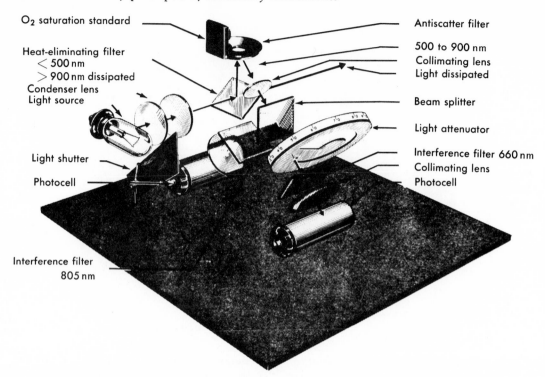

O₂ saturation standard

Heat-eliminating filter
$< 500 \, nm$
$> 900 \, nm$ dissipated
Condenser lens
Light source

Light shutter

Photocell

Interference filter
805 nm

Antiscatter filter

500 to 900 nm
Collimating lens
Light dissipated

Beam splitter

Light attenuator

Interference filter 660 nm
Collimating lens
Photocell

Fig. 13-18. Optical path of the AO Oximeter. Light from the exciter lamp is reflected, by the heat-eliminating mirror, to the bottom of the cuvette, which sits in the ring at top center. This filtered light is reflected by the blood, back through the collimating lens, to the beam splitter. At the beam splitter, half the light goes to the 660 filter and photocell while the other half goes to the 805 filter and photocell. The light attenuator blocks some of the light on the 660 side to null the photocurrents. The amount of light attenuated is obivously a function of oxyhemoglobin concentration, so values can be printed on the attenuator dial. (Courtesy American Optical Corp.)

cording to a predetermined time sequence. Small motors, gear assemblies, levers, and microswitches are the components that cause these to function. A few minutes of close observation will usually suffice for understanding the mechanics of any part of the system when it is open for observation. Problems usually involve the failure of microswitches or small motors. Occasionally lack of lubrication or long use may cause wear of a gear train or bearing, but in general these devices are well designed and capable of many years of hard service without excessive wear. Some comments about the checking of microswitches, fuses, small motors, etc. may be found in the next chapter.

A recent innovation of Technicon Corporation is the Autotechnicon Ultra, which adds heating of reagents, better agitation, and vacuum to the mechanics of the well-known models. It might be assumed, on the basis of past experience with Technicon's mechanical engineering, that there would be no significant problem with this system other than minor ones mentioned earlier.

Knife sharpeners. These are in use in nearly every histology laboratory. Although they are extremely simple devices, they seem to give trouble occasionally. There are several common designs. They are of either the flat-surface type or the honing-wheel type. The first moves the knife in a very concise position back and forth over a glass honing plate to which honing compound has been applied. Some provision is made for turning the knife occasionally, either automatically or manually. This process obviously produces a straight bevel on the knife. The wheel type of sharpener presents the knife edge to a honing wheel, which may be glass or smooth metal, to which honing compound is applied. This type of sharpener gives the bevel a slightly concave characteristic, which some microtomists prefer. Obviously, when a knife has been sharpened on one type sharpener, a great deal of time is required to reestablish the new bevel on the other type of machine. It should be equally obvious that changing the bevel angle can be disastrous and should be done only if absolutely necessary. Any significant change in the bevel should be done by the manufacturer or another service facility completely knowledgeable concerning microtome knife reconditioning.

Abrasive compound is designed to cut away metal. Its accidental presence in bearings and gears is certain to cause unusual wear, and care should be taken to keep it away from moving parts. Lubrication should be done regularly. Electric parts should be kept dry. All these points would seem to be obvious, but problems such as these contribute greatly to the maintenance of equipment of this sort.

There is much variation between instruments in the use of abrasives, oils, soaps, etc. in the sharpening process, and the only admonition appropriate is that the manufacturer's directions should be followed implicitly unless experience and careful observation have shown it safe to deviate from them. The same might be said about such details as turning cycles, bevel settings, etc.

Microtome Knife Sharpener (American Optical Corp., Analytical Instrument Division). The AO Knife Sharpener is in very common use and deserves special attention here. It moves the knife back and forth across a honing plate a few times and then raises and turns it to present the opposite side for the same cycle. This process saves considerable manual manipulation, and the instrument has produced very good cutting edges. Two characteristics have given some mechanical difficulty. (1) On earlier models the motor was rather unsatisfactory and caused considerable problem. Newer models have a heavier, better-designed motor that has worked quite well. The newer motor can be obtained from the company and used to replace the older one with a minimum of inconvenience. (2) If the adjustments having to do with cycling the mechanism are disturbed, the process of integrating all functions again can be very time-consuming. With some combinations of adjustments, the knife-elevating arm jams and locks the entire gear train. Unless it becomes absolutely necessary in the course of repair, no adjustments should be made.

Balances. Anyone working in a laboratory regularly has been exposed to many types of balances, and the principle of operation of some types is simple and obvious. In recent years a few new devices have been introduced in this area, and it seems worthwhile to make some mention of them. *Substitution balances* have come into common use. In these balances a weight in an air-damping chamber at one end of a beam is exactly balanced by a group of removable weights at the other end. When a sample is added to the latter end, weights are removed mechanically to maintain a constant balance. The weights removed represent the weight of the sample. Some of these balances have a small lens with a scale mounted in the beam in such a position that a slight imbalance moves the shadow of the scale into position along a pointer to indicate small errors in substitution. The air-damping chamber consists of a vane mounted around the weights in the nearly airtight chamber. As the weight moves, air slowly leaves the chamber, allowing the weight and vane on the beam to gradually assume the proper balance position. Magnetic damping is also used on some balances. Although the readout dial may be illuminated or an electric light may project the scale to show the imbalance and magnetic damping may be used, the substitution balance itself is still mechanical. In work on a balance of this sort, care in handling weights and protecting the ruby knife edges must be exercised, just as in a classic analytical balance.

Another concept is the *electrobalance,* which is capable of very accurate weighing of very small samples. The sample is weighed from a light metal beam attached to an electromagnetic coil that is suspended in a stronger electromagnetic field. Current through the field is automatically adjusted to counteract the torque caused by the object being weighed. The correcting electric current is calibrated against standard weights. The balance is quite versatile; different spans can be chosen to provide accurate weighings from tenths of a milligram to a few grams. Several sources of weighing error are eliminated in this instrument. The Cahn Division of Ventron Instruments Corp. has been a leader in developing electrobalances.

Pipetters and dilutors. A large number of devices for pipetting accurately measured quantities of fluid are now available. These vary from the hand-gun type mentioned in the discussion of the Bio-Quest Fibrometer, through the syringe variations, all the way to highly automated repetitive pipetters for moving tubes in a rack or drum and adding predetermined amounts of fluid to each. Two remarks might be appropriate here.

In general these devices are as good as their *seals.* Around the plunger, displacement element, or other device there must be some sort of seal to contain the fluid that is generally being displaced under some positive pressure. Constant use eventually causes wear or damage to these seals, and they begin to leak. Even glass on glass and stainless steel on glass are eventually

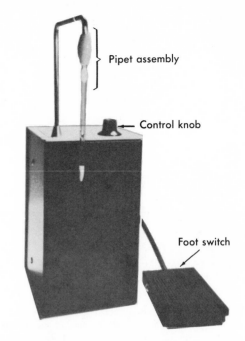

Fig. 13-19. Dade Dilutor. This is one of the most consistently accurate dilutors in its price class. (Courtesy Dade Reagents, Division of American Hospital Supply Corp.)

subject to this sort of wear. Small pieces of broken glass, sand, or other material can cause jamming and possibly considerable damage. Stainless steel on glass or heavy Teflon seems to be the most durable.

In general, motor-driven systems are more accurate than those operated by hand.

Motor-driven models seem to provide a consistent action that gives much more reproducible results. One motor-driven dilutor that has proved itself to be highly accurate and reproducible is the Dade Dilutor (Fig. 13-19). The addition of a motor drive has made the Auto-Dilutor a very good instrument (Fig. 13-20). It is now produced by **American Optical Corp.** and is called the **Power-Actuated Auto-Dilutor.**

Mixers, shakers, rotators, pumps, and other power-driven mechanical devices are all very simple in concept and need no elucidation. Some comments in the next

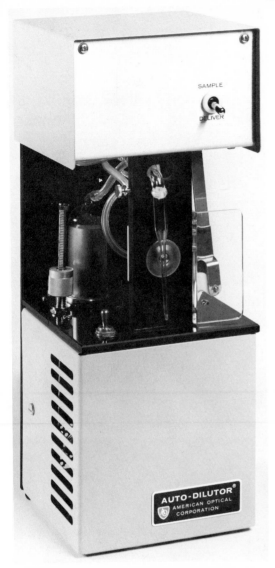

Fig. 13-20. Power-actuated Auto-Dilutor with motor-driven plungers. (Courtesy American Optical Corp.)

chapter may prove applicable to their maintenance and repair. The same is true, in general, about ovens, incubators, baths, hot plates, etc., which produce or control temperature.

OSMOMETRY AND OSMOMETERS

In some clinical laboratories and particularly in those involved with testing many patients with renal disease, the measurement of *osmolarity* has become common. Osmolarity is concerned with the measurement of the concentration of solute in a solvent. In clinical applications urine and blood serum are usually tested. One gram molecular weight of nonionizable material per kilogram of water equals 1 *osmol* or 1000 *milliosmols*. Sodium chloride, for example, ionizes almost completely, and a gram molecular weight is equal to 2 osmols. *Osmolality* is preferred as a standard unit of measurement. Whereas osmolarity refers to solute weight per kilogram of solvent, osmolality is solute weight per liter of solvent.

Specific gravity, total solids, and the refractive index do not give the same information as osmolality, since they are all concerned with the mass of the solute. Osmolality has specific value, since it is closely related to the colligative properties of body fluids, and it is these properties that determine thirst and stimulate diuresis and retention of water through their action on the osmoreceptors of the body.

The osmolality of serum depends, in large part, on sodium. The serum sodium in milliequivalents per liter times 2.1 should give the approximate milliosmols if the patient is normally healthy. Increases and decreases in serum sodium usually, but not always, cause changes in the osmolality. Abnormal osmolalities of serum should be immediately checked for sodium, sugar, and urea to determine the nature of the disturbance.

The ratio of serum to urine osmolality should be between 1:3 and 1:4 in first morning urine. A urine value of less than 600, after overnight fluid deprivation, strongly suggests renal disease.

As can be seen from the above random notes, the measurement of osmolality in serum is largely a screening procedure that quickly and easily points up certain abnormalities that might be missed without the testing of several parameters. In some situ-

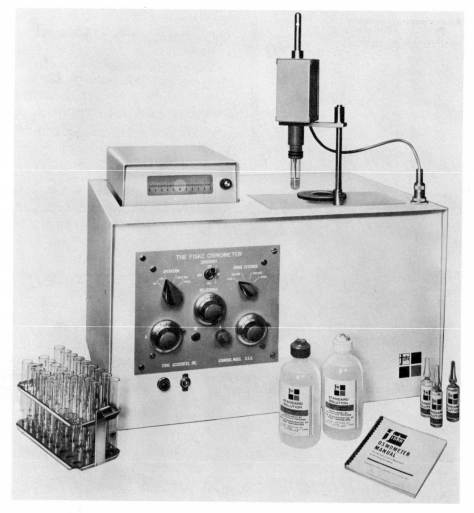

Fig. 13-21. Fiske Osmometer with galvanometric readout. (Courtesy Fiske Associates, Inc.)

ations it would seem to be a simple screening device with considerable value.

Several theoretically possible ways of measuring osmolality exist. All the commercially available devices depend on the measurement of *depression of freezing point,* since the freezing point of a liquid is dependent on its solute concentration. Fiske Associates, Inc., has pioneered in the development of osmometers, and its instrument is described here as representative. The **Fiske Osmometer** is shown in Fig. 13-21.

When a solution is cooled rapidly, it may not form ice even though the temperature is far below its freezing point. If a crystal or some impurity is added or if the solution is disturbed, ice formation quickly follows. An unfrozen solution that is colder than its normal freezing point is called a *supercooled liquid.*

When supercooled water produces ice, the temperature rises rather quickly to 0° C due to the fact that crystal formation of water produces heat. This temperature change is not instantaneous, since crystal formation is not an instantaneous process. The freezing point (0° C for water) is an *equilibrium point,* and the temperature will stay constant there for a few minutes.

The Osmometer is a device that supercools urine or serum, causes it to crystalize, and measures its freezing point by locating the equilibrium-point plateau. The freezing point, however, is read in milliosmols of solute rather than degrees of temperature.

The sample of serum or urine is placed in position, with the sensing probe tips immersed in the liquid. The sensing probe contains a tiny thermistor through which a small current is passed. As the temperature changes, the current is monitored by a galvanometer. The sample and probe are lowered into the coolant, where the refrigerator unit rapidly supercools the sample. A vibrator is activated, causing crystalization, and the temperature is watched on the galvanometer readout until the equilibrium-point plateau is reached. At this point resistance is applied to the Wheatstone balancing bridge to bring the galvanometer into balance. The resistance applied is relative to the temperature of the probe, which, of course, indicates the freezing point and osmolarity of the sample.

In general we could say that the instrument contains a refrigeration unit with circulating pump, a temperature probe that activates a galvanometer, a vibrator, and a Wheatstone bridge. There is also a precooling tank for lowering the temperature of the sample before the test.

Although the above is an oversimplification of this well-designed instrument, it should provide the student with some comprehension of the Osmometer's construction.

In operating the instrument, the student should follow the instruction of the manufacturer in detail, since this is a very exact procedure.

The Fiske Osmometer is well built and relatively trouble-free. There is little about the instrument that should give trouble in normal use.

Two other osmometers are in common use. One is the **Osmette,** manufactured by **Precision Systems,** and the other is manufactured by **Advance Instruments, Inc.**

REVIEW QUESTIONS

1. What determines relative centrifugal force?
2. How does a bimetallic thermostat work?
3. What is a strobe light?
4. What is deadband?
5. What is the isosbestic point for most hemoglobin forms?
6. How does a substitution balance work?
7. Explain the rationale used in osmolality measurement.
8. Name two devices used for temperature control.
9. What is the function of the commutator in a centrifuge?
10. Explain how the Disc Integrator, pictured in Fig. 13-8, sums up the area under a curve.
11. Explain the difference in principle between the Fibrometer clot detection system and that of the Electra 620.
12. List the heating and cooling devices, involved in laboratory analysis, in your laboratory. Do you understand, in general terms, how each works?

14
Care, maintenance, and repair

The foregoing chapters should have given some insight into the principles and ideas behind the equipment in use. A good understanding of electricity and electronics could involve study for many months, and any single chapter of this book could be the subject for a book or a small library. Hopefully the student has now attained some appreciation of the instruments he uses. The important problem of keeping valuable equipment working is yet to be considered.

Many of the devices in the laboratory are small, simple instruments: pumps, heaters, dilutors, simple spectrophotometers, etc. These should be understood by qualified laboratory personnel, and their failure or malfunction should be diagnosable and in many cases repairable. Often solutions to problems with simple equipment involve calm good sense more than profound knowledge. In the second edition of this book a chapter entitled "Shop Talk and Horse Sense" provided a long list of pretty simple problems and their solutions. It was included with some misgivings. Surprisingly, this feature has received considerable favorable comment from readers, and I have learned of quick courses, for instrument repairmen and engineers, designed to get people to logically define their problem before starting some heroic solution. One sign in a shop reads: IF IT WORKS DON'T FIX IT. This is another

way of saying, "Be sure there is a problem that would indicate the repair measures you are about to undertake." The same simple suggestions still make sense.

1. Are you sure it is *plugged in?* Maybe the cleaning lady pulled the plug.

2. Are you sure the *overload breaker* in the breaker panel is not thrown out? Try a desk lamp or a test light in the receptacle to be sure there is electricity available.

3. If there is no electricity at the plug, find the *breaker box* that furnishes your area of the building. It is probably a small metal door in the hallway close by.

4. In older buildings there may be screw-in fuses in the box. They are rated as to the number of amps they will carry. You can tell if the *fuse is blown* by looking at the mica front window. If it is smoked up and the little metal band under it is melted, the fuse is blown and must be replaced.

5. Do not replace the fuse or reset the breaker until you have looked around for the *cause* of the fuse blowing. It may have been a direct short from a broken wire or some obvious defect. It could also be from too much load on the line (too many heating devices, etc.). If no immediate cause is found, unplug as many items as possible, replace the fuse, and reconnect the devices one at a time until the new fuse blows. This will tell you which item is responsible for the overload. By taking everything else off the line and trying again, you can tell if the total load was too much for the fuse or if there was an electrical problem in the device last reconnected.

6. More than likely you will find rocker-type circuit breakers in the panel, instead of fuses of the older, screw-in type.

7. Rocker-type breakers have a small element that heats and expands, when overloaded, throwing out the breaker and thus

cutting off electricity to that circuit. When they are depressed to the right, they are usually "on" (depending on the mounting). At any rate they will be marked.

8. When breakers throw out, you cannot always easily tell by glancing at them. They may be pushed only slightly up from the "on" position. If you run a finger down the line of breakers, the one that is out will be slightly raised. Immediately after a circuit breaker throws out, it may feel warm or even hot. Other breakers that are heavily loaded may also feel warm, however.

9. To put the circuit back in use, push down on the off (or out) side and then depress the on (or in) side as far as it will go. If it throws out again and you cannot locate the problem, call an electrician.

10. If the instrument is still dead although plugged in and there is electricity in the line, check the instrument's fuse. Usually the fuse holder is a little black or brown knob close to the point where the power cable goes into the instrument. Some fuse holders have a cover with a milled edge that can be easily removed with the fingers. Other are threaded and must be screwed out, whereas still others have a bayonet lock that requires only a half-turn. Some fuse covers require a screwdriver to turn. The fuse holder is spring loaded so that the fuse will usually spring out, and one end may be clamped to the fuse cover.

11. Look at this small glass *minifuse* to see whether it is smoked up and whether the metal band or wire inside is melted. If it is a tiny wire, it may burn up completely. If you are not sure whether it is burned out, check it with a multimeter or replace it with another fuse of the same rating. The rating is engraved in the metal band at one end.

12. To check the fuse with a meter, set the meter to ohms and turn the selector knob to the lowest setting, which is usually marked × 1 (or simply 1). Touch the two meter leads together. The needle should move to the right side of the meter. (This shows that you are in the proper meter setting.) Now touch the two meter probes to either end of the fuse. If the needle responds, the fuse is all right.

13. If the fuse is good and the intrument still does not respond, check lamps. If an exciter lamp is out, a photometer will obviously not respond. Try a new exciter lamp. If the instrument has a galvanometer lamp and it is out, no light will appear on the scale even though the exciter lamp is on. It is probably best to unplug the instrument while checking and changing lamps, to avoid the possibility of shock. Never work with an instrument's wiring while standing on a wet floor or leaning against metal surfaces unless you are sure it is disconnected. Do not forget to plug it in again before trying it.

14. If the instrument still does not respond, remove the cover and start hunting for obvious problems such as the following: (A) A blackened spot may indicate a short-circuit. (B) A loose wire that goes no place may indicate a broken lead. See if you can tell where it should have been connected. If this is not apparent, do not just guess. This could cause damage. (C) Melted resin, smoke deposit, or a strong smell around a transformer or motor may indicate that it is burned out. (D) Look for resistors that are split open. Sometimes excess heat or humidity may destroy a resistor, leaving a circuit open. (E) Check for any rarely used switches on the back or inside the instrument that might cancel the function you are attempting to use. (F) With the multimeter on the ohms position, attach a lead to one prong of the power cable and touch the other lead to the point inside the instrument where the power comes in. Repeat with the other side of the cable. A little searching will show where terminals connect inside the instrument. One side of the power cord will almost certainly go to the fuse holder. If continuity cannot be demonstrated (if the nee-

dle will not move), there may be a break in the cable. While checking, it is a good idea to bend or flex the cable to be sure that the wires inside the insulation are not broken and only occasionally making contact. Also check between the two wires for shorts. (G) If a three-strand power cable is used, the round peg of the plug-in is the ground and it is probably attached to the frame of the instrument. Check this for continuity with the ohmmeter also. (H) Attach the meter leads (still on ohms) to the two sides of the main power switch and throw the switch. The meter should deflect in the "on" position and return to the peg in the "off" position. (I) If the instrument has vacuum tubes, replace them, being careful to replace with the proper type of tube. (J) Switch the meter to AC volts and set it on 110 v or higher to see whether, with the instrument plugged in and turned on, you can measure 110 v (more or less) at the point where the power cord enters the instrument. If you can, follow the two lines along to see how far you can trace the current. You may be able to find the defective element in this way after you have had a little experience and know the instrument. Be careful not to shock yourself or produce a short by touching two hot points with the same probe. Handle the probes on the insulated portion only. If the problem has not been solved by this time, you would be wise to turn the instrument over to a qualified repairman.

15. When a meter responds erratically and the controls do not produce a smooth response, the problem may be in a faulty potentiometer. Try turning the control, as evenly as possible, from one end of its travel to the other. If the meter needle does not respond smoothly, the pot may be defective. Try tapping the control knob with the ball of your finger and notice whether the meter needle remains relatively steady. If not, this is an additional indication of a defective pot. Try this latter test in several positions of the control knob. The defect of the pot may be at only one point. A pot is not difficult to change after a little practice with a soldering iron. Be sure to replace with the proper type of pot. The size indicates the wattage, whereas the ohms and the percent accuracy are usually stamped on the back. Be sure to note which lead goes to which contact of the pot. If you have wired it backward, the meter will move in the wrong direction when the knob is turned. Also be sure that all contacts are tightly soldered and that no loose drops of solder have fallen where they can cause shorts.

16. Soldering is not difficult, and you can become reasonably proficient, with a little practice. For instrument work a small *pencil-type iron* is to be preferred over a *solder gun*. The latter heats more quickly but produces more heat than is needed and is harder to get into small places without causing damage to delicate parts. Remove as much of the old solder as conveniently possible. Hook the wires to be soldered into the solder holes or otherwise secure them. Place the tip of the iron on the point to be soldered so that both the wire and the contact are heated. Touch the solder to the iron at the point of contact and let the solder fuse completely before withdrawing the iron. If the contact is not hot enough, the solder will not bond to it and a "cold-solder joint" may be made; this could result in a poor electrical connection. Avoid using an excess of solder and dripping hot drops of the metal onto other parts. A resin-core solder of about no. 20 G or 22 G is right for this sort of work. The soldering iron should not be left plugged in for extended periods of time. *Retinning* the tip of the iron occasionally helps to keep it in good shape. This is done by melting a drop of solder on the point and quickly wiping it over the hot surface with a piece of waste.

17. When electric motors will not function, the following checks may be made: (A) Is electricity getting to the motor? Check whether the motor is plugged in,

check the line circuit breaker, the instrument fuse, etc., as noted earlier. (B) Check whether the motor can be turned freely by hand. (C) If it can, unplug the device and check the *brushes.* They are accessible through small plastic caps on either side of the motor. Be sure that plenty of carbon is left on the brushes, that the brushes are actually touching the *armature* (is the lower edge worn shiny?), and that the spring or wire making electric contact in the brush holder is not broken. The brush should fit snugly in the brush holder. If it is so loose that the brush is worn off at an angle, it is probably the wrong size brush. If the brush does not slide easily into the holder, it may fail to feed down against the *commutator* as the carbon is worn away. This may be due to the brush being too large or to a deposit of carbon building up in the brush holder. Carbon may be cleaned out with a cotton-tipped applicator soaked in carbon tetrachloride or some simialr solvent. Dry out any excess solvent. Special solvents for cleaning motors are available. (D) If the motor turns but not easily, there is a good chance that a *bearing* has gotten so dry that it is impeding the motor and could result in burning the motor out. Work light oil into the bearings as well as possible and turn the motor back and forth on its bearings until the bearings are completely free and the motor will turn easily by hand. Try it under power to see whether the problem has been solved. Next time, oil the bearings before they get dry. (E) If the motor cannot be turned by hand, a bearing is probably "seized" or "frozen" from lack of lubrication and possibly too much heat. An attempt can be made to work the bearing loose with lubricants and a little carefully exercised force. If this does not work, the motor must be torn down and the bearings replaced. If the bearing has been frozen and under power for very long, it is possible that the motor is badly burned and will require extensive repair or re-

placement. (F) If the motor turns freely and the brushes are in good shape, it is quite possible that there is a break in either the *field coil* or *armature winding* and the motor will need to be sent to a shop for rewinding. (G) If the motor hums but does not move or moves only slightly, there may be a short, which condition will also require rewinding. (H) If the motor runs very noisily and occasionally hangs up, the bearings may be badly worn. To check end play, with the motor in a vertical position (as in a centrifuge), lift the shaft as much as possible and let it drop a few times. A little play with just a faint click can be heard as the shaft falls back into place. A barely perceptible end play is necessary for the motor to run smoothly. If considerable play exists or if a definite metallic clank can be heard, the bearing is probably getting rather badly worn. Some motors have a single ball bearing at the lower end of the shaft with a take-up screw beneath it for adjusting out any end play. If this does not exist, the motor will have to be removed and the bearing replaced. To check the top bearing, grasp the top of the shaft (or the centrifuge head) and attempt to work it from side to side. If any play is felt, the bearing is worn. If a definite metallic clank can be heard, the bearing is in bad condition and should be replaced before the motor binds and causes damage to the windings. Keep in mind that some motors are mounted on rubber grommets and the whole motor may move when you attempt to move the shaft in its bearings. (I) It is always possible that a switch, a rectifier, Variac, or some other component has failed. By using the multimeter and a little reasoning, you may possibly locate such a failure, but in any case a repairman may very possibly be needed to make the repair.

18. Heating equipment rarely fails except when cords are broken or switches defective, but heat control is often a problem. Heating elements seem to last about as long as the device in which they are in-

stalled. The thermostat may be a different matter. As discussed in Chapter 1, there are several types of thermostats. The type that actually makes and breaks the current to the heater through the thermostatic elements is very often subject to failure. The points may become so corroded and burned that contact can no longer be made. Burnishing the contacts with emery cloth may restore them temporarily. New points or a new thermostat may have to be installed. If the points arc and get hot enough to weld together, current will continue to flow until a fuse blows or the device actually burns. This type of thermostat is fortunately seldom used now. A more common type relies on a microswitch actuated by the thermostatic element, to make and break the circuit. These switches fail occasionally. In most cases the switch makes an audible click when switching occurs. If you cannot cause the switch to click by depressing and releasing its plunger, it is probably bad. It can be checked with an ohmmeter as described if there is any doubt about it. These switches are usually easy to replace if the correct replacement can be found. In water baths the sensing element (often a fluid-filled capsule and capillary) lies in the bottom of the bath. Corrosive reagents used around the bath may corrode the capillary until it leaks. The sensing element must then be replaced.

19. Laboratory power lines are often overloaded, since planners often do not realize the considerable amount of electricity used by the dozens of laboratory devices. Although there is usually at least one electrician or plant engineer who worries about such things, it is wise to keep an eye on overload problems. One danger signal is excessive heat at the circuit breaker panel. If a circuit is heavily loaded, that particular breaker will be hot, and, if the circuit is very much overloaded, the breaker will throw out occasionally. Sometimes it is possible to physically move some high-consumption devices to other circuits, or the electrician may move some circuits from one breaker to put them on a less-used position in the breaker box. When the entire lab load begins to be too heavy for the system supplied, voltage may drop. This may cause many serious problems with laboratory equipment. Voltage can be checked at the wall plug with a voltmeter. One of the wires at the receptacle is the hot wire and the other is essentially zero. For current to be quite adequate, the voltage difference between the two should be 117 v or close to it and fluctuations should not occur. Recording voltmeters are available to monitor voltage over a period of time if this seems desirable. Most laboratory instruments will compensate fairly well for drops to about 100 v, but some will not. A lower drop may cause motors to stall and burn. Surges of very high voltage, occasionally associated with overloading, can be very damaging to some components, including vacuum tubes. Voltage measured from the hot line to the ground line (the round hole of the receptacle on a three-wire system) should read essentially the same as the voltage from the high wire to the low wire. If there is no reading at all, the ground line is not grounded and the electrician should check it. When power requirement exceeds the potential of the system, unused 220 v lines may be split out to provide two 110 v circuits, or lines may be run in from adjacent areas.

20. The person responsible for the care and maintenance of laboratory equipment is seldom able to keep up with all the potential problems. If he develops an awareness of equipment and constantly looks and listens for items needing attention, he may be able to avoid many breakdown situations. The tools should be closely available, and loose screws should be tightened, dry bearings lubricated, dirty contacts cleaned, etc. as a normal part of housekeeping.

21. A listing and a diagrammatic rep-

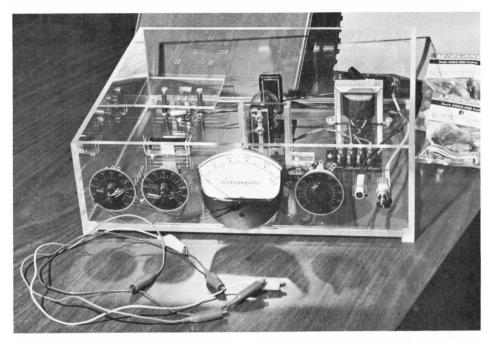

Fig. 14-1. Instra-Mentor, a training device with manual of experiments. (Courtesy Elementary Principles, Inc.)

resentation of the symbols used in wiring diagrams are presented on pp. 264 and 265. As experience is gained, you can pick up some comprehension of diagrams that will enable you to follow through some wiring plans and better understand their function and their potential problems. Some diagrams are presented throughout the book both for their practical value and for practice work. Study these in comparison with the instrument involved to gain more understanding of wiring diagrams.

22. It is quite possible to read extensively about instruments and still not know a transformer from a transistor. Experiments and experience with components help greatly. For the really serious student of the subject, a regular course in commercial electronics is suggested. Another approach to learning in this area is assembly of various Heathkits, sold by the Heath Co., or the use of training devices such as the Instra-Mentor (Fig. 14-1), made by Elementary Principles, Inc.

23. There are no instant electronics or instrument experts. Only experience, observation, and interest can develop the abilities necessary to cope with instrument failure. It is to be hoped that the information contained herein will help the student acquire some understanding and interest.

24. The following tools and supplies are suggested for any reasonably active laboratory.

Tools

Pliers—needle-nosed and ordinary
Wire cutter and stripper
Vise-grip wrenches
Files—crosscut, rattail, and triangular
Set of small end wrenches
Set of screwdrivers—small to large, and offset screwdriver
Phillips screwdrivers
Set of Allen wrenches
Small vise
Small soldering iron
Flashlight

Tools—cont'd
Mulitmeter
Test lamp
Small knife
Hemostats
Small hammer

Supplies

Solder
Spool of 18- or 20-gauge hook-up wire
Electrician's tape
Emery paper
Epoxy cement
Spade terminals or other types
Fuses for all instruments
Brushes for all motors
Didymium filter that will fit into appropriate spectrophotometer
Spare vacuum tubes for instruments in use
Replacement lamps for all instruments on hand
3-in-one oil and centrifuge lubricant
Instruction manuals for all instruments
Any repair or replacement parts recommended by manufacturer
Collection of miscellaneous hardware—nuts, bolts, etc.

As equipment becomes more sophisticated and automated, it becomes less possible for medical laboratory personnel to perform adequate repairs. Indeed, the maintenance problem is one that is shared with society in general. Cars, radios, TVs, refrigerators, etc. become less amenable to simple repair, and each year shows a larger proportion of the national work force involved in service and less in production. Also, the problem of getting competent repair is often next to impossible. Several solutions may be suggested. One of the simplest, intended to avoid serious repair problems, with down time, is to insist that all personnel who use equipment carefully read operating and maintenance instructions. All steps in care and maintenance should be posted (if complicated or detailed) and should be followed in all cases. Deviations

from normal instrument performance should be noted and investigated. A record should be kept of repairs, calibrations, and maintenance procedures. It may be expedient to keep operating records at the work bench and major repair records in an instrument maintenance section if one exists. Fig. 14-2 shows a sample of the computer printout of the record kept by the maintenance section in my laboratory.

Some source of repair service should be available at all times. Rarely is this a simple matter. Many instruments are on warranty or maintenance agreement. Some instruments cannot reasonably be repaired by any but factory personnel. The repair situation may be complex, and only the chief technologist can designate the individual to call when disaster strikes.

One solution is to have available a person with electronics background, trained to do some repairs and knowing what steps to take when the matter is beyond his competence. Finding the right man and establishing his limitations in a realistic manner may be a problem. Vocational schools and junior colleges are beginning to train men with a fair competence in instrumentation. The supply is improving, as is the quality of training. The person being introduced into this role should have immediate access to all manuals and operating instructions. Once he has familiarized himself with the equipment, he should set up an *adequate* and *realistic* inventory of repair parts (with help from a knowledgeable technologist). A regular schedule for checks and maintenance should be set up and followed.

Sometimes a local repair shop that is adequate to the situation can be found. In larger cities this is generally possible. In smaller towns it may be a problem. Radio and TV repairmen are generally not too helpful unless they are willing to take the time to learn laboratory equipment and be available when needed.

Recently several large companies have undertaken to train and equip persons to

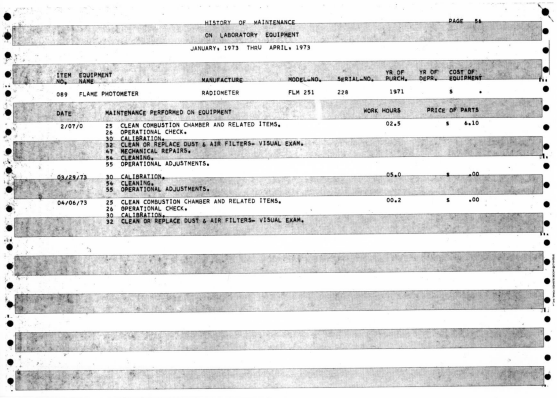

Fig. 14-2. Computer printout of instrument maintenance record.

meet the laboratory-wide or even hospital-wide repair problems. Honeywell Corp., through its Test Instruments Division, has set out to provide repair centers in many areas of the United States. These centers would be able to repair any hospital equipment and would have a complete library of maintenance and repair information on common equipment and a reasonable stock of repair parts. This company has made much progress, but the project is a much larger one that most people realize. Bendix Corp. also undertook a rather major effort along these lines a few years ago. This was apparently not a sustained national effort. A smaller company, On-Call Corp., has attempted to put together a chain of repair facilities in various areas. It has met with some success but lacks a great deal of having national coverage. This would seem to

be a potential opportunity for a large company but the problems are numerous.

Many companies offer service contracts on their equipment. Some do not. Some claim good repair capability but cannot actually furnish it. With major equipment systems, it is necessary that a company have an adequate, reliable repair capability. The more expensive a system is, the more critical it is that it can be kept in service. Some large companies have had very real problems with equipment that was reasonably good, because their repair backup was inadequate.

Most equipment is warranted in some way for a year. Larger equipment can then be put under a maintenance contract with the manufacturer in most instances. The prices for these maintenance contracts seem to be more realistic in the past year or so.

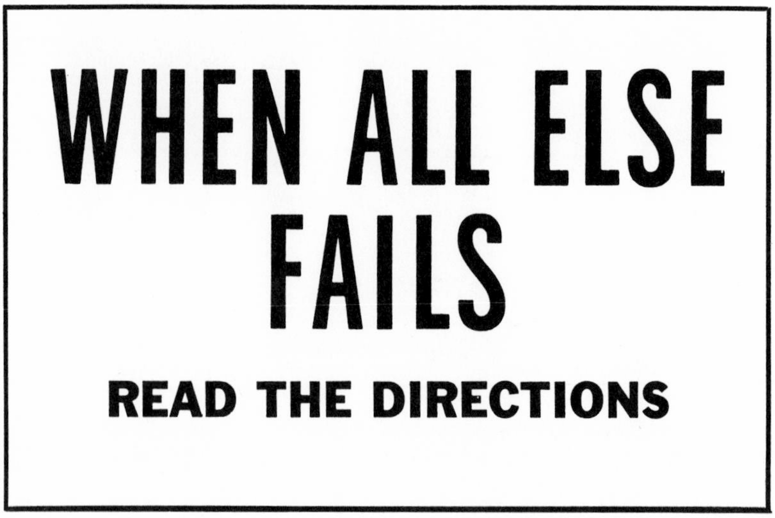

WHEN ALL ELSE FAILS

READ THE DIRECTIONS

Fig. 14-3. (Courtesy Cahn Division, Ventron Instruments Corp.)

To make an adequate judgment about the reasonableness of a maintenance proposal, one must have some idea about past repair costs, the existence of viable alternatives, etc.

The medical laboratory represents a considerable investment in equipment and a large on-going payroll and overhead expense. A thorough appreciation of equipment, its application, maintenance, repair, and replacement is crucial. Hopefully the time spent with this book has been profitable.

REVIEW QUESTIONS

1. Try to find the breaker box for the outlet nearest you. Find the breaker that controls that outlet.

2. Remove the fuse from an instrument and read the type and rating from the band at the end of the fuse.

3. Follow through the wiring diagram of the Coleman Flame Photometer pictured earlier.

4. Check a centrifuge for worn bearings. Find its lubrication points.

5. Check the brushes of a centrifuge.

6. Change an exciter lamp.

7. With a multimeter, check the line voltage in a plug close to you. Be careful. Be sure that the meter selector is on AC volts and that it is higher than 110 v. Exactly what is the voltage?

8. Take a desk light or similar device and check the continuity of the power cord.

Glossary of terms

absorbance Optical density of a substance expressed as negative log (base 10) of percent transmittance.

A-D converter Circuit or device for converting an analog signal to digits so that it can be expressed as a decimal number.

alphanumeric Including both alphabetical and numerical information.

ampere Unit of electric current; amount that will flow through resistance of 1 ohm when potential of 1 volt is applied.

amplifier Electrical circuit for amplifying or increasing strength of a signal; this is normally done by vacuum tubes or transistors; amplifier circuit is usually single system within entire circuitry of instrument; there may be more than one amplifier circuit (for example, a preamp circuit, signal amplifier, and high-voltage amplifier), in one instrument.

analog Physical variable, such as a photosignal, that is analogous to value being measured by system generating the signal.

angstrom unit (Å) Unit of length approximately 0.1 nm; identified as equal to wavelength of red line of cadmium.

anion Ion bearing negative charge; hence, ion that is attracted to anode.

anode Electrode having positive charge, to which stream of electrons will flow; also called *plate* in vacuum tubes.

armature Moving part of motor, generator, relay, or other magnetic circuit; commonly called *rotor*.

background Extraneous signal not related to parameter being measured.

band pass Section of spectrum allowed to pass through monochromator; Coleman 6C has band pass of 35 nm; Spectronic 20 has 20 nm band pass; Beckman DU can work effectively in some areas well under 5 nm.

barrier-layer cell Common type of photogenerative or photovoltaic cell.

BCD output Binary coded digital information is in a form that will allow most printers to print digital values without further signal conversion.

Beer's law Physical law that describes behavior of light; Beer's law states that intensity of light transmitted through chemical solution is inversely proportional to molar concentration of solution and that relationship is logarithmic. Not all solutions obey Beer's law and most vary at extreme concentrations.

bias Voltage applied to grid of vacuum tube to control flow of electrons between cathode and anode; grid voltage controls amplification factor of vacuum tube.

binary Having to do with number two; binary system used in computers allows only two choices in each situation—positive or negative, first or second, up or down, etc.

bit Single digit of computer information, which can be stored on one magnetic position.

blaze angle Angle of the grooves in the face of a diffraction grating; blaze angle determines which area of the spectrum is least distorted.

bolometer Instrument for measuring very small changes in radiated heat.

bridge Arrangement in which electrical measuring device is connected or bridged between two sides of circuit; bridge often arranged so as to measure resistance changes (see Wheatstone bridge); in physiological measurement resistance transducers and bridge arrangements of this sort are common.

byte Grouping of bits, of computer information, of a given size; may be thought of as a computer "word."

capacitance Measure of capacity for storage of electric charge; read in farads.

capacitor Electrical component with capacity of storing electrical energy for release at later time; stored energy is measured in farads; two conducting surfaces with known capacitance are separated by resistor of known resistance.

carousel A circular conveyor that presents samples or tests in a sequential pattern depending on their relative positions near the circumference of the conveyor.

cathode Negative electrode; emits electrons; often referred to as *emitter*.

cation Positive-charged ion that would be attracted to cathode or negative pole.

chopper Component for converting direct current into alternating current with minimum of distortion; this may be done mechanically or electronically or, in case of photocurrents, by interrupting light path.

coefficient of extinction Term sometimes used to denote optical density of a solution at a given wavelength under various conditions. Since it is ambiguous, its use is discouraged.

collimate To arrange into organized column or beam.

collimator Lens or other device for collimating energy into organized beam or path; in radioisotope work, lead shield allowing radiation to pass in only one pathway or in several more or less parallel pathways.

colorimeter Device for measuring color intensities; usually refers to filter colorimeter, which defines transmitted light in terms of color characteristics of filter used.

common mode Potential difference between the measuring circuit and ground; hopefully it is constant.

Compton effect Effect produced when a gamma ray collides with an electron, causing dissipation and scattering of the transmitted energies.

computer language Machine-readable codes by which the computer can be instructed as to what manipulations to perform; *low-level languages* are *assembly* or *machine languages* that devices can immediately follow; *higher-level languages* such as Fortran, Cobol, and ASCII are closer to standard English and require more complex equipment to utilize.

conductance Reciprocal of resistance, measured in terms of mho.

continuous-flow analyzer Analyzer in which the sample is moved along through consecutive analytical steps in a flowing stream; primarily, the Technicon AutoAnalyzer systems.

coulomb Unit of electric charge, equal to 6.28×10^{18} electrons.

CPU Central processing unit of a computer.

curie Measure of radioactivity, equal to 3.7×10^{10} disintegrations per second; this is a rather large unit, and the millicurie (one thousandth) and microcurie (one millionth) are more commonly used.

current Flow of electrons; when current measurement is referred to, it is in terms of amperes (that is, total number of electrons).

dark current Current flowing through light-measuring cell or tube when no light is striking its sensitive surface; most light-measuring instruments (except those with photogenerative cells) have control for cancelling out effect of dark current on readout of instrument; photogenerative cells have no appreciable dark current.

d'Arsonval movement Moving-coil movement that is heart of most ammeters; current to be measured is passed through coil that is delicately mounted between poles of magnet; electric field thus produced opposes magnetic field, producing torque, that moves coil and attached pointer clockwise; small spring attached to coil reorients it when no current is flowing.

deadband Range of voltage or amperage through which the input signal can vary without moving the recorder pen.

diffraction grating Surface bearing delicately etched or superimposed gridwork of very fine lines capable of scattering or diffracting light waves in such a way as to form spectrum.

digital readout Device for converting increments in electric current into digits in multiples of ten and decimal values.

diode Vacuum tube or transistor having only two electrodes or elements; since plate is always positive in relation to cathode, this arrangement allows only part of alternating current flowing in one direction to pass, since all electrons go from cathode to anode (that is, toward positive pole); other half of cycle is rejected and may be passed through another diode and inverted; two outputs then become direct current of regularly varying voltage (see discussion of vacuum tubes).

direct current Electric current in which electrons flow only in one direction; negative-charged electrons flow toward positive pole.

discrete analyzer Analyzer in which the sample maintains its identity in a separate, discrete reaction vessel or vessels throughout the analysis.

electrochemistry Study of interrelations of electricity and chemical change.

electromagnetic spectrum Spectrum of frequencies possessing radiant energy, including gamma rays, X rays, ultraviolet light, visible light, infrared heat waves, microwaves, and radio waves.

electromotive force (EMF) Potential difference between terminals or materials; measured in volts.

electron Smallest effective unit of electrical energy; theories differ over whether it possesses mass or is simply energy; quantum theory seems to indicate it does possess mass (9.1×10^{-28} gram).

electron volt Very fine measurement of power, equal to energy of 1 electron accelerated through potential difference of 1 volt, or 1.6×10^{-16} erg.

encoder Device for transferring coded information from one medium to another.

end point reactions Reactions in which the final change is measured after a given time, following a specific experimental protocol; the total change is significant rather than the rate of change.

error signal Difference between two opposing electrical impulses.

exciter lamp Source of light energy used in measurement of color intensity and fluorescence in colorimeters, photometers, fluorimeters, etc.

extrinsic conduction Conduction in a semiconductor due to the impurities added to the crystal to enhance conduction.

farad Unit of capacitance, equal to 1 coulomb under pressure of 1 volt.

feedback Utilization of fraction of output signal to make a correction electronically.

FET Field-effect transistor; a transistor designed to permit direct current to be amplified without being chopped.

filter In electronics, filter is component, such as induction coil, that eliminates or controls ripple or eliminates undesirable frequencies.

flip-flop circuit Circuit that may reverse direction of current flow each time it is brought into use to prevent polarization; in computers, term refers to components able to assume two different stable states in order to store information of binary nature.

flow cell The cuvette, in continuous-flow analysis, where the stream carrying individual tests passes for colorimetric determination.

fluorometer Instrument for measuring fluorescent light or light excited by stimulation of substance with light of lower wavelength.

frequency Number of times event occurs per time interval; for example, *cycles of alternating current per second is frequency* of alternating current; often expressed in hertz (Hz).

gain Expression of amplification factor of amplifier circuit or element; primarily dependent on grid bias.

galvanometer lamp Lamp used to provide light image reflected by galvanometer mirror.

galvanometer or string galvanometer Ammeter in which moving coil (see *d'Arsonval movement*) is suspended on thin string or wire that offers very little resistance to movement; more sensitive than ordinary ammeter; usually coil has small mirror attached that reflects beam of light (rather than pointer) to scale to indicate current value.

gamma energy Radiant energy having a wavelength of less than 1 Å, usually produced by nuclear transitions, as in radiactive isotopes.

ground Contact to earth, with zero potential.

ground state Normal state of an atom, in which no electron is in an elevated energy state.

half-life Time required for a radioactive substance to lose one half of its radioactivity.

half-life, biological Time required for half of a radioactive substance to disappear from a physiological system to organism by excretion, without regard to physical half-life.

half-life, physical Time required for an isotope to lose half of its radiant energy; radioactivity is lost exponentially; therefore not all energy is lost in two half-lives.

hardware In computer terminology, the actual instruments and devices forming the computer system.

heat filter Filter that allows light waves to pass but deflects or absorbs heat waves.

heat sink Metal radiator provided to dissipate heat around such components as power transistors.

henry Unit of inductance.

hertz Unit of frequency per second.

hollow cathode lamp Vapor lamp having a cathode charged with a specific element or elements; emission of the hollow cathode lamp will be the same as the emission of the element when heated in a flame; used in atomic absorption spectrophotometry.

ideal black body radiator Surface that would not reflect any light energy of any kind; statistically significant but nonexistent.

impedance Total opposition to flow of alternating current, which is offered by circuit or component; in complicated circuit its calculation can become quite complex, for it often varies with frequency and is sum of number of variables; impedance is measured in ohms and is represented by letter z in formulas.

incident light Light falling on sample.

inductance Resistance to change in current, caused by counter potential of field of induction; measured in henries.

induction Production of magnetic field around current-carrying conductor or production of current in a parallel wire.

infrared (IR) Region of spectrum having longer wavelengths than red light; these wavelengths are invisible; usually considered to be from about 700 to 5,000,000 nm or 0.5 cm; they may produce heat.

input Information that is received by an instrument or component, such as light striking phototube or photoelectric current fed to meter.

integrated circuit Component containing several semiconductor crystals in a configuration allowing that single component to perform multiple electronic functions.

intrinsic conduction Conduction in a semiconductor crystal that is due to naturally occurring carriers in the pure crystal.

ion Atom or molecule with electrostatic charge.

ionization Dissociation of any substance into its constituent ions.

isolating transformer Transformer used primarily to assure that the secondary current is protected from changes in the primary.

isosbestic point Wavelength at which two solutions of equal concentration have equal optical density.

kinetic reaction Reaction in which the rate of reaction or change is the significant variable; primarily enzyme reactions.

Lambert's law Physical law that states that transmitted light decreases exponentially as absorbing medium increases arithmetically in thickness.

LED Light-emitting diode; semiconductor diode capable of converting electrical energy into light; now widely used in digital readout devices.

limits of reliability (colorimetry) With most types

of colorimeters and spectrophotometers concentrations of solutions showing more than 85% transmittance, or less than 20%, give unreliable readings; limits will vary considerably with instrument, cuvettes, and handling of sample in question.

linear-log converter Device or circuit for converting linear numbers into log numbers. Since Beer's law indicates that concentration has a linear relationship to the log of the %T, this converter, in effect, makes it possible to read out photoelectric information in terms of concentration.

mechanical zero Device on most galvanometers and ammeters for mechanically adjusting meter to read zero with no current flow.

mho Unit of conductance; reciprocal of ohm.

millimicron (mμ) 10 Å or 1/10,000,000 (10^{-7}) cm; wavelength of light is often expressed in millimicrons.

mnemonics Shortened forms of words that are used in communicating with the computer.

molar absorptivity (ε) Absorbance of 1 molar solution when viewed in 1 cm light path.

monochromatic light Light of one color; composed of narrow band of wavelengths.

monochromator Filter, prism, or diffraction grating, along with slit and/or other parts necessary, that separates out narrow band of light, essentially of one color.

MOS detectors Detectors of radiation, utilizing the sensitivity of metal oxide semiconductors for radiant energy.

nanon Millimicron; newer and preferred terminology.

nephelometer Instrument for measuring light reflected or scattered by particles in solution.

neutral-density filter Filter capable of reducing total light transmitted without absorbing light of any given wavelength more than another.

noise In electronics, any unwanted electrical disturbance that interferes with signal one is attempting to read.

ohm (Ω) Unit of resistance used in electrical measurements; amount of resistance in which 1 volt maintains current of 1 amp; a 1-meter column of mercury 1 mm in diameter provides resistance of about 1 ohm.

optical density Characteristic of solution, defined in terms of ability to absorb light energy; it is log of reciprocal of transmittance; term is nearly synonymous with *absorbance;* since absorbance is somewhat more explicit, it is preferred.

ordinate Of graph, chart, or recording, its vertical axis.

parallax error Error caused by looking at meter needle at angle that makes pointer seem to be higher or lower on scale; parallax-correcting meters have mirrored panel on scale; if needle image is obscured by needle, there is no parallax error.

parameter Variable to be measured or considered in given situation.

percent transmittance Ratio of transmitted light to incident light, expressed as a percentage.

periodic Recurring in a definite sequence, as atoms recur in the same arrangement to form a crystal.

phase When two or more currents have same frequency and polarity, they are said to be "in phase."

photoconductive cell Component that does not conduct appreciable quantity of current in dark but transmits well when illuminated; resistance is inversely proportional to light.

photocurrent Current produced by photodetector when it is exposed to light energy.

photodetector Device that uses photoelectric effect to detect light energy.

photoelectric effect Effect produced when a gamma ray transmits all of its energy to an electron, which in turn produces a photocurrent analogous to the energy of the gamma ray.

photogenerative cell or photovoltaic cell Component made up of metal base (often iron) covered with layer of oxide or selenide capable of producing small direct current when exposed to light; electrons flow from coating to metal base through external circuit; actual construction somewhat more complex, but function remains quite simple; electricity produced is proportional to incident light; this is not linear but approaches linearity through working range.

photomultiplier tube Phototube with cathode, usually nine dynodes (each providing step-higher voltage), and anode; arrangement provides successive steps of amplification to original signal from cathode; mica shield prevents electrons from jumping to wrong dynode; photomultiplier tubes provide as high as 2,000,000 amplication factor.

photon Unit of measurement of light energy.

photosignal Electric signal generated or modified by light-detecting device.

phototube Vacuum or gas-filled tube with cathode capable of emitting stream of electrons when exposed to light and provided with appropriate plate voltage; with all other conditions constant, current is directly proportional to illumination; much larger current can be obtained with phototube than with photocell.

polarography Electronic measurement of the gain or loss of electrons in a chemical reaction.

potential Difference in EMF, or voltage difference between two bodies or portions of circuit.

potentiometer or pot Variable resistance.

power Change in energy per second; in electricity, usually expressed in watts (see *watt*).

power supply Electrical circuit or component designed to provide proper voltages, amperages, and frequencies to operate systems of instrument; may include transformers, batteries, diodes, capacitors, filters, etc.

precision Measure of repeatability, irrespective of accuracy.

premix burner In flame photometry, a burner in which only the thoroughly nebulized portion of the sample is burned, as it is drawn from an atomizer chamber in which heavier droplets fall out.

prism Piece of glass cut in such manner as to diffract light to form spectrum of good quality.

program In computer science, the set of instructions telling the computer what steps to take to accomplish a desired function.

programmer Person who converts problems from human-readable form to a program the computer can understand.

quantum efficiency In fluorescence measurement, relationship between the incident light and the emitted light.

radiant energy Energy of electromagnetic waves.

raster pattern Pattern produced by a scanner detector as it crosses a field, moves over a short distance, and returns on a line parallel and close to its previous excursion.

ratio recording Characteristic of a spectrophotometric instrument rendering it capable of recording ratio of light transmitted through reference tube to light transmitted through sample at each wavelength, without manual correction.

recorder Instrument for converting electric or physical signals to a graphic record; many types; most relate time as one coordinate to electrical impulse (such as absorbance from a spectrophotometer) as other coordinate.

relative centrifugal force (RCF) Measure of centrifugal force, expressed in relation to gravity; calculated by multiplying the square of the revolutions per minute $\times$ radius in cm $\times$ 0.00001118.

relay Electrically operated switch by means of which weak current may be made to open or close much heavier circuit.

resolution (colorimetry) Ability of a colorimetric instrument to faithfully record small bands of spectral absorption or transmission.

root mean square (rms) or effective voltage In sine wave, square root of sum of squares of infinite number of moment voltage is effective voltage.

scintillation detector Instrument for detecting radiation; radiation from radioactive isotope is absorbed by phosphor crystal that emits very small flashes of short duration that are detected by photomultiplier tube and amplified.

servomechanism Self-correcting feedback device; usually input signal is matched to reference signal, and error signal drives motor or other device to perform some function such as change of position, temperature, or other environmental factor or equalization of reference and input by slide-wire mechanism, with readout as analog of parameter providing input.

Severinghaus electrode The electrode used to measure P_{CO_2} by measuring the change in pH of a buffer as it is affected by absorbed CO_2 passing from blood to buffer across a semipermeable membrane.

shunt Secondary channel or bypass for current; in meter, for example, shunt carries larger fraction of current around measuring movement.

signal Information (usually electric in nature) arising from system or situation under measurement and analagous to change that is to be measured.

signal-to-noise ratio Ratio of extraneous current variations to variations of current being measured.

slit width Width of slit or opening through which section of spectrum falls on sample; determines band pass when other conditions remain fixed.

software Total of the coded instructions to the computer, necessary to make it functional.

solenoid Electromagnetically operated valve to control flow of liquids or gas.

"spec sheets" Specification sheets that give factual technical information in concise form. Most instrument specifications are given in uniformly acceptable terms and units of reference.

spectral emission Specific spectrum emitted by given light source; sun, for example, emits light generally accepted to be pure white light; other sources vary in spectral content; each element has characteristic spectral emission when heated to appropriate temperature.

spectral scanning Continuous sequential examination of solution with varying colors in light, to determine its absorbance at each wavelength; most conveniently done with the ratio-recording spectrophotometer, which automatically corrects for varying phototube characteristics at different wavelengths.

spectrophotometer Colorimeter in which monochromatic light is provided by creation of spectrum and isolation of one small band of color.

spectroscope Instrument designed to produce spectrum from light source or from light reflected from object; such spectrum defines emitted or reflected light, thereby identifying substance under examination.

spectrum Continuously varying band of color observed when stream of white light is passed through prism, which separates various components of light into their respective wavelengths; recognizable colors, from shortest to longest wavelength, are violet, blue, green, yellow, orange, and red.

stray light Light, of scattered wavelengths, that

passes (unwanted) through the cuvette of a photometer. The spectra of higher orders and small amounts of reflected light make up most of the stray light.

supercooled liquid Substance in its liquid state at temperature lower than its freezing point.

taut-band suspension Meter suspension in which moving coil is suspended on taut wire or other material in such way that no friction is involved in its rotation.

TC detectors Thermal conductivity or "hot wire" detectors used in gas chromatography.

thermal runaway Unfortunate situation in which heat increases conductivity of a semiconductor, and increased current flow increases heat until the component is destroyed by excessive heat.

thermistor Device working on principle of impedance varying with temperature in circuit; output unit of thermistor circuit may be a thermometer scale indicating temperature or an electronic device of any sort that might be operated on error signal.

thermocouple Bimetallic device capable of generating current whose potential varies with temperature; may be constructed to measure very small temperature changes in physiological situations.

thermoregulator Component that responds to change in temperature by opening and closing relay to put in motion heating or cooling device to correct change.

total-consumption burner In flame photometry, a burner in which all of the aspirated sample passes into the flame.

transducer Component designed to convert some physical signal—pressure, temperature, movement, etc.—into transmissible signal, usually electric in nature.

transformer Component designed to change voltage supply to voltage desired; step-up transformer increases voltage; step-down transformer diminishes voltage; change of voltage is effected by setting up induction current in coil parallel to coil carrying supply voltage; new voltage depends on relative number of turns of wire in coils.

transistor Solid-state component capable of most of functions of vacuum tubes.

transmittance Ability of solution to pass or transmit light of selected wavelength; usually expressed in percentage of light transmitted; this value has reciprocal relationship to absorbance.

turbidimetry Measurement of cloudiness or turbidity of solution by amount of light it is able to transmit or disperse.

turn-key operation Computer system in which the responsibilities for programming and operational details are the responsibility of the vendor.

ultraviolet (UV) Region of spectrum having shorter wavelengths than violet light; outside the visible range and generally considered between 5 and 400 nm (between X rays and violet light).

Venturi T-shaped tube for producing suction in side arm by rapid passage of stream of liquid or gas through straight portion.

volt (v) Unit of electromotive force (pressure) that will send 1 ampere through 1 ohm of resistance.

voltage stabilizer Device for preventing large fluctuations in current supplied to instrument; these vary from simple stabilizing transformers to complex electronic power supplies.

voltaic Producing difference in potential by chemical action or contact.

watt (w) Unit of electric power equivalent to work performed when 1 volt moves 1 ampere; this is 1 joule per second.

wavelength (λ) Distance between crests of consecutive waves of any sort; might apply to light, sound, radio waves, X rays, etc.

Wheatstone bridge Arrangement of four opposing resistances by which resistance can be measured; first pair of resistances acts to bring two currents to comparable levels; one of remaining resistors is unknown, and fourth is variable; if all resistor values are known, this device may be used to calculate voltage or amperage by applying Ohm's law.

Zener diode Semiconductor diode designed to carry a very specific current when reverse-biased at a given voltage. Generally used to control current very accurately.

Zener voltage Voltage required to cause a Zener diode to conduct when reverse-biased; also called "breakdown voltage"; indicated as V_z.

Periodic table of elements

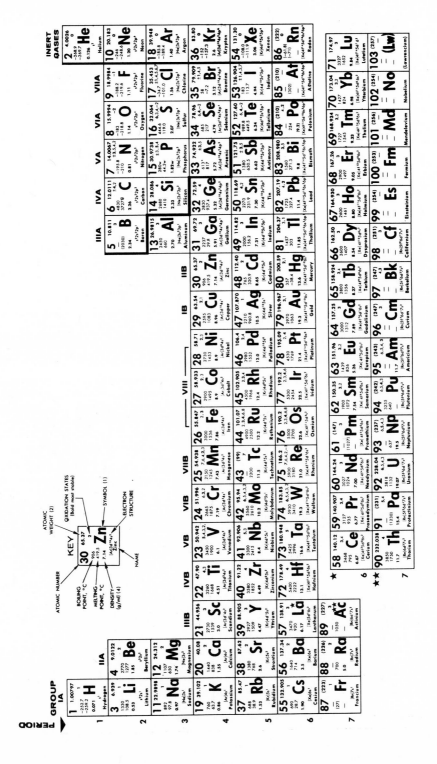

Units of electricity

counter electromotive force of 1 volt is generated by rate of change of current of 1 ampere per second.

hertz (Hz) Unit of frequency per second.

mho Unit of conductance; reciprocal of resistance; that is, relation between conductance G and resistance R is given by:

$$G = \frac{1}{R} \text{ mho}$$

ampere Practical unit of electric current; amount of current that will flow through resistance of 1 ohm when potential of 1 volt is applied across resistance; abbreviation is amp; amperage in formulas is I.

coulomb Charge containing 6.28×10^{18} electrons; 1 coulomb passing a point in 1 second is 1 ampere.

farad Unit of capacitance; circuit, or capacitor, is said to have capacitance of 1 farad when charge of 1 volt per second across it produces current of 1 ampere.

henry Unit of inductance; circuit, or inductor, is said to have self-inductance of 1 henry when

ohm Practical unit of resistance; amount of resistance that will permit 1 ampere to flow at potential difference of 1 volt. Usually designated on diagrams by Greek letter *omega* (Ω); in formulas R, for resistance, is used.

volt Practical unit of electromotive force (EMF) or electrical potential; potential that will cause current of 1 ampere to flow through resistance of 1 ohm; abbreviation is v; voltage or EMF in formulas is E.

watt Unit of electrical power defined as work performed when 1 volt moves 1 ampere; abbreviation is w (or, in formulas, W).

Table 5. Accepted nomenclature for photometry

Preferred nomenclature and symbols	Definition	Other terms used
Absorbance (A)	$\mathrm{Log}_{10}(1/T) = -\log_{10} T = 2 - \log_{10} \% T$	Optical density (OD) Density Extinction Absorbancy
Absorptivity (a)	Absorbance per unit concentration and thickness; i.e., specific absorbance	Extinction coefficient Specific absorption Absorbance index
Molar absorptivity	Absorptivity in moles per liter per light path; concentration in moles per liter and thickness in centimeters (usually 1 mole per liter in 1 cm light path)	Molar extinction coefficient Molar absorbancy index
Angstrom unit	Approximately 10^{-10} meter	Å or A
Frequency	Cycles of energy per unit of time	
Far UV	Radiant energy between 10 and 200 nanons	
Near UV	Radiant energy between 200 and 380 nanons	
Visible light	Radiant energy between 380 and 780 nanons	
Near IR	Radiant energy between 780 nanons and 2.5 microns	
Middle IR	Radiant energy between 2.5 and 25 microns	
Far IR	Radiant energy between 25 and 400 microns	
Transmittance (T)	Ratio of radiant energy transmitted by sample to radiant energy incident on sample under identical conditions	Transmission Transmittancy
Percent transmittance	Transmittance expressed as percent	$\% T$

262

Table 6. Greek alphabet as symbols*

A	Alpha	
α	Alpha	
B	Beta	
β	Beta	Van Slyke buffer value, beta particle
Γ	Gamma	
γ	Gamma	Gamma radiation
Δ	Delta	Symbol of finite change
δ	Delta	
E	Epsilon	
ε	Epsilon	Molar absorptivity or coefficient of extinction
Z	Zeta	
ζ	Zeta	
H	Eta	
η	Eta	
Θ	Theta	
θ	Theta	Angle of diffraction
I	Iota	
ι	Iota	
K	Kappa	
κ	Kappa	
Λ	Lambda	
λ	Lambda	Wavelength
M	Mu	
μ	Mu	Micron or micro
N	Nu	
ν	Nu	Frequency
Ξ	Xi	
ξ	Xi	
O	Omicron	
ο	Omicron	
Π	Pi	3.14
π	Pi	3.14
P	Rho	
ρ	Rho	Density
Σ	Sigma	Sum of
σ	Sigma	Standard deviation, also used for wave number
T	Tau	
τ	Tau	
Υ	Upsilon	
υ	Upsilon	Velocity or speed
Φ	Phi	
φ	Phi	
X	Chi	
χ	Chi	
Ψ	Psi	
ψ	Psi	
Ω	Omega	Ohm
ω	Omega	Energy per reciprocal centimeter

*Greek letters are used widely in the sciences as symbols. The same letter may have different meanings in different disciplines. A few of the very common usages are indicated above.

Table 7. Prefixes

Multiple or submultiple		Prefix	Symbol
1 000 000 000 000	10^{12}	tera	t
1 000 000 000	10^{9}	giga	g
1 000 000	10^{6}	mega	m
1 000	10^{3}	kilo	k (or K)
100	10^{2}	hecto	h
10	10^{1}	deka	dk
0.1	10^{-1}	deci	d
0.01	10^{-2}	centi	c
0.001	10^{-3}	milli	m
0.000 001	10^{-6}	micro	μ
0.000 000 001	10^{-9}	nano	n
0.000 000 000 001	10^{-12}	pico	p

Electrical symbols

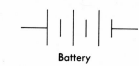
Battery

Capacitor, fixed

   Several of the more commonly used electrical symbols appear on this and the following page. There are, of course, many others. Some draftsmen use symbols that are slightly different from those shown here. Using these, however, you will find simple diagrams easy to follow. As you become more experienced you will recognize additional symbols, and practice will greatly increase your comprehension. If some diagrams are confusing or individual circuits seem hopeless, do not become discouraged. Follow the general outline and fill in the details as you puzzle them out.

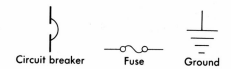
Circuit breaker   Fuse   Ground

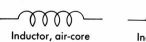
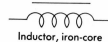

Inductor, air-core   Inductor, iron-core

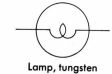
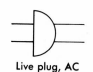

Lamp, tungsten   Live plug, AC

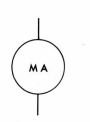

Meter (lettering in center tells type)

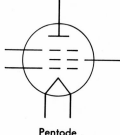

Pentode
vacuum tube

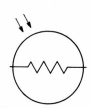

Photoconductive cell

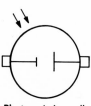

Photoemissive cell

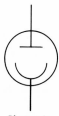

Phototube

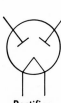

Rectifier,
full-wave,
vacuum tube

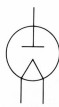

Rectifier,
half-wave,
vacuum tube

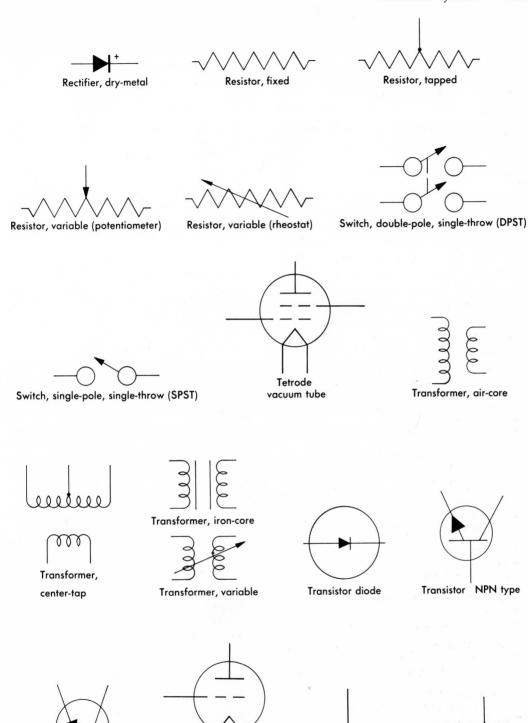

Rectifier, dry-metal

Resistor, fixed

Resistor, tapped

Resistor, variable (potentiometer)

Resistor, variable (rheostat)

Switch, double-pole, single-throw (DPST)

Switch, single-pole, single-throw (SPST)

Tetrode
vacuum tube

Transformer, air-core

Transformer,
center-tap

Transformer, iron-core

Transformer, variable

Transistor diode

Transistor   NPN type

Transistor PNP type

Triode
vacuum tube

Wires, crossed

Wires, joined

Manufacturers' addresses

For convenience the following company names and addresses are provided. All these companies are manufacturers of instruments discussed or mentioned earlier. More information on many technical matters relating to these instruments is available through the manufacturers' technical manuals, operating manuals, seminars, and training courses. Many of the companies have provided illustrations, consultations, data, and advice, for which I wish here to express my deep appreciation.

Abbott Scientific Products Division
820 Mission St.
South Pasadena, Calif. 91030

Addressograph Multigraph Corp.
1200 Babbitt Rd.
Cleveland, Ohio 44117

Advanced Instruments, Inc.
44B Kenneth St.
Newton Highlands, Mass. 02161

AGA Corp.
550 County Ave.
Secaucus, N. J. 07094

American Instrument Co., Inc.
8030 Georgia Ave.
Silver Springs, Md. 20910

American Monitor Corp.
P.O. Box 68505
Indianapolis, Ind. 46268

American Optical Corp.
Analytical Instrument Division
200 S. Garrard Blvd.
Richmond, Calif. 94804

Ames Co.
Division Miles Laboratories, Inc.
Elkhart, Indiana 46514

Antek Instruments, Inc.
6005 N. Freeway
Houston, Texas 77022

Artek Systems Corp.
275 Adams Blvd.
Farmingdale, N. Y. 11735

Baird Atomic, Inc.
125 Middlesex Turnpike
Bedford, Mass. 01730

Bausch & Lomb
820 Linden Ave.
Rochester, N. Y. 14625

Beckman Instruments, Inc.
2500 Harbor Blvd.
Fullerton, Calif. 92634

Becton, Dickinson & Co.
Bio-Quest Division
Cockeysville, Md. 21030

The Bendix Corp.
Galileo Park
Sturbridge Park, Mass. 01518

Berkeley Medical Instruments
1220 Tenth St.
Berkeley, Calif. 94710

Bio/Data Corp.
3615 Davisville Rd.
Hatboro, Pa. 19040

Bio-Dynamics, Inc.
9115 Hague Rd.
Indianapolis, Ind. 46250

Bio-Technology Instrument Corp.
10770 Talbert Ave.
Fountain Valley, Calif. 92708

Brinkmann Instruments, Inc.
Cantiague Rd.
Westburg, N. Y. 11590

CAPCO
Cary Instruments, Applied Physics Corp.
2724 S. Peck Rd.
Monrovia, Calif. 91016

Clay Adams
Division of Becton, Dickinson & Co.
Parsippany, N. J. 07054

Clifford Instruments, Inc.
15 Willow St.
Natik, Mass. 01760

Clinical Analysis Products Co.
599 N. Mathilda Ave.
Sunnyvale, Calif. 94086

Coleman Instruments Division
Perkin-Elmer Corp.
42 Madison St.
Maywood, Ill. 60154

Corning Scientific Instruments
Medfield, Mass. 02052

Coulter Electronics, Inc.
590 W. 20th St.
Hialeah, Fla. 33010

Dade Reagents
Division of American Hospital Supply Corp.
1851 Delaware Parkway
Miami, Fla. 33152

Digital Equipment Corp.
146 Main St.
Maynard, Mass. 01754

Disc Instruments, Inc.
2701 Halladay St.
Santa Ana, Calif. 92705

Diversified Numeric Applications
Division of AVNET, Inc.
9801 Logan Ave., South
Minneapolis, Minn. 55431

The Dow Chemical Co.
2030 Abbott Road Center
Midland, Mich. 48640

E. I. du Pont de Nemours & Co.
Wilmington, Delaware 19898

Electro-Nucleonics Laboratories, Inc.
4905 Del Ray Ave.
Bethesda, Md. 20014

Elementary Principles, Inc.
P.O. Box 1606
Orlando, Fla. 32802

Elron Electronics Industries
Haifa, Israel

Farrand Optical Co., Inc.
Commercial Products Division
535 S. Fifth Ave.
Mount Vernon, N. Y. 10550

Fisher Scientific Co.
711 Forbes Ave.
Pittsburgh, Pa. 15219

Fiske Associates, Inc.
Quaker Highway
Uxbridge, Mass. 01569

Gam Rad, Inc.
16825 Wyoming Ave.
Detroit, Mich. 48221

Gelman Instrument Co.
600 South Wagner Rd.
Ann Arbor, Mich. 48106

General Science Corp.
Subsidiary of J. T. Baker Co.
525 Broad St.
Bridgeport, Conn. 06604

Gilford Instrument Laboratories, Inc.
132 Artina St.
Oberlin, Ohio 44074

Harleco
60th & Woodland Ave.
Philadelpiha, Pa. 19143

Helena Laboratories
P.O. Box 752
Beaumont, Texas 77704

Hewlett-Packard
Route 41
Avondale, Pa. 19311

Honeywell, Inc.
Industrial Division
1100 Virginia Dr.
Fort Washington, Pa. 19034

Honeywell, Test Instruments Division
Second Street, Extended—Greenwood Acres
Annapolis, Md. 21404

Hycel, Inc.
P.O. Box 36329
Houston, Texas 77036

Hyland, Division of Travenol Laboratories, Inc.
3300 Hyland Ave.
Costa Mesa, Calif. 92626

IBM Corp.
Blood Cell Processor
P.O. Box 10
Princeton, N. J. 08540

Infotronics, Inc.
8500 Cameron Rd.
Austin, Texas 78753

Instrumentation Laboratory, Inc.
113 Hartwell Ave.
Lexington, Mass. 02173

International Equipment Co.
Division of Damon
300 Second Ave.
Needham Heights, Mass. 02194

International Sales Associates
115 E. Maple Ave.
Langhorne, Pa. 19047

International Technidyne Corp.
P.O. Box 2200
Menlo Park Station
Edison, N. J. 08817

Johnson Laboratories, Inc.
3 Industry Lane
Cockeysville, Md. 21030

Kiess Instruments, Inc.
8768 S.W. 131 St.
Miami, Fla. 33156

E. Leitz, Inc.
468 Park Ave. South
New York, N. Y. 10016

Lipshaw Manufacturing Co.
7446 Central Ave.
Detroit, Mich. 48210

The London Co.
811 Sharon Dr.
Cleveland, Ohio 44145 (Representative in USA
for Radiometer of Denmark)

Medical Laboratory Automation, Inc.
520 Nuber Ave.
Mt. Vernon, N. Y. 10550

Medi-Computer Corp. (Vickers Distributor)
581 W. Putnam Ave.
Greenwich, Conn. 06830

Millipore Corp.
Ashby Rd.
Bedford, Mass. 01730

Nuclear Data, Inc.
100 W. Golf Rd.
P.O. Box 451
Palatine, Ill. 60067

Ohio Nuclear, Inc.
6000 Cochran Rd.
Solon, Ohio 44139

Orion Research, Inc.
11 Blackstone St.
Cambridge, Mass. 02139

Ortho Diagnostic Instruments
Raritan, N. J. 08869

Packard Instrument Sales Corp.
2200 Warrenville Rd.
Downers Grove, Ill. 60515

Perkin-Elmer Corp.
723G Main Ave.
Norwalk, Conn. 06856

Philips Electronic Instruments
750 S. Fulton Ave.
Mount Vernon, N. Y. 10550

Photovolt Corp.
1115 Broadway
New York, N. Y. 10010

Picker X-ray Corp.
25 S. Broadway
White Plains, N. Y.

Polaroid Corp.
Cambridge, Mass. 02139

Precision Systems
6 Cornell Rd.
Framingham, Mass. 01704

Process & Instruments Corp.
1943 Broadway
Brooklyn, N. Y. 11207

Radio Corporation of America, Electronic
Components
Harrison, N. J. 07029

Sargent-Welch Scientific Co.
10558 Metropolitan Ave.
Kensington, Md. 20795

Schoeffel Instrument Corp.
15 Douglas St.
Westwood, N. J. 07675

Searle Analytic, Inc.
Subsidiary of G. D. Searle & Co.
2000 Nuclear Dr.
Des Plaines, Ill. 60018

Serosonic Laboratories, Inc.
1644 Locust Ave.
Bohemia, N. Y. 11716

Sherwood Medical Industries, Inc.
1831 Olive St.
St. Louis, Mo. 63103

Smith Kline Instrument Co.
1500 Spring Garden St.
Philadelphia, Pa. 19101

Sony Corp. of America
47-47 Van Dam St.
Long Island, N. Y. 11101

Ivan Sorvall, Inc.
Norwalk, Conn.

Spear Medical Systems
Division of Becton, Dickinson & Co.
335 Bear Hill Rd.
Waltham, Mass. 02154

Technicon Instruments Corp.
Tarrytown, N.Y. 10502

Tech/Ops Instruments
Distributors for Joyce Loebel
Northwest Industrial Park
Burlington, Mass. 01803

Texas Instruments, Inc.
P.O. Box 66029
Houston, Texas 77006

Transidyne General Corp.
462 Wagner Rd.
Ann Arbor, Mich. 48106

T & T Technology
813 Stewart St.
Madison, Wis. 53713

G. K. Turner Associates
2524 Pulgas Ave.
Palo Alto, Calif. 94303

Union Carbide Corp.
Tarrytown, N.Y. 10591

Varian Techtron
3939 Hillcroft Ave., Suite 180
Houston, Texas 77027

Ventron Instruments Corp.
Cahn Division
7500 Jefferson St.
Paramount, Calif. 90723

Vickers Instruments, Inc.
15 Waite Ct.
Malden, Mass. 02148

Yallen Instruments, Inc.
160 Pleasant St.
Brocton, Mass. 02401

Bibliography

Ackerman, P. G.: Electronic instrumentation in the clinical laboratory, Boston, 1972, Little, Brown & Co.

Adler, R. B., Smith, A. C., and Longini, R. L.: Introduction to semiconductor physics, New York, 1964, John Wiley & Sons, Inc.

Astrup, P., Jorgensen, K., Siggaard Andersen, O., and Engel, K.: The acid-base metabolism. A new approach, Lancet 1:1035, 1960.

Bauman, R. P.: Absorption spectroscopy, New York, 1962, John Wiley & Sons, Inc.

Bennett, C. E.: College physics, ed. 6, New York, 1965, Barnes & Noble, Inc.

Burns, P.: Identification of microorganisms using computer programs, unpublished Master's thesis, submitted Oct., 1972, Mississippi State University.

Coulter, W. H.: High speed automatic blood cell counter and cell size analyzer, Hialeah, Fla. 1956, Coulter Electronics, Inc.

Edisbury, J. R.: Practical hints on absorption spectrometry, New York, 1967, Plenum Publishing Corp.

Gambino, S. R.: Workshop manual on blood pH, P_{CO_2}, oxygen saturation, and P_{O_2}, 1963, ASCP Council on Clinical Chemistry.

Malmstadt, H. V., and Enke, C. G.: Electronics for scientists, New York, 1962, W. A. Benjamin, Inc.

Mann, G. B.: ABC's of transistors, Indianapolis, 1968, Bobbs-Merrill Co., Inc.

Meloan, C. E.: Instrumental analysis using physical properties, Philadelphia, 1968, Lea & Febiger.

Meloan, C. E.: Instrumental analysis using spectroscopy, Philadelphia, 1968, Lea & Febiger.

Naval Training Course: Basic electricity, Washington, D. C., 1960, U. S. Government Printing Office.

Philco Techrep Division: Electronic and electrical fundamentals, vol. 3, Philadelphia, 1960, Philco-Ford Corp.

Pollack, H.: Photoelectric control, New York, 1962, John F. Rider Publisher, Inc.

Severinghaus, J. W., and Bradley, A. F: Electrodes for blood P_{O_2} determination, J. Appl. Physiol. 13:515, 1958.

Sisler, H. H.: Electronic structure, properties, and the periodic law, New York, 1963, Reinhold Publishing Corp.

Slurzberg, M., and Osterheld, W.: Essentials of electricity-electronics, ed. 3, New York, 1965, McGraw-Hill Book Co.

Smith, I.: Chromatographic and electrophoretic technics, New York, 1960, Interscience Publishers, Inc.

Suprynowiez, V. A.: Introduction to electronics, Reading, Mass., 1966, Addison-Wesley Publishing Co., Inc.

Tammes, A. R.: Electronics for medical and biology laboratory personnel, Baltimore, 1971, The Williams & Wilkins Co.

Timbie, W. H., and Pike, A. L.: Essentials of electricity, ed. 3, New York, 1958, John Wiley & Sons, Inc.

Ward, P. F., Polanyi, M. L., Mehir, R. M., Stapleton, J. F., Sanders, J. I., and Kocot, S. L.: A new reflection oximeter, J. Thorac. Cardiovasc. Surg. 42:580, 1961.

White, W. L., Erickson, M. M., and Stevens, S. C.: Practical automation for the clinical laboratory, ed. 2, St. Louis, 1972, The C. V. Mosby Co.

Willard, H. H., Merritt, L. L., Jr., and Dean, J. S., Instrumental methods of analysis, ed. 4, Princeton, N. J., 1965, D. Van Nostrand Co., Inc.

Yanof, H. M.: Biomedical electronics, Philadelphia, 1965, F. A. Davis Co.

Index